The Digital Pillbox: Integrating AI, IoT, and Pharma Solutions

(Part 1)

Edited by

Akhil Sharma
R.J. College of Pharmacy
Raipur, Gharbara, Tappal, Khair
Uttar Pradesh, India

Neeraj Kumar Fuloria
Department of Pharmaceutical Chemistry, Faculty of
Pharmacy, AIMST University
Semeling Campus
Bedong, Kedah, Malaysia

Pankaj Kumar Singh
Institute of Biomedicine, University of Turku
Turku, Finland

&

Shaweta Sharma
School of Medical and Allied Sciences
Galgotias University
Greater Noida, Uttar Pradesh
India

The Digital Pillbox: Integrating AI, IoT, and Pharma Solutions *(Part 1)*

Editors: Akhil Sharma, Neeraj Kumar Fuloria, Pankaj Kumar Singh & Shaweta Sharma

ISBN (Online): 978-981-5324-45-7

ISBN (Print): 978-981-5324-46-4

ISBN (Paperback): 978-981-5324-47-1

need for a court order if at any point you breach any terms of this License Agreement. In no event will any delay or failure by Bentham Science Publishers in enforcing your compliance with this License Agreement constitute a waiver of any of its rights.

3. You acknowledge that you have read this License Agreement, and agree to be bound by its terms and conditions. To the extent that any other terms and conditions presented on any website of Bentham Science Publishers conflict with, or are inconsistent with, the terms and conditions set out in this License Agreement, you acknowledge that the terms and conditions set out in this License Agreement shall prevail.

Bentham Science Publishers Pte. Ltd.
No. 9 Raffles Place
Office No. 26-01
Singapore 048619
Singapore
Email: subscriptions@benthamscience.net

BENTHAM SCIENCE

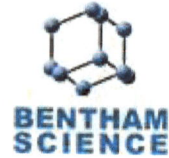

CONTENTS

FOREWORD

The healthcare sector stands at the cusp of a profound transformation. With the rapid advancement of digital technologies, traditional models of care are evolving into interconnected ecosystems that prioritize precision, efficiency, and patient empowerment. Among the most impactful developments in this journey is the fusion of Artificial Intelligence (AI), the Internet of Things (IoT), and pharmaceutical innovation, a convergence that holds immense promise for tackling longstanding challenges in medication management and beyond.

The Digital Pillbox: Integrating AI, IoT, and Pharma Solutions (Part 1) delves into this very intersection, offering a timely and insightful exploration of how these cutting-edge technologies are reimagining healthcare delivery. From addressing the persistent issue of medication non-adherence to enabling real-time tracking and personalized treatment plans, this volume presents both the urgency and the opportunity inherent in this digital transformation.

What sets this work apart is its holistic approach combining theoretical insights with real-world applications to illuminate how AI and IoT are not just tools, but enablers of a more responsive, data-driven, and patient-centric care model. The emphasis on smart pillboxes, remote monitoring, and predictive analytics is particularly noteworthy, showcasing how integrated digital solutions can improve clinical outcomes while enhancing the daily lives of patients.

This book is the result of a collaborative effort by forward-thinking researchers and professionals who recognize the necessity of embracing innovation to drive sustainable healthcare improvements. It offers a roadmap for clinicians, pharmacists, technologists, policymakers, and other stakeholders who are navigating the digital health frontier.

As we move forward into an era of smarter medicine, the Digital Pillbox stands as both a guide and a call to action inviting us to rethink, retool, and revolutionize the way we approach care in the 21st century.

Shelly Pathania
Senior Researcher
Institute of Biomedicine
University of Turku
Turku, Finland

PREFACE

In today's dynamic healthcare landscape, the convergence of Artificial Intelligence (AI), the Internet of Things (IoT), and pharmaceutical innovation marks a pivotal transformation. The Digital Pillbox: Integrating AI, IoT, and Pharma Solutions (Part 1) explores this evolution, focusing on how these technologies are reshaping medication adherence, personalized medicine, and healthcare delivery.

This volume begins by addressing the root challenges of medication non-adherence, followed by an in-depth analysis of AI's role in tailoring treatments and enhancing pharmaceutical care. It highlights how IoT-enabled solutions like smart pillboxes and remote monitoring are empowering both patients and providers. Through chapters dedicated to real-time tracking, predictive analytics, and smart integration, the book outlines a forward-thinking framework for improving outcomes and optimizing therapy.

This work is a collaborative effort by dedicated researchers and professionals, aiming to guide healthcare stakeholders in embracing this digital revolution to foster smarter, more connected, and patient-centric care systems.

Akhil Sharma
R.J. College of Pharmacy
Raipur, Gharbara, Tappal, Khair
Uttar Pradesh, India

Neeraj Kumar Fuloria
Department of Pharmaceutical Chemistry, Faculty of Pharmacy, AIMST University
Semeling Campus
Bedong, Kedah, Malaysia

Pankaj Kumar Singh
Institute of Biomedicine, University of Turku
Turku, Finland

Shaweta Sharma
School of Medical and Allied Sciences
Galgotias University
Greater Noida, Uttar Pradesh
India

List of Contributors

Akanksha Sharma	R.J. College of Pharmacy, Raipur, Gharbara, Tappal, Khair, Uttar Pradesh, India
Akhil Sharma	R.J. College of Pharmacy, Raipur, Gharbara, Tappal, Khair, Uttar Pradesh, India
Ashish Verma	Mangalmay Pharmacy College, Greater Noida, Uttar Pradesh, India
B. Rama Mohana Reddy	Department of Civil Engineering, Aditya University, Surampalem, India
B. Rama Sagar	Department of Civil Engineering, Aditya University, Surampalem, India
Dimple Singh Tomar	Kharvel Subharti College of Pharmacy, Swami Vivekanand Subharti University, Meerut, India
Gaddam Dinesh	Department of Civil Engineering, Aditya University, Surampalem, India
K.K. Yashwanth	Department of Civil Engineering, Aditya University, Surampalem, India
Neeraj Kumar Fuloria	Department of Pharmaceutical Chemistry, Faculty of Pharmacy, AIMST University Semeling Campus, Bedong, Kedah Darul Aman, Malaysia
N. Bhaskara Rao	Department of Civil Engineering, Aditya University, Surampalem, India
P. Lakshmi	Department of Civil Engineering, Aditya University, Surampalem, India
P. Siva Kumar	Department of Civil Engineering Aditya University, Surampalem, India
P. Ravi Kishore	Department of Civil Engineering, Aditya University, Surampalem, India
Shaweta Sharma	School of Medical and Allied Sciences, Galgotias University, Greater Noida, Uttar Pradesh, India
Sunita	Metro College of Health Sciences and Research, Greater Noida, Uttar Pradesh, India
Shekhar Singh	Faculty of Pharmacy, Babu Banarasi Das Northern India Institute of Technology, Lucknow, Uttar Pradesh, India
S. Govindarajan	Department of Civil Engineering, Aditya University, Surampalem, India
Sumit Chowdary Mukund	Department of Civil Engineering, Aditya University, Surampalem, India
S. Ananda Kumar	Department of Civil Engineering, Aditya University, Surampalem, India
Shivkanya Fuloria	Department of Pharmaceutical Chemistry, Faculty of Pharmacy, AIMST University Semeling Campus, Bedong, Kedah, Malaysia

CHAPTER 1

Understanding Medication Adherence Challenges

Akanksha Sharma[1], Shaweta Sharma[2], Sunita[3], P. Lakshmi[4] and **Akhil Sharma[1,*]**

[1] *R.J. College of Pharmacy, Raipur, Gharbara, Tappal, Khair, Uttar Pradesh, India*

[2] *School of Medical and Allied Sciences, Galgotias University, Greater Noida, Uttar Pradesh, India*

[3] *Metro College of Health Sciences and Research, Greater Noida, Uttar Pradesh, India*

[4] *Department of Civil Engineering, Aditya University, Surampalem, India*

Abstract: Despite its relevance in managing different health conditions, medication adherence remains difficult for diverse reasons. This abstract details the complicated nature of medication adherence difficulties, which involve patient-related factors and healthcare system complexities, as well as specific issues related to medications. For medical practitioners seeking to make outcomes better for their patients, it is important to know how these three factors interact with each other. These factors include socioeconomic status, illness literacy, and psychological obstacles. Socio-economic barriers such as financial incapability and lack of insurance often affect the capability of patients to adhere to given prescriptions. Lack of awareness about certain drugs leads to confusion about recommended treatment, while depression and anxiety are examples of some psychological aspects that increase non-adherence. Communication breakdowns in the healthcare system, prescription complexity, and limited access to care have become problematic within the field today. Inadequate communication between patient-provider relationships and lack of clarity in drug instructions lead to misunderstanding or non-compliance. That aside, a range of complex prescription processes combined with accessibility barriers increase these challenges, predominantly among those individuals who are at higher risk due to social exclusion. Additionally, whether due to side effects observed or perceived, efficacy declines regimen complications and further complicates adherence efforts. Patients can stop taking their medications because they cannot stand the side effects experienced; they may also find it difficult to follow complex dosing schedules or lose interest if they do not see any improvement after all. Whereas family dynamics may be responsible for this behavior in some instances, cultural beliefs coupled with social networks influence patients' attitudes toward medication continuity. The culture-sensitive healthcare environment promotes adherence, while stigma and cultural barriers undermine the process. In brief, handling medication non-compliance takes into account the inter-connectedness among patients' characteristics of healthcare systems, medicines, and environmental features. This way, healthcare providers enhance their patients' ability to

---

* **Corresponding author Akhil Sharma:** R.J. College of Pharmacy, Raipur, Gharbara, Tappal, Khair, Uttar Pradesh, India; E-mail: xs2akhil@gmail.com

take drugs in the long term and ensure that equitable distribution is upheld by addressing such hindrances.

Keywords: Anxiety, Adherence, Depression, Health, Medication, Non-adherence, Patient, Psychology, Regimens, Record, Socioeconomic, Technology, Treatment.

INTRODUCTION

Medication adherence is an important pillar of effective healthcare management that encompasses the level to which patients stick to their prescribed drug plans. It is a crucial institution in terms of ensuring that individuals get all the curative benefits contained in their presumed medication scripts. Nevertheless, even with its undeniable relevance, medical non-adherence remains a widespread and complicated matter globally, leading to many hardships for healthcare systems as well as individual patients [1].

In recent years, healthcare specialists, policymakers, and scholars have paid increasing attention to medication non-adherence as a serious issue. The profoundness of its effects justifies this increased level of consciousness. Nonadherence is thus closely linked with a range of negative health effects, including disease advancement, morbidity, and mortality rates, and high healthcare costs. Besides, it weakens interventions for different medical conditions, from chronic diseases like diabetes and hypertension to acute illness and mental health conditions [2].

The multifaceted nature of the challenges linked to adherence means that understanding such problems would require a deeper knowledge of what causes non-adherence. These factors cover a wide range, including those related to patients, pharmaceutical and health services systems, and socio-environmental ones. For instance, patients' socioeconomic status, health literacy, and psychological barriers like depression and anxiety can have great impacts on their medication-taking behaviors. Moreover, healthcare systems are complex, with communication breakdowns and limited access to care, which further worsen adherence issues, especially among vulnerable populations [3, 4].

In addition, medication-specific aspects such as adverse effects, treatment burden, and perceived effectiveness can be highly influential in determining the behavior of patients when following prescriptions. In this regard, patients may stop using their drugs due to adverse reactions that have become unbearable or find it difficult to stick to a complex dosage regimen, thus compromising therapeutic outcomes. Additionally, socio-environmental factors like family dynamics, social support systems, and cultural beliefs are key determinants of adherence to medication, necessitating tailored approaches aimed at addressing these contextual factors [5].

Medication adherence is one challenge that seems unbeatable. However, things are not entirely hopeless. Medical practitioners have the necessary tools and expertise to develop targeted interventions that boost medication adherence, thereby leading to better patient outcomes. Ideally, it is multidisciplinary and incorporates evidence-based strategies derived from various fields such as medicine, psychology, and public health. With technologies like mobile health applications and telemedicine platforms in place, health providers can improve patient involvement and also monitor their medication adherence through them [6].

Moreover, it is through encouraging patient-centered care approaches that prioritize shared decision-making and customized treatment plans that patients will be equipped to be actively involved in their healthcare journey. Equally important is building effective communication between patients and the health providers as well as intervening for a better understanding of health literacy, which often leads to misunderstandings relating to drugs, hence a partnership aimed at treating patients. Besides, dealing with structural impediments such as the availability of affordable medicines and healthcare facilities is crucial in ensuring there is equal access as well as reducing gaps in medication adherence [7].

PATIENT-RELATED FACTORS

Patient-related factors for medication adherence are summarized in Fig. (**1**).

Socioeconomic Status

Financial Constraints

Among people with low socioeconomic status, financial constraints are a major issue when it comes to taking medicine as directed. Patients' capacity to follow their prescribed treatments closely is dependent on their ability to pay for the drugs themselves, which has an effect on health results and general welfare. Among individuals who do not have much money, high prices of medications can make them fail to take them regularly. Many chronic diseases need continuous treatment, hence the higher expenses in the long run with regard to these drugs. Inadequate earnings may hinder patients' ability to buy prescription medicines; lack of insurance coverage or expensive co-payments could force individuals into making tough choices about which bills they should prioritize over buying drugs [8, 9].

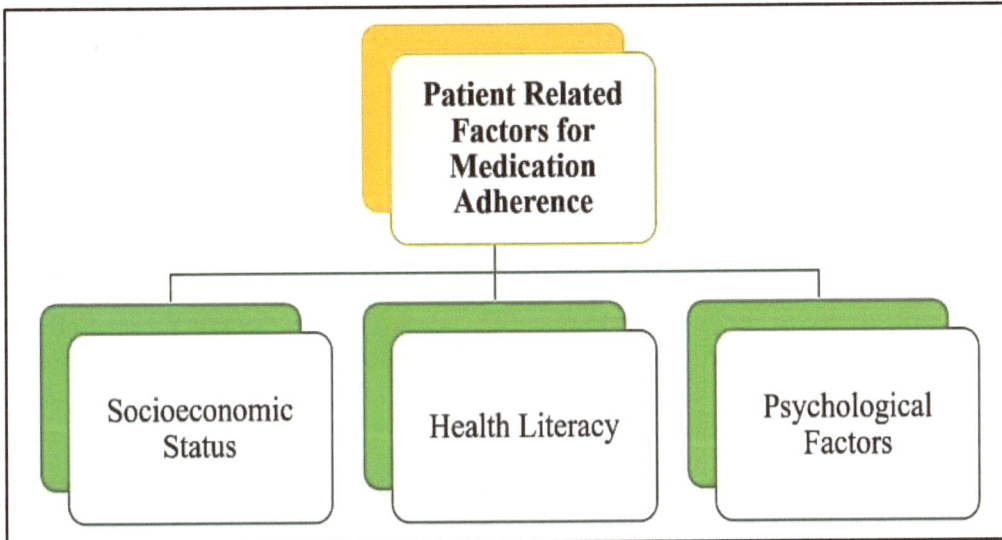

Fig. (1). Patient-related factors for medication adherence.

Financial limitations frequently create a situation in which the cost of drugs is not followed as it should be such that individuals change the way they take medicine to cut expenditures. This might mean skipping doses, dividing tablets, or postponing restocking them so that one pack can be used for a longer time. Failing to follow treatment procedures due to expense concerns may undermine its efficacy, thereby worsening health conditions and increasing medical care utilization and long-term costs. When people cannot pay for their prescriptions adequately, managing illnesses becomes impossible leading to bad health outcomes. Inadequate adherence to treatment can cause patients' ailments to progress further; symptoms become more severe while at the same time bringing about higher chances of having complications from these disorders [10].

To avoid problems and stay healthy, long-term illnesses like diabetes, high blood pressure, or asthma need continuous medication. When people cannot stick to their treatment because of money shortages, they risk getting sick beyond control, which will negatively impact their lives. Pharmaceutical Assistance Programs (PAPs), Patient Assistance Programs (PAPs), and drug discount cards are some ways that can ease the financial strain of drugs for those who qualify. As much as they can, healthcare professionals should always recommend cheaper drugs, such as generic substitutes, when writing prescriptions so that patients do not spend too much out-of-pocket [11].

To enable patients to minimize costs effectively, education on prescription drug affordability through techniques such as splitting pills, making large purchases, and comparing prices is important. Policy reforms advocating for reduced drug costs, increased insurance coverage, and improved access to affordable healthcare can help overcome socio-economic barriers to medication adherence [12].

Lack of Insurance Coverage

People who do not have enough money are the ones who are affected most by the lack of insurance coverage, which makes adherence to medication difficult. Patients without health insurance are usually faced with financial difficulties that prevent them from getting drugs that were prescribed for them, and this is because they have to pay for everything themselves. Due to this fact, many people find it impossible to buy necessary medicines and hence start using cost-related non-adherence methods like skipping doses or reducing the amount taken in order to ease their budgets. Another thing is when you do not have insurance cover; some medications may become hard to get, especially if one does not work since retail prices can be quite high [13].

This restriction bars patients from receiving important care and makes them resort to other, possibly less successful treatments. The consequences of being uninsured go further than just money problems; it can also greatly affect health. Those without coverage are more likely to suffer from negative health outcomes as a result of unattended or poorly controlled illnesses caused by not taking prescribed medicines. Uninsured portions of the population will see an increase in health disparities for chronic ailments like diabetes, which need regular adherence to drugs leading to the use of medical services among such groups [14].

This challenge can be tackled in many ways, such as widening healthcare coverage through government insurance programs, setting up safety net clinics and community health centers, making policy changes that will make healthcare more affordable, and reducing the prices of prescribed drugs. Health systems could promote better health outcomes among vulnerable groups through the reduction of disparities in care between insured and uninsured patients, which might be achieved if they decrease the number of people who don't take their drugs because they are not covered by insurance [15].

Limited Access to Healthcare Resources

The reason behind not following prescribed medications is the lack of enough healthcare resources due to differences in incomes, which makes them difficult to get. The inability to reach healthcare facilities due to distance, low medical structures, and issues with transport all combine leading to the failure of patients to take drugs as required by doctors. People living in remote regions or areas without enough health services find it hard to visit hospitals and drug stores, which worsens their situation since they do not take medicine as directed [16].

Moreover, barriers with regard to transport and logistics could hold patients back from making it to medical appointments, refilling prescriptions, or even getting essential healthcare services. These challenges worsen the current disparities in healthcare access based on socioeconomic status thus putting more pressure on underprivileged groups. As a result, patients who do not have enough opportunities for health care provision are very likely to suffer negative health effects caused by failure to take medicine as required, which leads to uncontrolled treatment of their illnesses [17].

To eliminate these obstacles, there should be a general strategy, which includes making better the healthcare infrastructure, widening the transport industry and introducing telemedicine programs that can help fill in the distance between people living in different regions. Moreover, community-centered actions like mobile clinics or outreach schemes may come into play so as to reach out to those who are underserved and ensure they get medication. Health systems should address themselves towards reducing the lack of access to resources; this way, they will also be dealing with non-compliance with drugs as well as creating equal opportunities for all individuals irrespective of their social standing [18].

Health Literacy

Understanding of Treatment Regimen

Medicine adherence is highly dependent on health literacy because it refers to the patient's understanding and compliance with their prescribed treatment. In order to fully adhere to a regimen for optimum health outcomes, patients need to know how complex such plans can be, including drug directions, dosage timings, and possible adverse reactions, among other things [19].

People who have limited health literacy can have a lot of trouble understanding their treatments. This often leads to them not taking their medicine and it is not working as well as it should. They might not understand what the doctor tells them, they have trouble reading, or they can't figure out when to take how much of what medicine. Because of this, patients may misinterpret medication instructions by either over- or under-dosing themselves at the wrong times; or they may simply ignore adherence altogether without realizing its significance toward treatment success thus failing to achieve therapeutic targets [20].

Medication misconceptions can make it difficult for people with inadequate medical knowledge to take medicine as directed. They may think it is unnecessary, have wrong ideas about side effects, or misunderstand how much they control their disease. All these beliefs can cause doubt or unwillingness to follow through with treatments that were prescribed thereby reducing their effectiveness [21].

Patients who cannot speak English properly because it is not their first language face many problems in understanding instructions for medication when they are sick and have no knowledge about health. They may not be able to comprehend how much medicine should be taken or what time, thus leading them into a serious condition that could have been avoided if only they understood the prescription given by their doctor. These people also find it hard to express themselves when something goes wrong with regard to treatment, mainly because of miscommunication that arises from using unfamiliar languages [22].

In order to deal with obstacles related to health literacy, interventions must be designed specifically with the intention of helping patients comprehend their treatment regimens. Healthcare providers must facilitate patient education and communication, which involves using accessible language when explaining medication instructions and treatment plans. Patients' understanding can be improved through interactive educational materials, visual aids as well as tools used for managing medicines, thus enabling them to take charge of their health [23].

Additionally, it is important to consider patient participation in shared decision-making as well as the involvement of patients in their treatment plans because these practices can make people feel more responsible for what happens to them health-wise. To overcome language obstacles and ensure that different communities comply with prescriptions, medical practitioners must employ patient education programs that are sensitive to culture such as hiring interpreters who understand various languages and using appropriate materials [24].

Misconceptions about Medication

Misconceptions about medications present a huge problem among people with poor health education, hindering compliance. These erroneous beliefs may stem from different sources, including false information, cultural traditions, and ignorance of what drugs are meant for or how they work. A common misunderstanding is the supposed indispensability of medicines; patients may doubt their necessity because they think their state will improve without any help or that drugs do not help in dealing with symptoms [25].

As a result, patients may neglect their recommended course of therapy, which puts their health at risk. In addition, they could have wrong ideas about the side effects of drugs based on overblown fears or misunderstanding of what could go wrong. People may opt not to take medicines because they prioritize evading imagined dangers as opposed to realizing their advantages. Also, an inadequate grasp of health knowledge can lead to misconstruing medication involvement in disease control; for example, many individuals do not know that drugs are meant to keep symptoms under control or prevent further deterioration by breaking down illnesses [26].

To deal with such mistaken ideas, we have to educate patients in specific ways; one such way is by providing them with adequate information about the objectives, advantages, and possible adverse reactions of their medicines as prescribed for them. This can be achieved through giving out written materials and using visual aids. At the same time involving patients in shared decision-making will enable them to understand better what this entails on their part, too. Moreover, it may involve adopting culturally sensitive approaches towards educating patients so that any wrong beliefs arising from culture are dealt with appropriately, as well as ensuring that knowledge is passed across different cultural backgrounds efficiently. To sum up, getting rid of misconceptions about drugs plays a crucial role in enhancing compliance among people who have a little understanding of health matters and also helps in improving their well-being [27].

Language Barriers

Among people who have a poor ability to read, language serves as a barrier that hinders them from taking their medication on time. This makes it difficult for doctors and patients to understand each other well enough, thus leading to ineffective communication. When the patient and doctor do not share common languages, it becomes tough for them to comprehend drug prescriptions, treatment plans, or even likely side effects, which can result in misuse of drugs as well as non-adherence. Still, these same barriers might stop people from sharing their worries about medicine with healthcare professionals if they do not speak the same language as them [28].

Moreover, patients with limited access to language are likely to have difficulty managing their medications because they do not have enough resources in the language they understand. It is recommended that medical professionals overcome this issue by using qualified interpreters or translation services and giving drug instructions in plain words. Furthermore, the provision of translated written materials, as well as the adoption of culturally sensitive care practices, is necessary for supporting adherence to medicines among people from different linguistic backgrounds. Health workers should strive to ensure that there are no communication hindrances between them and the patients, which will help in following prescriptions correctly, leading to better health results for all, irrespective of the language used [29, 30].

Psychological Factors

Depression and Anxiety

Among those with chronic diseases, depression as well as anxiety are among the most serious psychological factors that may significantly affect adherence to medication. Such psychiatric problems create unique problems for sticking to prescribed medicine regimens, which often lead to less-than-ideal outcomes in treatment. One of the main issues caused by these two conditions is they decrease motivation levels and involvement in self-care activities. Apathy, lack of hope, and tiredness that accompany such illnesses usually reduce a person's desire to follow a timetable or even visit doctors regularly [31].

Furthermore, depression and anxiety can disrupt cognitive abilities such as memory, concentration, and decision-making. This dysfunction of cognition may cause unintended non-adherence as patients try hard to recall taking drugs or understand complicated dosing directions. Another thing is that individuals who have depression together with anxiety could start avoiding drugs which they think remind them about being sick or giving rise to undesirable effects that make them emotionally uncomfortable. Such a dislike may lead to deliberate non-compliance when people intentionally fail to take medicine prescribed in order to relieve themselves from pain or anxiety [32].

In addition, depression and anxiety often take the form of not being treated and unwillingness to cooperate with health care providers, complicating efforts to ensure adhesion to medication. Fear of criticism or stigma attached to mental health can interfere with a person's decision to seek assistance or follow through on treatment plans. Dealing with these emotional issues calls for a comprehensive strategy that involves screening and treating mental illnesses in primary healthcare centers, encouraging joint decisions between primary care physicians and psychologists; as well as evidence-based practices like teaching patients about their condition (psychoeducation) and helping them manage it themselves through cognitive-behavioral therapy [33].

Also, it improves treatment if there is a supportive and unconditionally evaluative alliance between patients and healthcare providers. In conclusion, to support the treatment of chronic ailments, the impact of depression and anxiety on medication adherence should be recognized and dealt with accordingly [34].

Stigma Associated with Medication

Medication usage is burdened with a heavy psychological load, which is responsible for the poor adherence to medicines by patients with various health problems. Rooted in social stereotypes and prejudices, this attitude mostly affects people suffering from mental disorders like depression, anxiety, or schizophrenia. The way medication is seen negatively by society could make those affected feel humiliated and even judge themselves, lowering their adherence [35].

Fear of social isolation and stigmatization is one of the main consequences of medication stigmatization. Stigma prevents people from talking about their medicines freely or seeking help; they do not want to be labeled as outcasts or discriminated against. This fear increases isolation, making it hard for individuals to deal with their health issues effectively. Additionally, such stigma may be internalized by patients, forcing them to think negatively about themselves and self-stigma when in need of medications. The above effects can lead to individuals feeling useless and guilty, thus reducing motivation to stick to prescribed doses [36].

As a result, the stigma of medication often leads to non-compliance with treatment because people may refuse to take their drugs deliberately so that they do not have to appear as "different" or "weak." In some instances, a number of individuals even go to the extent of hiding taking medicines and altogether stop using drugs for fear of being judged or discriminated against. Similarly, medication stigmatization can pose a challenge when it comes to seeking assistance from healthcare service providers who deal with psychological issues. Due to stigma, delayed help-seeking behavior can lead to late diagnosis, insufficient therapy, and deteriorated mental health indications. Tackling drug stigmatization necessitates an array of interventions, such as education, advocacy, and support [37].

Stigmatization of medication use can be minimized by means of education and awareness campaigns that challenge stereotypes and increase dialogue. Medical treatment centers, the general public, and individualized medical care settings are able to offer a supportive backdrop for patients, making them feel safe when seeking help and following their prescription drug regimens without apprehension of stigma. Besides, those organizations advocating for mental health and other peer support communities can be invaluable in terms of providing essential assistance and combating misconceptions associated with drug use [38].

Fear of Side Effects

The major psychological barrier to medication adherence among people managing health conditions is the fear of side effects from medication. Such fear often arises from worries about possible allergic responses, risks that seem real or unreal, and their influence on daily activities and lifestyle. A number of difficulties come about in relation to drug compliance due to apprehension over side effects. Anxiety increases for those who are anxious about taking medications because they are scared of possible adverse results. This anxiety may result in a person's lack of willingness to start treatment or continue it as long as they view the harm as outweighing any good given by medicine [39].

Additionally, people may be afraid of various side effects that can arise from consuming particular drugs, thus avoid taking them completely. However, in an effort to escape possible harm and danger, individuals may fall into the avoidance behavior. Another factor that contributes to intentional non-adherence is when some people choose short-term anxiety reduction against long-term disease control and symptom management. The fear of any reaction associated with medication leads to increased body monitoring concerning perceived adverse effects leading to skipping doses of medicine. This heightened awareness increases worries and leads to non-compliance with prescriptions as they may wrongly associate harmless symptoms or natural body feelings with medicine-induced damage [40].

Moreover, the fear of side effects can also ruin the trust people have in health care professionals and how medication functions; hence individuals will begin to doubt their safety and appropriateness of the prescribed treatment plan. As a result, they may opt for other forms of treatments or even try out self-medication as this is believed to help them reduce their anxiety levels, thus making it difficult for them to stick to drugs and recover better from illnesses. Eradicating fear of any side effect requires a client-centered approach that focuses on teaching, talking, and supporting patients. Health providers must deal with patients' concerns and give the right information about drug benefits and risks while explaining misconceptions or worries concerning side effects [41].

Dialogue should be opened, and individuals must be allowed to make decisions together with others. It helps people actively engage in their treatment-related decision-making processes, overcoming their fear. This, in the long run, promotes adherence to medication, thus improving health outcomes. Additionally, by providing reassurance and support as well as access to resources, including patient support groups or counseling services, individuals can learn how to cope with their fears and develop strategies for coping with drug-related anxiety. To conclude, the fear of side effects acts as a major psychological impediment that hinders patients from adhering to medication, which further emphasizes the need for addressing patients' worries and giving holistic care in order to enhance the successful management of illnesses [42].

FACTORS AFFECTING HEALTHCARE SYSTEM

Factors affecting medication adherence in the healthcare system are summarized in Fig. (**2**).

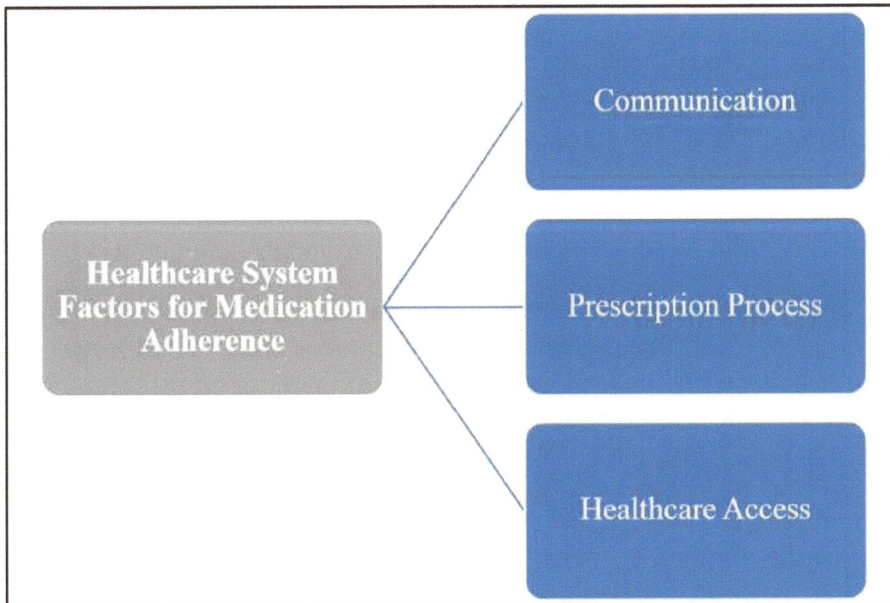

Fig. (2). Healthcare system factors for medication adherence.

Communication

Patient-Provider Communication

A cornerstone of effective healthcare delivery is patient-provider communication which significantly influences patient satisfaction, treatment adherence, and health outcomes. This exchange involves information sharing, concerns, and a collective process of decision-making between patients and health providers. The transparent transfer of medical information, starting from medical history to treatment alternatives, is critical in this interaction. Patients are well educated about their health condition and its treatment through access to clear and all-inclusive information, which allows them to actively involve themselves in their care plan [43].

Active listening is also very important to healthcare providers in enabling them to understand patients' feelings, choices, and ambitions with empathy. In addition, when clinicians carefully listen to clients, they can adapt their communication styles so as to meet individual requirements, thus promoting patient participation in decision-making. Further, trust and therapeutic relationships are built on a foundation of empathy and emotional support. Through showing empathy and compassion for the patients, the healthcare providers foster an environment that allows open communication and patient disclosure [44].

The importance of shared decision-making in patient-provider communication is further emphasized, enabling coordinated talks that result in treatment plans that match the patients' value systems and aspirations. This way, it helps patients take responsibility for their own health thereby leading to better medication adherence and satisfaction. Also, the mode of language used has a big role to play as clear communication is needed for patients to understand medical information or instructions. When using plain language and avoiding medical terms, all clients with different health literacy levels are able to participate actively in care [45].

Finally, respecting patient self-determination is the most important thing; which can be done by enabling patients to make choices that are informed by their values and beliefs. In medical practice, practitioners employ shared decision-making models in which patient autonomy is a priority yet expert medical recommendations are given. Thus, better training for health care providers regarding how to communicate appropriately with the patients as well as executing effective methods and tools of communication is necessary alongside recognizing the importance of patient feedback and promoting an organizational culture characterized by excellent communication practices. Eventually, concern for transparent, compassionate, and cooperative conversation promotes reliance leading to an improved level of satisfaction among patients while it enables individuals to access their desired health expectations [46].

Clarity of Medication Instructions

Patient adherence to medication directions and treatment outcomes are largely influenced by how well the medication instructions have been communicated. The patient must be able to understand what it means and how to take the medicines as prescribed- dose, frequency, route of administration, and what side effects could be expected. For healthcare providers to communicate effective medication instructions, they should use simple language that would not contain medical jargon but would make it easy for patients to know exactly what is being talked about. By making complicated medical terms simpler and putting explanations in a few words that every patient will comprehend, clinicians will enable their clients to appreciate why they were given such prescriptions [47, 48].

To make sure that the patient has grasped the information, healthcare providers should use a teach-back method where patients are asked to repeat the given instructions in their own words while taking drugs . Beyond medical offices, medication labels, prescription inserts, and patient education tools are included since they concern clear communication of medication instructions. It is important to present such materials in a readable manner with instructions that can be easily seen and organized for easy reference. Having bilingual or multilingual materials as well as translating services for patients who cannot understand English well will also improve accessibility and understanding of medication directions [49].

In order to increase sincerity in the provision of instructions for drugs, healthcare institutions should adopt efforts aimed at enhancing quality such as standardized labeling protocols for drugs, electronic prescribing systems that have patient education modules embedded in them, and interdisciplinary communication strategies among caregivers. Doctors can make patients take full responsibility for their health by emphasizing clarity on the use of medication thus increasing compliance with medications and eventually leading to improved patient results and better care [50].

Follow-up Mechanisms

Within the healthcare system, a resilient monitoring system is needed to maintain care coordination, patient safety, and outcome improvements. This routine entails structured exchanges between medical practitioners and patients after surgeries, appointments, or changes in therapy. Follow-up communication serves several crucial purposes, including monitoring patient progress, addressing concerns or complications, reinforcing treatment adherence, and facilitating coordination of care. Healthcare providers use such follow-up channels as telephone calls, electronic mail, e-portals, and telemedicine applications to track patients' post-visit conditions [51].

Prompt follow-up after visits lets the doctor or nurse review what happened during a visit, measure if medicines are taken correctly, and fix problems as soon as they arise. Also, follow-up communication is an opportunity for patients to ask about their prescriptions, understand how to take them better, and share any symptoms that have shown afterward. This helps in engaging more patients actively by encouraging trust amongst them thus increasing the level of care provided in general. In addition, mechanisms of follow-up are important in the coordination of care which acts as a platform for effective communication among healthcare teams as well as ensuring appropriate referral or other ancillary services for further management [52].

Furthermore, structured follow-up protocols help identify patients at higher risk of treatment failure or adverse events, allowing for timely intervention and personalized care adjustments. Healthcare organizations can implement standardized follow-up procedures, including automated reminder systems, electronic health record alerts, and quality improvement initiatives, to enhance the efficiency and effectiveness of follow-up communication. By prioritizing systematic follow-up mechanisms, healthcare providers can improve patient outcomes, reduce healthcare disparities, and promote patient-centered care delivery [53].

Prescription Process

Complexity of Medication Regimen

As a matter of fact, within healthcare systems, the intricacy of medication regimens in the prescription process is a major problem affecting patient adherence, treatment efficacy, and safety. Drug regimes as a matter of fact can be extremely varied because they are influenced by such factors as the number of drugs prescribed, dosing periods, methods of administration, and times for taking them. As regimens for medicines become more complicated, it may be hard for patients to understand and strictly follow their prescriptions. In any case, complex medicinal routines usually require patients to manage multiple medications at once which have unique dosing instructions as well as possible interactions with other drugs. Remembering when and how to take each medication is difficult for certain patients leading to mistakes or even missed doses [54, 55].

In addition, hard-to-follow programs intensify the chances that a patient may not adhere to medication schedules because they might feel dragged or confounded by the number of drugs and how to use them. Healthcare providers also face problems with regard to medication regimens being complex as they have to prescribe accurately and communicate treatment instructions effectively. It is necessary that the regimen design incorporates factors such as patient medical history, comorbidities, medicine tolerance, *etc.* when defining the regimen; otherwise, poor results will be received as a consequence thereof. Also, clinicians must ensure that medication regimes are suitable for each individual patient taking into consideration their age, and cognitive ability among other lifestyle preferences [56].

Healthcare organizations can adopt tactics for simpler prescriptions that facilitate medication adherence in light of complex medication regimens. This may involve the employment of tools for drug reconciliation, e-prescribing systems, and providing information to patients as a way of smoothening communication and issuing unambiguous guidelines. Also, collaboration between healthcare professionals, pharmacists, and patients in terms of interdisciplinary can lead to optimized medication regimens with less complexity. Complex medication regimes pose challenges that health systems must surmount to better patient outcomes, improve drug security, and allow effective management of chronic diseases [57].

Inadequate Prescription Refill System

An inadequate prescription renewal system is a real problem in healthcare. One of the difficulties it causes is breaks in patients' treatment, problems with taking prescribed drugs as scheduled, and even harm to these individuals. The continuation of medication access by patients who have continuous therapy or chronic illnesses would depend on the re-prescription procedure. Nevertheless, when there are deficiencies in this refilling system; it may result in delays, errors, and wastage which affect the health status of the patient negatively. Problems come about because refill processes are not streamlined properly; whereby customers meet barriers such as long waits, heavy documentation, or unclear instructions regarding prescription renewals. Such obstacles are frustrating and leave one unhappy with the services offered within a hospital [58].

Moreover, poor communication among healthcare providers, pharmacies, and patients can lead to delays in refilling prescriptions and misunderstandings about the medications required and their use. Patients may be perplexed or puzzled when it comes to requesting refills thus leading to missed doses or treatment interruptions. Additionally, inconsistency in prescription renewal approaches by medical practitioners complicates the process of refilling thereby creating discrepancies in medication availability and dosing instructions. Poor systems for prescription refills are also not safe as patients may find themselves engaging in harmful coping mechanisms such as rationing drugs or resorting to alternative sources due to drug scarcity. These practices heighten the risk of adverse drug events, medication errors, and non-compliance with therapy [59].

To tackle issues related to refill systems that are not sufficient, healthcare organizations could find ways of making their refill processes more straightforward, improving communication and coordination between individuals involved, and employing technology to make electronic prescribing easier as well as automated refill reminders more viable. Also, patients can be taught and mobilized in such a way that they participate actively in self-administration of drugs and calling for timely refills. Through improved prescription refill systems, healthcare systems can improve satisfaction among patients while optimizing medication adherence thus leading to safer and more effective service delivery [60].

Availability of Generics vs. Branded Medications

The availability of generic *vs.* branded medications with different aspects is shown in Table **1**.

Table 1. Availability of generic *vs.* branded medications with different aspects.

Aspect	Generics	Branded Medications
Cost	Generally more affordable	Often more expensive [61].
Accessibility	Widely available	Availability may vary [62].
Insurance Coverage	Often covered by insurance	Coverage may vary [63].
Quality and Safety	Subject to regulatory standards	Subject to regulatory standards [64].
Therapeutic Equivalence	Bioequivalent to branded versions	Original formulation [65].
Perception	Sometimes perceived as less effective or inferior	Perceived as premium or superior [66].
Appearance	May differ from branded counterparts	Consistent appearance and packaging [67].
Inactive Ingredients	May differ from branded counterparts	Consistent with branded formulation [68].
Market Competition	Encourages competition and lowers prices	May face limited competition leading to higher prices [69, 70].

Healthcare Access

Geographic Barriers

Healthcare accessibility difficulties resulting from geographical barriers are more severe for those people living in remote or rural areas with limited proximity to health facilities. These obstacles consist of various elements of the landscape that can hinder a person's access to medical care within a short period. The first challenge is poor infrastructure and the absence of healthcare facilities in remote regions, which results in limited contact with primary care providers, specialists as well as medical centers. Moreover, this problem is worsened by the insufficient number of healthcare professionals in rural areas since patients have to spend a lot of time travelling and waiting before they can receive basic medical assistance [71].

Furthermore, these geographic barriers often cross socio-economic barriers like poverty and transportation shortages thus minimizing their access to healthcare. For individuals living in rural areas with limited cash or who are immobile, fewer public transport options and poor road networks present major challenges for them while getting to health facilities. Moreover, there may be limitations on the availability of emergency medical services due to geographical factors mainly in areas where the population density is low and the terrain is roughly rugged hence leading to late ambulance response times. In addition, people without available health facilities may depend on informal caregivers or even do self-care for minor illnesses thereby, increasing health inequities and delaying early identification as well as treatment of diseases [72, 73].

There are many strategies that can be used to overcome geographic barriers to healthcare access such as telemedicine, mobile clinics, and community health outreach programs in order to extend healthcare services to underserved rural populations. Moreover, the expansion of telecommunication networks, enhancing transportation infrastructure, and motivating health workers to provide healthcare services in rural areas will enable residents living in remote places to have an opportunity to have access to these services. If geographical obstacles could be countered with improved accessibility, then health delivery systems would become more fair and equal for people irrespective of their localities, thereby aiding in the promotion of better health outcomes [74].

Long Waiting Times

Healthcare access may be impaired by long waiting times, which are an obstacle to those who require prompt and efficient medical attention. Consultations, tests, appointments, or surgeries involving waiting times could result in delayed diagnosis of diseases preventing their treatment, hence managing them in order to restore normal health status for patients. One of the main causes for these endless waits is the mismatch between the number of patients and the amount of resources available to provide healthcare provision such as inadequate health infrastructure, shortages in the workforce, and insufficient funding. The demand for healthcare services has increased due to population increase, aging populations as well as an escalation in incidence rates of chronic illnesses that further worsens this situation, leading to overpopulated Outpatient Departments (OPDs), emergency units (EUs), and medical wards [75].

The use of inefficient healthcare workflows, administrative bottlenecks, and outmoded scheduling systems can also lengthen waiting periods as patients work through complicated pathways to get medical attention. The danger in long waiting times is that it not only affects the patients but also hampers equity among those with limited resources or competing obligations who may struggle more in accessing care on time. Furthermore, prolonged wait times lead to patient dissatisfaction, frustration, and anxiety, which impact overall health experiences and trust in the health system. Therefore, strategies such as optimizing appointment schedules; enhancing workflow productivity as well as better resource allocation can be used by healthcare organizations to address long waiting times [76].

This might involve embracing technology solutions including electronic health records, telemedicine platforms, and patient appointment reminder systems for process improvement and administrative burden reduction. Moreover, increasing healthcare capacity through workforce expansion, infrastructure investment, and service innovation could help meet the growing patient demand and address waiting times. By prioritizing efforts to reduce waiting times, healthcare systems can enhance patient access to timely and equitable care, improve patient satisfaction, and ultimately promote better health outcomes for all individuals [77].

Availability of Specialized Care

In order to address such medical cases and be able to cater to the different health needs of the patients, access to specialized care is necessary. Specialized care refers to a variety of medical services provided by healthcare professionals who have received specific training and have expertise in various areas or subspecialties. Such services may comprise but are not limited to sophisticated diagnostic approaches, cutting-edge treatment techniques, surgical procedures and multidisciplinary team management meant for rare or complex ailments. The lack of even distribution of specialized health providers and facilities contributes to the unequal availability of specialty care across different regions [78].

There are limited options for individuals in rural or underserved areas to access specialized care because of an insufficient supply of specialized healthcare providers, long travel distances, and lack of appropriately developed health facilities. In addition, socioeconomic factors such as income, insurance coverage, and social support networks can contribute to disparities in accessing specialist care including financial barriers and navigating the health system among low-income populations. Healthcare organizations can apply strategies that will enhance the availability and accessibility of specialized care in order to address these challenges. This may involve extending telemedicine services, setting up regional referral networks, and investing in mobile healthcare units that deliver specialty services to communities that are disadvantaged [79].

Moreover, workforce development initiatives such as employee recruitment incentives, training programs, and interdisciplinary collaborations can enlarge the pool of specialized healthcare providers and increase the capacity of healthcare systems to deliver specialized care. By concentrating on improving access to specialized care, health delivery systems can ensure that patients get timely access to quality treatment based on evidence, regardless of where they live or their earnings. Doing this not only leads to improved patient outcomes and satisfaction but also helps in reducing disparities in healthcare and achieving health equity across diverse populations [80].

MEDICATION-SPECIFIC FACTORS

Medication-specific factors for medication adherence are summarized in Fig. (**3**).

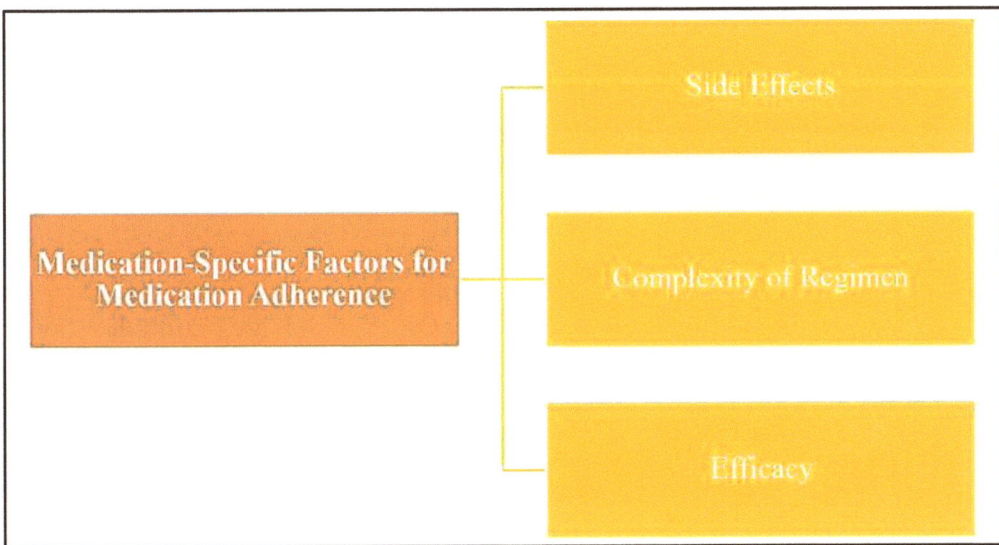

Fig. (3). Medication-specific factors for medication adherence.

Side Effects

Severity of Side Effects

Medication-specific side effects influence medication compliance and patient outcomes. Medications are meant to relieve symptoms or manage medical conditions, but they can also cause harmful consequences, which may vary in intensity from minor to severe. Nausea, dizziness, fatigue, and gastrointestinal disturbances are some of the most frequent side effects that commonly lower patients' ability to bear them and risk their commitment to a therapy regimen. The gravity of these side effects, on the other hand, also shapes how patients react and make choices regarding adherence to drugs. Mild side effects may be tolerable by others so much as they endure treatment in spite of pain [81].

Still, mild and observable side effects, for instance, allergic reactions, cardiovascular events, or even neurological complications, can cause severe health issues and require patients to stop taking medicine. The complexity of the effect of side effects on adherence is diverse because it depends on different things like how severe symptoms are believed to be by patients, their ability to cope with side effects, and trust in medical practitioners' leadership. Healthcare providers can also tackle medication-specific factors by discussing potential side effects with them ahead of time, providing anticipatory guidance, and offering strategies to manage adverse reactions [82].

Monitoring patients for side effects during their treatment and dealing with any worries, concerns, or complications that arise will also reduce the effect on patient adherence and safety. The impact of adherence to medication through enhanced treatment outcomes, improved health outcomes and patient satisfaction can be enhanced by addressing the medication-specific factors such as side effects in terms of how severe they are [83].

Perception of Side Effects

Medication adherence and patient outcomes are heavily influenced by the perception of side effects, which affect patients' behaviors, attitudes toward treatment, and their experiences with it. Personal beliefs, past experience, information given by health care providers, and the media and cultural norms influence how patients perceive side effects. Positive perceptions of side effects, such as regarding them as indicators of drug effectiveness or being inherent in healing processes can enhance acceptance and adherence to treatment [84].

On the other hand, patients' belief in negative perceptions can reduce their reliance on prescribed drugs due to the fear, anxiety, or anticipation of adverse reactions. The subjective nature of perception means that individuals may interpret identical side effects differently; some may have minimal disruption to ordinary life while others find them unbearable. Also, the nocebo effect happens when people experience bad feelings due to their expectation of harm as a result of side effects which complicates medication adherence and treatment outcomes even more [85].

To address patients' perceptions of side effects, it is important for providers to offer correct information, maintain open lines of communication, and handle wrong notions or concerns that come with medication use. Empowering patients to take part in their own care through the provision of continuous support and reassurance is one way of reducing apprehension about adverse reactions, making adherence to treatment better, and improving overall satisfaction among patients thereby leading to improvement in health outcomes [86, 87].

Frequency of Dosing

The frequency of dosing, is the rate at which a drug needs to be taken within a given period, like daily, many times a day, weekly, or as needed. This is a critical aspect of medication administration because it affects treatment compliance, convenience, and therapeutic efficacy. Patients and healthcare providers may face distinct difficulties and concerns with medications having different dosing schedules. For example, drugs that need to be taken more often (*e.g.*, several times per day) can be problematic for patients who have to organize their time around the medication schedule or remember when every dose should be taken [88].

The drugs with less frequent dosing regimens like once-daily or weekly treatment plans could be more convenient for patients, thereby increasing compliance and adherence to therapy by reducing the pill burden. However, less frequent dosing may hinder maintaining constant therapeutic drug levels in the blood, especially for medications with a short half-life or narrow therapeutic range. Furthermore, patient preferences, satisfaction, and acceptability are influenced by the frequency of dosing. For some patients, simplicity and ease of use are important so they would prefer fewer doses per day while others would prioritize effectiveness as well as tolerability over dosing frequency [89].

Various factors are taken into account by healthcare professionals in prescribing medications such as the pharmacokinetics of the drug, treatment goals, patient preferences, and possible side effects in determining the most appropriate dosing frequency for individual patients. As a means of ensuring adherence and getting the best results from treatment, educating patients concerning medication dosing schedules using techniques like pill organizers, reminders, and written instructions is essential [90].

Complexity of Regimen

Number of Medications

The medication number of a person is an important determinant for medication administration, adherence to treatment, and patient outcomes. Polypharmacy is the use of various medications concurrently to manage multiple medical conditions, prevent complications, or achieve therapeutic goals. This may be essential for individuals with complex or multiple comorbidities as well as older adults who face numerous challenges . The multiplicity of drugs to be taken causes errors, adverse drug reactions, drug interactions, and nonadherence to treatment more likely than ever before [91, 92].

Incidentally, keeping numerous medications in memory cannot be an easy thing for patients to do. Moreover, cases of polypharmacy contribute to a rise in healthcare costs, hospitalizations as well as medication-related complications. Apart from that the contribution of polypharmacy leads to higher levels of health care expenses, increased utilization rates, and the possibility of hospitalization due to medication-related problems. In this regard, it is important that the healthcare providers take up their role effectively by carrying out comprehensive medication reviews; reconciling medication lists, and optimizing treatment regimens based on individual patient needs and goals [93, 94].

This may mean that we have to eliminate some drugs from the list of medications prescribed and fewer drugs while giving our patients education regarding their health. Furthermore, interdisciplinary collaboration among healthcare providers such as doctors, chemists, and nurses is very important for coordinating care, monitoring medication safety, and preventing adverse outcomes associated with polypharmacy. Patient-centered approaches that prioritize shared decision-making, communication, and continuity of care can help minimize the negative impacts of polypharmacy while optimizing medication therapy and improving overall patient well-being [95, 96].

Specific Administration Requirements

The administration requirements contain specific instructions and guidelines for safe and effective medication delivery. These requirements differ depending on factors like the drug's route of administration, formulation, and the patient's unique situation. For example, oral medications may necessitate directives regarding timing in relation to food intake taking a glass of water when taking them, or avoiding some substances that hinder their absorption. Topical drugs may need exact ways to be used such as not getting into contact with mucosa or used with applicators or gloves if necessary [97].

In addition, it is important to note that extended-release formulations are not recommended to be crushed or chewed as this may alter their pharmacokinetic properties. The intravenous route of administration requires careful dosing, dilution, and infusion rate calculations to avoid undesirable reactions and complications. Furthermore, the age, weight, renal or hepatic functions, and other medicines taken concurrently by a patient influence the modality required for giving medications. Healthcare providers should use these aspects in selecting the best dose of medicine implementation and what time should a medical practitioner administer a particular drug. To ensure the safety of medication, therapeutic outcomes' optimization, and minimizing instances of adverse effects, adherence to specific administrative requirements is mandatory. Proper communication regarding administration instructions to patients or their caregivers is vital in ensuring comprehension and adherence. By adhering strictly to administration guidelines as well as offering thorough patient education, healthcare professionals can foster drug compliance, thereby improving patient results [98].

Efficacy

Perceived Effectiveness of Medication

The perceived effectiveness of a medication is an individual's judgment of how effectively the intended therapeutic effects are achieved by a medication. Efficacy, which is the ability of a medication to achieve the desired clinical outcomes in controlled settings, is a critical factor in drug development and regulation. On the other hand, the perception of effectiveness takes into account what patients have gone through and their beliefs concerning the advantages of treatment. Several factors determine patients' perceptions about how effective drugs are, such as their expectations, previous encounters with them, symptom relief, and responses from health workers or others on whom they rely for information. Confidence, satisfaction with healthcare provider consultations as well as adherence to prescribed therapy can be enhanced by positive experiences about drug efficacy while negative ones may breed doubtfulness about its usefulness [99].

The influence of perception on treatment response is highlighted by the placebo effect, which is a condition where patients get better in symptoms or outcomes because they believe in a therapeutic intervention. Furthermore, perceptions regarding medications are influenced by the nocebo effect where a person falls ill or their symptoms worsen due to having pessimistic views about drugs. The severity and duration of the disease, the patient's perception of shared objectives and personal values associated with therapy, as well as the degree to which patients trust their physicians' recommendations, all affect patients' beliefs about drug efficacy [100].

The communication, education, and participation of health workers have a lot to do with how patients perceive the efficacy of prescribed medications. The confidence of patients in their medication can be boosted by doctors clarifying what potential risks and benefits may arise from taking the treatment as well as answering any concerns that are raised. Good results come when medical practitioners monitor reactions, give support and feedback depending on how patients respond to therapy, and plan their remedy accordingly [101, 102].

Time to Symptom Relief

The time for the symptoms to get away from us is called how long it takes for a drug to get rid of or improve the main indications of sickness or condition. Such an aspect is very important for both patients and healthcare providers since it determines treatment expectations, patient satisfaction, and overall disease control. The onset of symptom relief has a wide range based on factors like; mechanism of action, dosage, route of administration, and nature of the treated ailment. Certain drugs produce quick action, with observable responses being felt within minutes to hours after taking [102, 103].

These drugs are commonly prescribed to patients with acute conditions characterized by discomfort, inflammation, or pyrexia. In contrast, it may take a longer time before medicines for chronic ailments show signs of improvement in symptoms, typically lasting from days to weeks or even months. Individuals suffering from persistent illnesses like diabetes, hypertension and psychiatric disorders may have to wait until such time when therapeutic drug concentrations are achieved as well as underlying pathology resolves gradually for symptom relief that matters. When the symptoms start disappearing completely, it also affects how much a patient will comply with their treatment and how satisfied they are with it [104 - 106].

Due to the long time it takes for symptoms of COVID-19 to end and be managed, many patients tend not to stick to taking drugs. When patients suffer from the pains of COVID-19 for a very long duration, they easily get discouraged or disappointed, which ultimately leads to a lack of medication adherence and to discontinuation. It is paramount for healthcare providers to manage patient expectations properly, provide realistic timelines for symptom relief, and offer support as well as reasonable assurances at different stages of treatment. Hereby, dealing with patient concerns, monitoring progress on therapy, and making necessary adjustments when required; can help optimize the timing of symptom relief, leading to overall better outcomes in patients [107].

SOCIAL SUPPORT AND ENVIRONMENT

Family Dynamics

Influence of Family Members on Adherence

The role that members of a family play in influencing the adherence to medication and other health behaviors of individuals who have chronic diseases or are on medical treatment is large. Medication adherence can either be supported or impeded by the way a family works; this depends mainly on communication patterns, social support, and shared beliefs about health and illness. These kinds of families are often characterized by open expression, helping one another out, and making decisions together. Adherence rates improve and better outcomes are realized when families have good communication channels, support each other's decisions as well as discuss matters openly. In nurturing environments, close ones act as pill boxes reminding the sick person when to take medicine to help him with drug administration while also giving emotional encouragement or practical assistance during navigation through complicated schedules for therapy [108].

Besides, family members can be there for patients during healthcare visits so that their concerns are met, and their medical plans are personalized to suit their personal needs and tastes. On the other hand, a poorly functioning family may make it difficult for medication compliance to take place and intensify hindrances in treatment. Stress or anxiety can arise from intense family criticism or constant disagreement, thereby leading to non-adherence as they try to cope with such situations. Furthermore, opposing opinions or perceptions of drug use within the home may stain the patient's trust in his/her medication schedule, leading to resistance towards medication and eventually discontinuation [109].

Healthcare providers should discern the effect of family dynamics on medication adherence and include in their care processes a family-centered approach. This implies that healthcare providers should engage the family in treatment discussions, address barriers to adherence related to the family as well as educate and support them to improve communication within the family and cohesion within it. In so doing, healthcare providers will be able to empower patients and families with knowledge that will enhance collaboration in chronic condition management hence promoting health and self-care [110].

Supportive vs. Unsupportive Environments

The environment in which individuals live and interact is important for shaping their health behaviors, medication adherence inclusive. Facilitating medication adherence and enhancing general well-being are factors of supportive environments that promote it. In supportive settings, family members, friends, and caregivers support individuals who have chronic illnesses or are undergoing medical treatments by encouraging them, reminding them of their prescriptions, and offering practical help. They offer emotional support, understanding, and empathy to enable the individual to deal with difficulties encountered when adhering to complex drug regimens [111].

A sense of belonging and connectedness is encouraged by supportive environments, which foster a collaborative approach to healthcare decision-making while reducing feelings of isolation. Furthermore, supportive environments allow for persons to engage in health-promoting activities like working out together, planning meals together as well as managing medication, all of which reinforce positive health behaviours as well as adherence to treatment plans. On the other hand, non-supportive environments typified by negativity, conflict, or lack of understanding can inhibit drug compliance and worsen treatment obstacles [112].

Under such circumstances, one is likely to be criticized or laughed at by relatives, comrades, and acquaintances who will perceive him as disgraced for being infected with a disease or using medications. Inadequate sociological interactions and strains in the immediate environment can compound mental disturbance, nervousness, or despair that may spoil an individual's adherence to prescribed drugs. Besides, suppose a negative environment does not provide constructive mediums of exchange and agreement on the objectives and expectations of therapy. In that case, it may leave patients confused about personal medical options, so they do not know whether to go for treatment [113].

Social Networks

Peer Influence

Social networks are sources of peer influence. This means that there is an impact on a person's health behavior, including medication adherence. These peers are individuals of the same age or background or those with shared experiences, and they have to be understood because they utilize different platforms in their operation, for instance, social support, normative influence, and modeling behavior, among others. Positive influences that come from one's friends may give support to ensure that someone adheres to his or her medical prescriptions, is accountable for oneself, and even provide him or her with some other life events that may relate to long-term care or any treatment procedure. They may act as a role model by showing how they adhere to medication timings and carry out healthy activities, thus encouraging others also to do so [114].

Additionally, peer support networks give individuals a chance to share information, ideas, and ways of dealing with problems related to taking medicine. Sharing victories, pitfalls, and practical hints are activities that make friends come together in order to help each other develop resistance and self-efficacy necessary for managing wellbeing. Contrariwise, medication non-compliance can also be promoted by bad peer influence through social media, resulting from different reasons such as peer pressure or even unhealthy habits among the said circles. Peer pressure to conform or engage in risky behaviors can cause people to care more about fitting into their groups than properly following the directions given, concerning their medications, particularly in adolescents and young adults [115, 116].

Besides, false information or misconceptions about drugs that are spread among friends can make the rumors or stigma persist, which results in skepticism and avoidance of treatment programs. Among other things, negative engagement with peers, like blame, mockery, or dismissal by friends, may perpetuate shame, guilt, or loneliness, thereby making it difficult for these individuals to comply with their prescribed treatment plans. Healthcare providers should acknowledge peer influence on medication adherence and advocate for peer support interventions in their practice. Consequently, through utilizing positive peer pressure, advocating for peer-led counseling groups, and providing knowledge plus materials combating adverse peer pressure, health providers will enable persons to handle social influences, hence ensuring that they achieve the best medicine compliance as well as good health outcomes [117, 118].

Social Stigma

The willingness of persons to obey their recommended medical routines can be interrupted by the social stigma that accompanies health conditions and drug utilization. Stigma is caused by negative attitudes, beliefs, or stereotypes about health conditions or medications, thus resulting in discrimination, marginalization, and social exclusion. Among these stigmatized individuals include people who feel shame, embarrassed, or scared of being looked down upon, thus making it difficult for them to talk openly about their health problems or seek necessary medical attention [119].

Social stigma surrounding health conditions such as HIV/AIDS, mental illness, substance abuse, or certain chronic diseases can create barriers to medication adherence. Fear of being labeled, stereotyped, or ostracized by society may lead individuals to conceal their condition or avoid seeking treatment altogether. Additionally, stigma may undermine individuals' confidence in their ability to adhere to their medication regimen, as they may perceive themselves as being judged or shamed for their health condition or medication use [120].

It may also corrupt their interactions with people whom they know in their social networks, like families, colleagues, and friends so that the relationships get strained, they become socially withdrawn, or even lose support. Misconceptions among peers regarding medication use can deepen the issue of stigma, thus deterring individuals from seeking help and complying with treatment regimens [121, 122].

Social stigma is one of the challenging issues that healthcare providers must grapple with in their pursuit of improved medication adherence. By being able to make people understand, teach them, and have a voice against stigmatization, healthcare providers can build a supportive environment where individuals can freely talk about their health issues, pursue appropriate treatment, and take medicine as prescribed without worrying about prejudice or stigmatization. Furthermore, integrating patient-centered care methods such as client education programs, counseling services, and peer support groups into an anti-stigma program will help alleviate the consequences of stigma on medication compliance and thus enhance general health [123, 124].

Cultural Beliefs

Traditional Remedies vs. Prescribed Medications

People's attitudes and actions in terms of treatment alternatives are always influenced by their beliefs about health and welfare, including cultural opinions on traditional medicine or prescribed drugs. Traditional treatments such as herbal remedies, homeopathic medicines, or cultural therapy procedures play a huge part in the belief system of many cultures. They are seen to be natural cures that appeal to all aspects of health that people believe in, hence providing them with comfort whenever they seek medical attention. Additionally, these treatments can be administered through guidance from religious leaders or healers who support people emotionally during the recovery period [125, 126].

On the other hand, prescribed drugs could be regarded as alien, fake, or intrusive in relation to someone's traditional medicinal background despite having valid scientific and medical bases. Some of these beliefs may include mistrust of Western medicine, fear of side effects, and spiritual beliefs concerning diseases and healing. Also, people may not use medicines that are prescribed for them by doctors because they see the whole thing as Western. However, apart from this, there are several other factors where language becomes a barrier to patient care, such as limited access to health care services or disparities in health care provision, and only traditional remedies can be trusted in such cases [127].

Culturally appropriate interventions imply that cultural beliefs about traditional remedies and prescribed medications are being addressed while considering an individual's cultural background, values, and preferences. To understand the culture of patients and their medical choices, healthcare providers must interact with them in a non-judgmental manner. They can also work together with traditional healers or community leaders to foster better healthcare practices. This will enable the integration of various healthcare systems, such as traditional and modern ones, leading to culturally diverse communities promoting trust as well as respecting each other's diversity, thus resulting in better healthcare outcomes [128, 129].

Religious Beliefs Impacting Adherence

Medication adherence can be significantly affected by Religious beliefs since they influence peoples' attitudes, conducts, and choices about healthcare practices and therapies. For several persons, spiritual faiths are vital in enlightening their knowledge of well-being, illness, and healing, as well as in deciding on pharmaceutical drugs and treatment adherence. Some spiritual beliefs could encourage belief in divine healing or supernatural interventions, thereby leading patients to opt for prayer, traditional ritualism, or other alternative curative methods instead of regular medical treatments. In such instances, people may view prescribed medicines as unimportant or against their religious beliefs, thus making them hesitant or unwilling to follow the prescription doses [130, 131].

Religious beliefs emphasize the stewardship of one's body and the sanctity of life. On the other hand, a religious duty or moral obligation may influence healthcare-seeking behaviors. Religious communities can also increase medication adherence by acting as social support networks, encouragers, and enforcers for those who consume these drugs [132].

Healthcare providers need to be sensitive about their patients' religious beliefs when discussing medication adherence. They must take into account how the patients' faith influences treatment decisions and avoid being insensitive. Healthcare professionals can recognize the potential reasons that might hinder adherence and support shared decision-making by having open conversations with patients on how religion affects their medical choices in a non-judgmental way. Religious leaders and spiritual advisors can also be involved in order to work well with providers so as to solve patients' problems, teach them the significance of following prescriptions, and use cultural approaches for healthcare provision. By incorporating religious beliefs into care plans, healthcare providers can build trust, improve patient-provider communication, and increase treatment compliance as well as health outcomes among patients from different religions [133, 134].

CONCLUSION

Healthcare providers ought to comprehend the complex problems relating to compliance with medication in order to help them devise better ways of helping patients. Among many issues that prevent people from adhering to prescriptions are factors such as patient socio-economic status, health literacy, psychological variables, and health system ones like communication and care access. Moreover, cultural and religious beliefs, as well as stigma around health issues and treatment, also influence people's attitudes toward medicine adherence. Healthcare providers can overcome these hurdles by acknowledging them and finding unique ways of providing support to their patients. In addition, this can be achieved by fostering an environment where open communication, trustworthiness, and partnership are upheld between patients and service providers. Additionally, making use of community resources, including cultural competence in care provision and fostering a strong social network, can also result in better medication adherence and health. In order to effectively address the challenges of medication adherence and to advance patient-centered care within healthcare settings, there is a need to approach it holistically by taking into account individualistic, cultural, and systemic factors that have a bearing on this issue.

REFERENCES

[1]   B. Jimmy and J. Jose, "Patient medication adherence: measures in daily practice," *Oman Med J*, vol. 26, no. 3, pp. 155–159, Mar. 2011.
       [http://dx.doi.org/10.5001/omj.2011.38]

[2]   P. Kardas, E. Aarnio, T. Agh, J.F.M. van Boven, A.L. Dima, C.M. Ghiciuc, F. Kamberi, G.I. Petrova, U. Nabergoj Makovec, and I. Trečiokienė, "New terminology of medication adherence enabling and supporting activities: ENABLE terminology", *Front. Pharmacol.*, vol. 14, p. 1254291, 2023.
       [http://dx.doi.org/10.3389/fphar.2023.1254291] [PMID: 37900155]

[3]   S. Yoon, Y.H. Kwan, W.L. Yap, Z.Y. Lim, J.K. Phang, Y.X. Loo, J. Aw, and L.L. Low, "Factors influencing medication adherence in multi-ethnic Asian patients with chronic diseases in Singapore: A qualitative study", *Front. Pharmacol.*, vol. 14, p. 1124297, 2023.
       [http://dx.doi.org/10.3389/fphar.2023.1124297] [PMID: 36969865]

[4]   K. Kvarnström, A. Westerholm, M. Airaksinen, and H. Liira, "Factors contributing to medication adherence in patients with a chronic condition: A scoping review of qualitative research," *Pharmaceutics*, vol. 13, no. 7. , p. 1100, Jul 2011.
       [http://dx.doi.org/10.3390/pharmaceutics13071100]

[5]   C. Nakata, L.K. Sharp, J. Spanjol, A.S. Cui, E. Izberk-Bilgin, S.Y. Crawford, and Y. Xiao, "Narrative arcs and shaping influences in long-term medication adherence", *Soc. Sci. Med.*, vol. 285, p. 114264, 2021.
       [http://dx.doi.org/10.1016/j.socscimed.2021.114264] [PMID: 34329922]

[6]   S. Hogervorst, M. Vervloet, R. Janssen, E. Koster, M.C. Adriaanse, C.L. Bekker, B.J.F. van den Bemt, M. Bouvy, E.R. Heerdink, J.G. Hugtenburg, M. van Woerkom, H. Zwikker, C. van de Steeg-van Gompel, and L. van Dijk, "Implementing medication adherence interventions in four Dutch living labs; context matters", *BMC Health Serv. Res.*, vol. 23, no. 1, p. 1030, 2023.
       [http://dx.doi.org/10.1186/s12913-023-10018-4] [PMID: 37752529]

[7]   A.H Krist, S.T Tong , R.A Aycock, D.R Longo. Engaging patients in decision-making and behavior change to promote prevention. *Info. Ser. Use*, vol. 37, no. 2, 105-122, 2017.
       [http://dx.doi.org/10.3233/ISU-170826]

[8]   A. Gast and T. Mathes, "Medication adherence influencing factors - An (updated) overview of systematic reviews," *Systematic Reviews*, vol. 8, no. 1. May 10, 2019.
       [http://dx.doi.org/10.1186/s13643-019-1014-8]

[9]   F.H Briggs, N.E. Adler, S.A. Berkowitz, M.H. Chin, T.L. Gary-Webb, A. Navas-Acien, P.L. Thornton, and D. Haire-Joshu, "Social determinants of health and diabetes: A scientific review," *Diabetes Care*, vol. 44, no. 1. American Diabetes Association Inc., pp. 258-279, Jan, 2021.

[http://dx.doi.org/10.2337/dci20-0053]

[10]   B.A. Briesacher, J.H. Gurwitz, and S.B. Soumerai, "Patients at-risk for cost-related medication nonadherence: a review of the literature", *J. Gen. Intern. Med.,* vol. 22, no. 6, pp. 864-871, 2007.
[http://dx.doi.org/10.1007/s11606-007-0180-x] [PMID: 17410403]

[11]   M. Rezaei, S. Valiee, M. Tahan, F. Ebtekar, and R. Ghanei Gheshlagh, "Barriers of medication adherence in patients with type-2 diabetes: a pilot qualitative study", *Diabetes Metab. Syndr. Obes.,* vol. 12, pp. 589-599, 2019.
[http://dx.doi.org/10.2147/DMSO.S197159] [PMID: 31118722]

[12]   E. M. Smale, T. C. G. Egberts, E. R. Heerdink, B. J. F. van den Bemt, and C. L. Bekker, "Waste-minimising measures to achieve sustainable supply and use of medication," *Sust. Chem. Pharm*, vol. 20, p. 100400, May 2021.
[http://dx.doi.org/10.1016/j.scp.2021.100400]

[13]   S. Panahi, N. Rathi, J. Hurley, J. Sundrud, M. Lucero, and A. Kamimura, "Patient Adherence to Health Care Provider Recommendations and Medication among Free Clinic Patients", *J. Patient Exp.,* vol. 9, p. 23743735221077523, 2022.
[http://dx.doi.org/10.1177/23743735221077523] [PMID: 35155751]

[14]   S. Sriram, and M.M. Khan, "Effect of health insurance program for the poor on out-of-pocket inpatient care cost in India: evidence from a nationally representative cross-sectional survey", *BMC Health Serv. Res.,* vol. 20, no. 1, p. 839, 2020.
[http://dx.doi.org/10.1186/s12913-020-05692-7] [PMID: 32894118]

[15]   M. E. Kruk *et al.*, "High-quality health systems in the Sustainable Development Goals era: time for a revolution," *The Lancet Global Health* vol. 6, no. 11. Elsevier Ltd, pp. e1196-e1252, 2018.
[http://dx.doi.org/10.1016/S2214-109X(18)30386-3]

[16]   Jose A. Morais, "Chapter-18, Limited access to healthcare resources," 2021.

[17]   C. Giebel, K. Hanna, H. Tetlow, K. Ward, J. Shenton, J. Cannon, S. Butchard, A. Komuravelli, A. Gaughan, R. Eley, C. Rogers, M. Rajagopal, S. Limbert, S. Callaghan, R. Whittington, L. Shaw, and M. Gabbay, "A piece of paper is not the same as having someone to talk to: accessing post-diagnostic dementia care before and since COVID-19 and associated inequalities", *Int. J. Equity Health,* vol. 20, no. 1, p. 76, 2021.
[http://dx.doi.org/10.1186/s12939-021-01418-1] [PMID: 33706774]

[18]   C. Giebel, "The future of dementia care in an increasingly digital world," *Aging and Mental Health* vol. 27, no. 9. pp. 1653-1654, 2023.
[http://dx.doi.org/10.1080/13607863.2023.2172139]

[19]   T. A. Miller, "Health literacy and adherence to medical treatment in chronic and acute illness: A meta-analysis," *Patient Education and Counseling*, vol. 99, no. 7. pp. 1079-1086, Jul, 2016.
[http://dx.doi.org/10.1016/j.pec.2016.01.020]

[20]   T. A. Parnell, *Health Literacy in Nursing: Providing Person-Centered Care*, 1st ed. Burlington, MA: Jones & Bartlett Learning, 2015.

[21]   H. Al Shamsi, A. G. Almutairi, S. Al Mashrafi, and T. Al Kalbani, "Implications of language barriers for healthcare: A systematic review," *Oman Medical Journal* vol. 35, no. 2, pp. 1-7, 2020.
[http://dx.doi.org/10.5001/omj.2020.40]

[22]   L. Kahler, and J. LeMaster, "Understanding Medication Adherence in Patients with Limited English Proficiency", *Kans. J. Med.,* vol. 15, no. 1, pp. 345-350, 2022.
[http://dx.doi.org/10.17161/kjm.vol15.15912] [PMID: 35106121]

[23]   P. Allen-Meares, B. Lowry, M. L. Estrella, and S. Mansuri, "Health Literacy Barriers in the Health Care System: Barriers and Opportunities for the Profession," *Health and Social Work*, vol. 45, no. 1. National Association of Social Workers, pp. 62-64, 2020.
[http://dx.doi.org/10.1093/hsw/hlz034]

[24]   M. Galletta, M.F. Piazza, S.L. Meloni, E. Chessa, I. Piras, J.E. Arnetz, and E. D'Aloja, "Patient Involvement in Shared Decision-Making: Do Patients Rate Physicians and Nurses Differently?", *Int. J. Environ. Res. Public Health,* vol. 19, no. 21, p. 14229, 2022.
[http://dx.doi.org/10.3390/ijerph192114229] [PMID: 36361109]

[25]   W. F. Gellad, C. T. Thorpe, J. F. Steiner, and C. I. Voils, "The myths of medication adherence," *Pharmacoepidemiology and Drug Safety*, vol. 26, no. 12. John Wiley and Sons Ltd, pp. 1437-1441, 2017.
[http://dx.doi.org/10.1002/pds.4334]

[26]   E.A. Belachew, A.K. Sendekie, S.A. Wondm, E.M. Ayele, and A.K. Netere, "Misunderstanding of dosing regimen instructions among patients with chronic diseases receiving polypharmacy at the University of Gondar comprehensive specialized hospital", *PLoS One,* vol. 18, no. 1, p. e0280204, 2023.
[http://dx.doi.org/10.1371/journal.pone.0280204] [PMID: 36634103]

[27]   P.B. Bhattad, and L. Pacifico, "Empowering Patients: Promoting Patient Education and Health Literacy", *Cureus,* vol. 14, no. 7, p. e27336, 2022.
[http://dx.doi.org/10.7759/cureus.27336] [PMID: 36043002]

[28]   A. Ohtani, T. Suzuki, H. Takeuchi, and H. Uchida, "Language barriers and access to psychiatric care: A systematic review," *Psychiatric Services*, vol. 66, no. 8. American Psychiatric Association, pp. 798-805, 2015.
[http://dx.doi.org/10.1176/appi.ps.201400351]

[29]   S. Khan, D.S. Arora, A. Mey, and S. Maganlal, "Provision of pharmaceutical care in patients with limited English proficiency: Preliminary findings", *J. Res. Pharm. Pract.,* vol. 4, no. 3, pp. 123-128, 2015.
[http://dx.doi.org/10.4103/2279-042X.162358] [PMID: 26312251]

[30]   X. Ji *et al.*, "Utility of mobile technology in medical interpretation: A literature review of current practices," *Patient Education and Counseling* vol. 104, no. 9. Elsevier Ireland Ltd, pp. 2137-2145, Sep. 01, 2021.
[http://dx.doi.org/10.1016/j.pec.2021.02.019]

[31]   X. Chai, Y. Liu, Z. Mao, and S. Li, "Barriers to medication adherence for rural patients with mental disorders in eastern China: a qualitative study", *BMC Psychiatry,* vol. 21, no. 1, p. 141, 2021.
[http://dx.doi.org/10.1186/s12888-021-03144-y] [PMID: 33685432]

[32]   D. L. Hare, S. R. Toukhsati, P. Johansson, and T. Jaarsma, "Depression and cardiovascular disease: A clinical review," *European Heart Journal*, vol. 35, no. 21. Oxford University Press, pp. 1365-1372, Jun. 01, 2014.
[http://dx.doi.org/10.1093/eurheartj/eht462]

[33]   R.C. Waumans, A.D.T. Muntingh, S. Draisma, K.M. Huijbregts, A.J.L.M. van Balkom, and N.M. Batelaan, "Barriers and facilitators for treatment-seeking in adults with a depressive or anxiety disorder in a Western-European health care setting: a qualitative study", *BMC Psychiatry,* vol. 22, no. 1, p. 165, 2022.
[http://dx.doi.org/10.1186/s12888-022-03806-5] [PMID: 35247997]

[34]   L. B. Dixon, Y. Holoshitz, and I. Nossel, "Treatment engagement of individuals experiencing mental illness: review and update," *World Psychiatry*, vol. 15, no. 1, pp. 13-20, 2016.
[http://dx.doi.org/10.1002/wps.20306]

[35]   S.E. Hadland, T.W. Park, and S.M. Bagley, "Stigma associated with medication treatment for young adults with opioid use disorder: a case series", *Addict. Sci. Clin. Pract.,* vol. 13, no. 1, p. 15, 2018.
[http://dx.doi.org/10.1186/s13722-018-0116-2] [PMID: 29730987]

[36]   S. Kansra, R. Calvert, and S. Jones, "Stigma from medication use: An under-recognized burden of care," *Breathe*, vol. 17, no. 1, 2021.
[http://dx.doi.org/10.1183/20734735.0002-2021]

[37] N. Hodson, M. Majid, I. Vlaev, and S. P. Singh, "Can incentives improve antipsychotic adherence in major mental illness? A mixed-methods systematic review," *BMJ Open*, vol. 12, no. 6. BMJ Publishing Group, 2022.
[http://dx.doi.org/10.1136/bmjopen-2021-059526]

[38] A.A. Ahad, M. Sanchez-Gonzalez, and P. Junquera, "Understanding and Addressing Mental Health Stigma Across Cultures for Improving Psychiatric Care: A Narrative Review", *Cureus,* vol. 15, no. 5, p. e39549, 2023.
[http://dx.doi.org/10.7759/cureus.39549] [PMID: 37250612]

[39] L. E. Smith, R. K. Webster, and G. J. Rubin, "A systematic review of factors associated with side-effect expectations from medical interventions," *Health Expectations*, vol. 23, no. 4. Blackwell Publishing Ltd, pp. 731-758, 2020.
[http://dx.doi.org/10.1111/hex.13059]

[40] S. Lyubomirsky, L. King, and E. Diener, "The benefits of frequent positive affect: does happiness lead to success?", *Psychol. Bull.,* vol. 131, no. 6, pp. 803-855, 2005.
[http://dx.doi.org/10.1037/0033-2909.131.6.803] [PMID: 16351326]

[41] I.A. Kretchy, F.T. Owusu-Daaku, S.A. Danquah, and E. Asampong, "A psychosocial perspective of medication side effects, experiences, coping approaches and implications for adherence in hypertension management", *Clin. Hypertens.,* vol. 21, no. 1, p. 19, 2015.
[http://dx.doi.org/10.1186/s40885-015-0028-3] [PMID: 26893929]

[42] A. Fiorillo, C. De Rosa, R. Del Vecchio, V. Jurjanz, M. Schnall, G. Onchev, V. Alexiev, A. Ojeda, M. Giugliano, A. Rega, and A. Volpe, "The role of shared decision-making in improving adherence to pharmacological treatments in patients with schizophrenia: a clinical review," *Ann. Gen. Psychiatry*, vol. 19, no. 1, 2020. [Online].
[http://dx.doi.org/10.1186/s12991-020-00293-4]

[43] K.K. Spooner, J.L. Salemi, H.M. Salihu, and R.J. Zoorob, "Disparities in perceived patient-provider communication quality in the United States: Trends and correlates", *Patient Educ. Couns.,* vol. 99, no. 5, pp. 844-854, 2016.
[http://dx.doi.org/10.1016/j.pec.2015.12.007] [PMID: 26725930]

[44] C.W. Duclos, M. Eichler, L. Taylor, J. Quintela, D.S. Main, W. Pace, and E.W. Staton, "Patient perspectives of patient-provider communication after adverse events", *Int. J. Qual. Health Care,* vol. 17, no. 6, pp. 479-486, 2005.
[http://dx.doi.org/10.1093/intqhc/mzi065] [PMID: 16037100]

[45] Beers E, Nilsen ML, Johnson JT. "The role of patients: shared decision-making". *Otolaryngologic Clinics of North America.* 2017 Aug 1;50(4):689-708.
[http://dx.doi.org/10.1016/j.otc.2017.03.006]

[46] P. Hudelson, "Improving patient-provider communication: insights from interpreters", *Fam. Pract.,* vol. 22, no. 3, pp. 311-316, 2005.
[http://dx.doi.org/10.1093/fampra/cmi015] [PMID: 15805131]

[47] E. L. López, A. R. Ferreras, A. P. López, L. V. Roces, and A. L. Blázquez, "4CPS-256 Linezolid usage and cost analysis after a hospital transfer," *BMJ*, vol. 26, Suppl. 1, pp. A188.1-A188, 2019.
[http://dx.doi.org/10.1136/ejhpharm-2019-eahpconf.405]

[48] M. G. Katz, S. Kripalani, and B. D. Weiss, "Use of pictorial aids in medication instructions: A review of the literature," *American Journal of Health-System Pharmacy*, vol. 63, no. 23. pp. 2391-2397, 2006.
[http://dx.doi.org/10.2146/ajhp060162]

[49] R. J. Mullen, J. Duhig, A. Russell, L. Scarazzini, F. Lievano, and M. S. Wolf, "Best-practices for the design and development of prescription medication information: A systematic review," *Patient Education and Counseling*, vol. 101, no. 8. pp. 1351-1367, 2018.
[http://dx.doi.org/10.1016/j.pec.2018.03.012]

[50] Y.M. Huang, L.J. Chen, L.L. Hsieh, H.Y. Chan, K.C.S. Chen-Liu, and Y.F. Ho, "Evaluation of use, comprehensibility and clarity of over-the-counter medicine labels: Consumers' perspectives and needs in Taiwan", *Health Soc. Care Community,* vol. 30, no. 2, pp. 753-761, 2022.
[http://dx.doi.org/10.1111/hsc.13190] [PMID: 33034423]

[51] P. Cramer, "Freshman to senior year: A follow-up study of identity, narcissism, and defense mechanisms," *Journal of Research in Personality*, vol. 32, no. 1, pp. 156-172, 1998.

[52] H. Calkins, K. H. Kuck, R. Cappato, J. Brugada, A. J. Camm, S. A. Chen, H. J. Crijns, R. J. Damiano Jr., D. W. Davies, J. DiMarco, J. Edgerton, K. Ellenbogen, M. D. Ezekowitz, D. E. Haines, M. Haïssaguerre, G. Hindricks, Y. Iesaka, W. Jackman, J. Jalife, P. Jais, J. Kalman, D. Keane, Y. H. Kim, P. Kirchhof, G. Klein, H. Kottkamp, K. Kumagai, B. D. Lindsay, M. Mansour, F. E. Marchlinski, P. M. McCarthy, J. L. Mont, F. Morady, K. Nademanee, H. Nakagawa, A. Natale, S. Nattel, D. L. Packer, C. Pappone, E. Prystowsky, A. Raviele, V. Reddy, J. N. Ruskin, R. J. Shemin, H. M. Tsao, and D. Wilber, "2012 HRS/EHRA/ECAS expert consensus statement on catheter and surgical ablation of atrial fibrillation: Recommendations for patient selection, procedural techniques, patient management and follow-up, definitions, endpoints, and research trial design," *Europace*, vol. 14, no. 4, pp. 528-606, Apr. 2012.
[http://dx.doi.org/10.1093/europace/eus027]

[53] K.E. Kurkul, and K.H. Corriveau, "Question, Explanation, Follow-Up: A Mechanism for Learning From Others?", *Child Dev.,* vol. 89, no. 1, pp. 280-294, 2018.
[http://dx.doi.org/10.1111/cdev.12726] [PMID: 28128445]

[54] L.L. Pantuzza, M.G.B. Ceccato, M.R. Silveira, L.M.R. Junqueira, and A.M.M. Reis, "Association between medication regimen complexity and pharmacotherapy adherence: a systematic review", *Eur. J. Clin. Pharmacol.,* vol. 73, no. 11, pp. 1475-1489, 2017.
[http://dx.doi.org/10.1007/s00228-017-2315-2] [PMID: 28779460]

[55] J. George, Y.T. Phun, M.J. Bailey, D.C.M. Kong, and K. Stewart, "Development and validation of the medication regimen complexity index", *Ann. Pharmacother.,* vol. 38, no. 9, pp. 1369-1376, 2004.
[http://dx.doi.org/10.1345/aph.1D479] [PMID: 15266038]

[56] M.V. McDonald, T.R. Peng, S. Sridharan, J.B. Foust, P. Kogan, L.E. Pezzin, and P.H. Feldman, "Automating the medication regimen complexity index", *J. Am. Med. Inform. Assoc.,* vol. 20, no. 3, pp. 499-505, 2013.
[http://dx.doi.org/10.1136/amiajnl-2012-001272] [PMID: 23268486]

[57] D. Stange, L. Kriston, A. von Wolff, M. Baehr, and D.C. Dartsch, "Medication complexity, prescription behaviour and patient adherence at the interface between ambulatory and stationary medical care", *Eur. J. Clin. Pharmacol.,* vol. 69, no. 3, pp. 573-580, 2013.
[http://dx.doi.org/10.1007/s00228-012-1342-2] [PMID: 22828657]

[58] K.T. Stroupe, M.D. Murray, T.E. Stump, and C.M. Callahan, "Association between medication supplies and healthcare costs in older adults from an urban healthcare system", *J. Am. Geriatr. Soc.,* vol. 48, no. 7, pp. 760-768, 2000.
[http://dx.doi.org/10.1111/j.1532-5415.2000.tb04750.x] [PMID: 10894314]

[59] K. Andersson, A. Melander, C. Svensson, O. Lind, and J.L.G. Nilsson, "Repeat prescriptions: refill adherence in relation to patient and prescriber characteristics, reimbursement level and type of medication", *Eur. J. Public Health,* vol. 15, no. 6, pp. 621-626, 2005.
[http://dx.doi.org/10.1093/eurpub/cki053] [PMID: 16126746]

[60] A.D. Müller, H.B. Jaspan, L. Myer, A. Lewis Hunter, G. Harling, L.G. Bekker, and C. Orrell, "Standard measures are inadequate to monitor pediatric adherence in a resource-limited setting", *AIDS Behav.,* vol. 15, no. 2, pp. 422-431, 2011.
[http://dx.doi.org/10.1007/s10461-010-9825-6] [PMID: 20953692]

[61] T. Gronde, C.A. Uyl-de Groot, and T. Pieters, "Addressing the challenge of high-priced prescription drugs in the era of precision medicine: A systematic review of drug life cycles, therapeutic drug

markets and regulatory frameworks", *PLoS One,* vol. 12, no. 8, p. e0182613, 2017.
[http://dx.doi.org/10.1371/journal.pone.0182613] [PMID: 28813502]

[62]   Available from: https://oig.hhs.gov/reports/all/2022/part-d-plan-preference-for-higher-cost-hep-titis-c-drugs-led-to-higher-medicare-and-beneficiary-spending/

[63]   A. Tungol, C.I. Starner, B.W. Gunderson, J.A. Schafer, Y. Qiu, and P.P. Gleason, *Generic Drug Discount Programs: Are Prescriptions Being Submitted for Pharmacy Benefit Adjudication?,* 2019. Available from: www.amcp.org

[64]   S.S. Dunne, and C.P. Dunne, "What do people really think of generic medicines? A systematic review and critical appraisal of literature on stakeholder perceptions of generic drugs", *BMC Med.,* vol. 13, no. 1, p. 173, 2015.
[http://dx.doi.org/10.1186/s12916-015-0415-3] [PMID: 26224091]

[65]   G. Boehm, L. Yao, L. Han, and Q. Zheng, "Development of the generic drug industry in the US after the Hatch-Waxman Act of 1984", *Acta Pharm. Sin. B,* vol. 3, no. 5, pp. 297-311, 2013.
[http://dx.doi.org/10.1016/j.apsb.2013.07.004]

[66]   S. Dunne, B. Shannon, C. Dunne, and W. Cullen, "A review of the differences and similarities between generic drugs and their originator counterparts, including economic benefits associated with usage of generic medicines, using Ireland as a case study," *Journal of Generic Medicines*, vol. 14, no. 1, pp. 1-9, 2013.
[http://dx.doi.org/10.1186/2050-6511-14-1]

[67]   Available from: https://www.nber.org/sites/default/files/2022-09/WhitePaper-Fowler10.2017.pdf

[68]   Congress.gov. *CRS Products from the Library of Congress.* Available from: https://crsreports.congress.gov

[69]   B. Latwal, and A. Chandra, "Authorized generics vs. branded generics: A perspective", *J. Generic Med.,* vol. 17, no. 1, pp. 5-9, 2021.
[http://dx.doi.org/10.1177/1741134320947773]

[70]   R. J. Wolf, "FDA 'New Drug' Approval Procedures: The Impact of Judicial Intervention on Public and Pharmaceutical Company Interests," *Seton Hall Law Review*, vol. 11, no. 4, pp. 879-915, 1981. Available: https://scholarship.shu.edu/shlr/vol11/iss4/5/

[71]   A. F. Howard, K. Smillie, K. Turnbull, C. Zirul, D. Munroe, A. Ward, P. Tobin, A. Kazanjian, and R. Olson, "Access to medical and supportive care for rural and remote cancer survivors in Northern British Columbia," *J. Rural Health*, vol. 30, no. 1, pp. 10-18, 2014.
[http://dx.doi.org/10.1080/22423982.2019.1571385]

[72]   T.A.H. Rocha, N.C. da Silva, P.V. Amaral, A.C.Q. Barbosa, J.V.M. Rocha, V. Alvares, D.G. de Almeida, E. Thumé, E.B.A.F. Thomaz, R.C. de Sousa Queiroz, M.R. de Souza, A. Lein, D.P. Lopes, C.A. Staton, J.R.N. Vissoci, and L.A. Facchini, "Addressing geographic access barriers to emergency care services: a national ecologic study of hospitals in Brazil", *Int. J. Equity Health,* vol. 16, no. 1, p. 149, 2017.
[http://dx.doi.org/10.1186/s12939-017-0645-4] [PMID: 28830521]

[73]   N. Douthit, S. Kiv, T. Dwolatzky, and S. Biswas, "Exposing some important barriers to health care access in the rural USA," *Public Health*, vol. 129, no. 6, pp. 611-620, 2015.
[http://dx.doi.org/10.1016/j.puhe.2015.04.001]

[74]   M.V. Evans, T. Andréambeloson, M. Randriamihaja, F. Ihantamalala, L. Cordier, G. Cowley, K. Finnegan, F. Hanitriniaina, A.C. Miller, L.M. Ralantomalala, A. Randriamahasoa, B. Razafinjato, E. Razanahanitriniaina, R.J.L. Rakotonanahary, I.J. Andriamiandra, M.H. Bonds, and A. Garchitorena, "Geographic barriers to care persist at the community healthcare level: Evidence from rural Madagascar", *PLOS Glob. Public Health,* vol. 2, no. 12, p. e0001028, 2022.
[http://dx.doi.org/10.1371/journal.pgph.0001028] [PMID: 36962826]

[75]   D. McIntyre and C. K. Chow, "Waiting Time as an Indicator for Health Services Under Strain: A

Narrative Review," *Inquiry (United States)*, vol. 57. SAGE Publications Inc., 2020.
[http://dx.doi.org/10.1177/0046958020910305]

[76] T. Zayas-Cabán, T. H. Okubo, and S. Posnack, "Priorities to accelerate workflow automation in health care," *J. Am. Med. Inform. Assoc.*, vol. 30, no. 1. pp. 195-201, 2023.
[http://dx.doi.org/10.1093/jamia/ocac197]

[77] A. Haleem, M. Javaid, R. P. Singh, and R. Suman, "Telemedicine for healthcare: Capabilities, features, barriers, and applications," *Sensors International*, vol. 2. 2021.
[http://dx.doi.org/10.1016/j.sintl.2021.100117]

[78] J. Zeisel, N.M. Silverstein, J. Hyde, S. Levkoff, M.P. Lawton, and W. Holmes, *Environmental Correlates to Behavioral Health Outcomes in Alzheimer's Special Care Units*, 2003. Available from: https://academic.oup.com/gerontologist/article/43/5/697/633882
[http://dx.doi.org/10.1093/geront/43.5.697]

[79] T. Guimarães, K. Lucas, and P. Timms, "Understanding how low-income communities gain access to healthcare services: A qualitative study in São Paulo, Brazil", *J. Transp. Health,* vol. 15, p. 100658, 2019.
[http://dx.doi.org/10.1016/j.jth.2019.100658]

[80] H. Alderwick, A. Hutchings, A. Briggs, and N. Mays, "The impacts of collaboration between local health care and non-health care organizations and factors shaping how they work: a systematic review of reviews", *BMC Public Health,* vol. 21, no. 1, p. 753, 2021.
[http://dx.doi.org/10.1186/s12889-021-10630-1] [PMID: 33874927]

[81] A. Pearce, M. Haas, R. Viney, S.A. Pearson, P. Haywood, C. Brown, and R. Ward, "Incidence and severity of self-reported chemotherapy side effects in routine care: A prospective cohort study", *PLoS One,* vol. 12, no. 10, p. e0184360, 2017.
[http://dx.doi.org/10.1371/journal.pone.0184360] [PMID: 29016607]

[82] V. Venditti, E. Bleve, S. Morano, and T. Filardi, "Gender-Related Factors in Medication Adherence for Metabolic and Cardiovascular Health," *Metabolites, Multidisciplinary Digital Publishing Institute (MDPI)*, vol. 13, no. 10, 2023.
[http://dx.doi.org/10.3390/metabo13101087]

[83] A. J. Gelenberg, M. L. Freeman, A. H. Markowitz, D. C. Rosenbaum, M. A. Thase, J. A. Dunner, J. S. M. Kupfer, M. E. Schatzberg, S. A. Hirschfeld, and A. L. Nemeroff, "Practice guideline for the treatment of patients with major depressive disorder, third edition: Work group on major depressive disorder," *Am. J. Psychiatry*, vol. 167, no. 10, pp. 1-56, 2010. Available: http://www.psychiatryonline.com/pracGuide/pracGuideTopic_7.aspx

[84] M. De Boer-Dennert, J. J. L. Jansen, P. A. A. de Haes, M. J. M. L. V. de Vries, E. M. G. P. J. A. Blijham, and J. A. L. M. M. Huitema, "Patient perceptions of the side-effects of chemotherapy: The influence of 5HT3 antagonists," *Eur. J. Cancer*, vol. 33, no. 12, pp. 2149-2153, 1997.

[85] M. DiBonaventura, S. Gabriel, L. Dupclay, S. Gupta, and E. Kim, "A patient perspective of the impact of medication side effects on adherence: results of a cross-sectional nationwide survey of patients with schizophrenia", *BMC Psychiatry,* vol. 12, no. 1, p. 20, 2012.
[http://dx.doi.org/10.1186/1471-244X-12-20] [PMID: 22433036]

[86] National Cancer Institute (NCI), Division of Cancer Control and Population Sciences (DCCPS), and the Agency for Research and Policy (ARP), "Patient-centered communication in cancer care: Promoting healing and reducing suffering," *National Cancer Institute*, 2007. Available: https://www.cancer.gov

[87] A. Kwame and P. M. Petrucka, "A literature-based study of patient-centered care and communication in nurse-patient interactions: barriers, facilitators, and the way forward," *BMC Nursing, BioMed Central Ltd*, vol. 20, no. 1, 2021.
[http://dx.doi.org/10.1186/s12912-021-00684-2]

[88] K. Patel, V.S. Sudhir, S. Kabadi, J.C. Huang, S. Porwal, K. Thakkar, and J.M. Pagel, "Impact of

dosing frequency (once daily or twice daily) on patient adherence to oral targeted therapies for hematologic malignancies: a retrospective cohort study among managed care enrollees", *J. Oncol. Pharm. Pract.,* vol. 25, no. 8, pp. 1897-1906, 2019.
[http://dx.doi.org/10.1177/1078155219827637] [PMID: 30823852]

[89]   K.S. Ingersoll, and J. Cohen, "The impact of medication regimen factors on adherence to chronic treatment: a review of literature", *J. Behav. Med.,* vol. 31, no. 3, pp. 213-224, 2008.
[http://dx.doi.org/10.1007/s10865-007-9147-y] [PMID: 18202907]

[90]   S. R. Maxwell, "CMJv16n5-CME_Maxwell.indd," *Clinical Medicine Journal*, vol. 16, no. 5, pp. 1-10, 2016.

[91]   J. Krska, S.A. Corlett, and B. Katusiime, "Complexity of Medicine Regimens and Patient Perception of Medicine Burden", *Pharmacy (Basel),* vol. 7, no. 1, p. 18, 2019.
[http://dx.doi.org/10.3390/pharmacy7010018] [PMID: 30717323]

[92]   J. George, M. A. C. Bissett, S. N. K. McEwan, and S. M. Ross, "Medication regimen complexity and adherence in patients at risk of medication misadventure," *Int. J. Clin. Pharm.*, vol. 28, no. 3, pp. 183-189, 2006.
[http://dx.doi.org/10.1002/j.2055-2335.2006.tb00580.x]

[93]   Sciacovelli M, Gonçalves E, Johnson TI, Zecchini VR, Da Costa AS, Gaude E, Drubbel AV, Theobald SJ, Abbo SR, Tran MG, Rajeeve V. Fumarate is an epigenetic modifier that elicits epithelial-t--mesenchymal transition. Nature. 2016 Sep 22;537(7621):544-7. https://doi.org/10.1038/nature19353

[94]   A.M. Advinha, S. de Oliveira-Martins, V. Mateus, S.G. Pajote, and M.J. Lopes, "Medication regimen complexity in institutionalized elderly people in an aging society", *Int. J. Clin. Pharm.,* vol. 36, no. 4, pp. 750-756, 2014.
[http://dx.doi.org/10.1007/s11096-014-9963-4] [PMID: 24906719]

[95]   A.M. Libby, D.N. Fish, P.W. Hosokawa, S.A. Linnebur, K.R. Metz, K.V. Nair, J.J. Saseen, J.P. Vande Griend, S.P. Vu, and J.D. Hirsch, "Patient-level medication regimen complexity across populations with chronic disease", *Clin. Ther.,* vol. 35, no. 4, pp. 385-398.e1, 2013.
[http://dx.doi.org/10.1016/j.clinthera.2013.02.019] [PMID: 23541707]

[96]   M. Carollo, V. Boccardi, S. Crisafulli, V. Conti, P. Gnerre, S. Miozzo, E. Omodeo Salè, F. Pieraccini, M. Zamboni, A. Marengoni, G. Onder, G. Trifirò, R. Antonioni, M. Selleri, G. Vitturi, A. Filippelli, S. Corrao, G. Medea, A. Nobili, L. Pasina, E.O. Salé, F.M. Petraglia, E. Poluzzi, A. Valle, A. Vercellone, and N. Veronese, "Medication review and deprescribing in different healthcare settings: a position statement from an Italian scientific consortium", *Aging Clin. Exp. Res.,* vol. 36, no. 1, p. 63, 2024.
[http://dx.doi.org/10.1007/s40520-023-02679-2] [PMID: 38459218]

[97]   H. Udono, D. L. Levey, and P. K. Srivastava, "Cellular requirements for tumor-specific immunity elicited by heat shock proteins: Tumor rejection antigen gp96 primes CD8+ T cells in vivo," *Proc. Natl. Acad. Sci. USA*, vol. 91, no. 13, pp. 5452-5456, 1994. Available: https://www.pnas.org

[98]   G. A. Shabir, "Validation of high-performance liquid chromatography methods for pharmaceutical analysis. Understanding the differences and similarities between validation requirements of the US Food and Drug Administration, the US Pharmacopeia and the International Conference on Harmonization," *J. Chromatogr. A*, vol. 987, no. 1–2, pp. 57–66, Feb. 2003.

[99]   J.B. O'Keefe, L.C. Newsom, and T.H. Taylor Jr, "A Survey of Provider-Reported Use and Perceived Effectiveness of Medications for Symptom Management in Telemedicine and Outpatient Visits for Mild COVID-19", *Infect. Dis. Ther.,* vol. 10, no. 2, pp. 839-851, 2021.
[http://dx.doi.org/10.1007/s40121-021-00432-8] [PMID: 33748931]

[100] F. Wolters, K.J. Peerdeman, and A.W.M. Evers, "Placebo and Nocebo Effects Across Symptoms: From Pain to Fatigue, Dyspnea, Nausea, and Itch", *Front. Psychiatry,* vol. 10, p. 470, 2019.
[http://dx.doi.org/10.3389/fpsyt.2019.00470] [PMID: 31312148]

[101] Y. Tu, L. Zhang, and J. Kong, "Placebo and nocebo effects: from observation to harnessing and clinical application," *Translational Psychiatry*, vol. 12, no. 1, 2022.

[http://dx.doi.org/10.1038/s41398-022-02293-2]

[102] C. M. Bate, S. J. Smith, R. J. McConnell, and A. J. Wilson, "Reflux symptom relief with omeprazole in patients without unequivocal oesophagitis," *Aliment. Pharmacol. Ther.*, vol. 10, no. 5, pp. 677-684, 1996.
[http://dx.doi.org/10.1046/j.1365-2036.1996.44186000.x]

[103] S. Wilkinson, K. Barnes, and L. Storey, "Massage for symptom relief in patients with cancer: systematic review", *J. Adv. Nurs.*, vol. 63, no. 5, pp. 430-439, 2008.
[http://dx.doi.org/10.1111/j.1365-2648.2008.04712.x] [PMID: 18727744]

[104] M. Robinson, R. J. N. S. Baker, S. P. Johnson, and C. A. White, "Onset of symptom relief with rabeprazole: A community-based, open-label assessment of patients with erosive oesophagitis," *Aliment. Pharmacol. Ther.*, vol. 15, no. 4, pp. 587-594, 2001.

[105] S.C. Kim, Y.S. Jo, I.H. Kim, H. Kim, and J.S. Choi, "Lack of medial prefrontal cortex activation underlies the immediate extinction deficit", *J. Neurosci.*, vol. 30, no. 3, pp. 832-837, 2010.
[http://dx.doi.org/10.1523/JNEUROSCI.4145-09.2010] [PMID: 20089891]

[106] A. Luz, M. Santos, R. Magalhães, J. Silveira, S. Cabral, V. Dias, F. Oliveira, S. Pereira, A. Leite-Moreira, H. Carvalho, and S. Torres, "Lack of benefit of ischemic postconditioning after routine thrombus aspiration during reperfusion: Immediate and midterm results", *J. Cardiovasc. Pharmacol. Ther.*, vol. 20, no. 6, pp. 523-531, 2015.
[http://dx.doi.org/10.1177/1074248415578171] [PMID: 25818931]

[107] J.T. Cortez, D.D. Oglesby, C. Kyriakopoulos, B. Wu, K. Chaudhuri, A. Ghosh, and R. Douilly, "On the Rupture Propagation of the 2019 M6.4 Searles Valley, California, Earthquake, and the Lack of Immediate Triggering of the M7.1 Ridgecrest Earthquake", *Geophys. Res. Lett.*, vol. 48, no. 4, p. e2020GL090659, 2021.
[http://dx.doi.org/10.1029/2020GL090659]

[108] T. A. Miller and M. R. DiMatteo, "Importance of family/social support and impact on adherence to diabetic therapy," *Diabetes, Metabolic Syndrome and Obesity*, vol. 6. pp. 421-426, 2013.
[http://dx.doi.org/10.2147/DMSO.S36368]

[109] C. C. Affusim and E. Francis, "The influence of family/social support on adherence to diabetic therapy," *Int. J. Adv. Sci. Res. Eng.*, vol. 5, no. 5, pp. 1-7, 2018.

[110] T. A. Miller and M. R. DiMatteo, "Importance of family/social support and impact on adherence to diabetic therapy," *Diabetes Metab. Syndr. Obes.*, vol. 6, pp. 421-426, 2013.
[http://dx.doi.org/10.2147/DMSO.S36368]

[111] P.A. Hall, C. Zehr, J. Paulitzki, and R. Rhodes, "Implementation intentions for physical activity behavior in older adult women: an examination of executive function as a moderator of treatment effects", *Ann. Behav. Med.*, vol. 48, no. 1, pp. 130-136, 2014.
[http://dx.doi.org/10.1007/s12160-013-9582-7] [PMID: 24500080]

[112] J. Frangieh, V. Hughes, A. Edwards-Capello, K. G. Humphrey, C. Lammey, and L. Lucas, "Fostering belonging and social connectedness in nursing: Evidence-based strategies: A discussion paper for nurse students, faculty, leaders, and clinical nurses," *Nurs. Outlook*, vol. 72, no. 4, p. 102174, Jul.–Aug. 2024.

[113] B. K. Ahmedani, "Mental health stigma: Society, individuals, and the profession," *J. Soc. Work Values Ethics*, vol. 8, no. 2, pp. 41–416, Fall 2011.

[114] X. Xu, W. Han, and Q. Liu, "Peer pressure and adolescent mobile social media addiction: Moderation analysis of self-esteem and self-concept clarity", *Front. Public Health*, vol. 11, p. 1115661, 2023.
[http://dx.doi.org/10.3389/fpubh.2023.1115661] [PMID: 37113179]

[115] J. Nesi, S. Choukas-Bradley, and M.J. Prinstein, "Transformation of Adolescent Peer Relations in the Social Media Context: Part 2—Application to Peer Group Processes and Future Directions for Research", *Clin. Child Fam. Psychol. Rev.*, vol. 21, no. 3, pp. 295-319, 2018.

[http://dx.doi.org/10.1007/s10567-018-0262-9] [PMID: 29627906]

[116] L. E. Sherman, "Social media use and peer influence in adolescence: Perspectives from neuroimaging," *UCLA Electronic Theses and Dissertations*, 2016. Available: https://escholarship.org/uc/item/2m547718

[117] A.K. Lane, J. Skvoretz, J.P. Ziker, B.A. Couch, B. Earl, J.E. Lewis, J.D. McAlpin, L.B. Prevost, S.E. Shadle, and M. Stains, "Investigating how faculty social networks and peer influence relate to knowledge and use of evidence-based teaching practices", *Int. J. STEM Educ.*, vol. 6, no. 1, p. 28, 2019.
[http://dx.doi.org/10.1186/s40594-019-0182-3]

[118] C.M. Wegemer, "Service, Activism, and Friendships in High School: A Longitudinal Social Network Analysis of Peer Influence and Critical Beliefs", *J. Youth Adolesc.*, vol. 51, no. 1, pp. 1-15, 2022.
[http://dx.doi.org/10.1007/s10964-021-01549-2] [PMID: 34894343]

[119] Liamputtong P, Rice ZS. Stigma, discrimination, and social exclusion. InHandbook of social inclusion: Research and practices in health and social sciences 2021 Dec 24 (pp. 1-17). Cham: Springer International Publishing.
[http://dx.doi.org/10.1007/978-3-030-48277-0_6-2]

[120] T. Ramaci, M. Barattucci, C. Ledda, and V. Rapisarda, "Social stigma during COVID-19 and its impact on HCWs outcomes", *Sustainability (Basel)*, vol. 12, no. 9, p. 3834, 2020.
[http://dx.doi.org/10.3390/su12093834]

[121] J. Crocker and B. Major, "Social stigma and self-esteem: The self-protective properties of stigma," *Psychol. Rev.*, vol. 96, no. 4, pp. 608–630, 1989.

[122] K. Hofstraat and W. H. Van Brakel, "Social stigma towards neglected tropical diseases: A systematic review," *International Health*, vol. 8. pp. i53-i70, 2015.
[http://dx.doi.org/10.1093/inthealth/ihv071]

[123] Torres MC, Herman D, Montano S, Love L. Pharmacy assistance programs in a community health center setting. Journal of the National Medical Association. 2002 Dec;94(12):1077. Available: https://pmc.ncbi.nlm.nih.gov/articles/PMC2568413/pdf/jnma00172-0087.pdf

[124] B. Pickett, T.R. Shin, and M. Norton, "Utilizing clinical pharmacists and a medication assistance program to improve medication access for indigent and underserved patients in primary care", *Explor. Res. Clin. Soc. Pharm.*, vol. 9, p. 100211, 2023.
[http://dx.doi.org/10.1016/j.rcsop.2022.100211] [PMID: 36582998]

[125] H. Yuan, Q. Ma, L. Ye, and G. Piao, "The traditional medicine and modern medicine from natural products", *Molecules*, vol. 21, no. 5, p. 559, 2016.
[http://dx.doi.org/10.3390/molecules21050559] [PMID: 27136524]

[126] A.N. Welz, A. Emberger-Klein, and K. Menrad, "Why people use herbal medicine: insights from a focus-group study in Germany", *BMC Complement. Altern. Med.*, vol. 18, no. 1, p. 92, 2018.
[http://dx.doi.org/10.1186/s12906-018-2160-6] [PMID: 29544493]

[127] B.U. Chali, A. Hasho, and N.B. Koricha, "Preference and Practice of Traditional Medicine and Associated Factors in Jimma Town, Southwest Ethiopia", *Evid. Based Complement. Alternat. Med.*, vol. 2021, pp. 1-7, 2021.
[http://dx.doi.org/10.1155/2021/9962892] [PMID: 34194530]

[128] P. Zagożdżon and M. Wrotkowska, "Religious beliefs and their relevance for treatment adherence in mental illness: A review," *Religions*, vol. 8, no. 8. 2017.
[http://dx.doi.org/10.3390/rel8080150]

[129] S. Joos, K. Glassen, and B. Musselmann, "Herbal Medicine in Primary Healthcare in Germany: The Patient′s Perspective", *Evidence-Based Complementary and Alternative Medicine*, vol. 2012, no. 1, p. 294638, 2012.

[130] B. Ali, Z. Nazar, N. Barnes, and P. Rutter, "The impact of religious beliefs on adherence to medication

in the Muslim population: A systematic scoping review," *Int. J. Pharm. Pract.*, vol. 30, no. Supplement 1, pp. i26-i35, 2022. Available: https://academic.oup.com/ijpp/article/30/Supplement_1/i26/6562353

[131] J. Hartog, E. A. Hartog, and S. Francisco, "Cross-cultural medicine: Cultural aspects of health and illness behavior in hospitals," 1983.

[132] F. J. Bekker, U. Hentschel, and M. Fujita, "Basic cultural values and differences in attitudes towards health, illness, and treatment preferences within a psychosomatic frame of reference," *Psychother. Psychosom.*, vol. 65, no. 2, pp. 97-104, 1996.
[http://dx.doi.org/10.1159/000289074]

[133] M.H. Kahissay, T.G. Fenta, and H. Boon, "Beliefs and perception of ill-health causation: a socio-cultural qualitative study in rural North-Eastern Ethiopia", *BMC Public Health,* vol. 17, no. 1, p. 124, 2017.
[http://dx.doi.org/10.1186/s12889-017-4052-y] [PMID: 28122606]

[134] T. Nilchaikovit, J. M. Hill, and J. C. Holland, "The effects of culture on illness behavior and medical care: Asian and American differences," *Psychosom. Med.*, vol. 55, no. 5, pp. 462-469, 1993.

CHAPTER 2

AI's Role in Personalized Medication Management

Sunita[1], Akhil Sharma[2], Akanksha Sharma[2], P. Siva Kumar[3] and Shaweta Sharma[4],*

[1] *Metro College of Health Sciences and Research, Greater Noida, Uttar Pradesh, India*

[2] *R.J. College of Pharmacy, Raipur, Gharbara, Tappal, Khair, Uttar Pradesh, India*

[3] *Department of Civil Engineering Aditya University, Surampalem, India*

[4] *School of Medical and Allied Sciences, Galgotias University Plot No. 2, Yamuna Expy, Opposite Buddha International Circuit, Sector 17A, Greater Noida, Uttar Pradesh, India*

Abstract: Healthcare has gone through a paradigm change, specifically in personalized medicine, due to the development of Artificial Intelligence (AI) technology. This chapter will discuss how AI is transforming healthcare delivery in general, particularly through precision medicine. Such AI technologies such as machine learning, deep learning, natural language processing, predictive analytics, robotics, and automation can utilize extensive databases that include patient genomics, medical history and real-time health monitoring, as well as patient demographics. By using AI to integrate data from Electronic Health records along with other patient sources, genomic data, and wearable IoT devices, it provides a holistic profiling of patients to predict their responses to drugs and identify possible adverse effects. Besides, AI also fast tracks drug discovery and development by target identification to drug repurposing, reducing time frames for research and development. Advances in Clinical Decision Support Systems (CDSS) enhance the decision-making process, providing real-time insights that guide healthcare professionals. However, the implementation of AI in personalized medicine comes with its own set of challenges. However, there are ethical issues associated with data privacy, biases in AI algorithms, regulatory considerations, and more. When it comes to the adoption of AI, the integration with existing infrastructure, training, and educating health professionals become key elements. There is a lot of potential for the future, as technology is constantly advancing and is sure to remove barriers preventing us from a more efficient, patient-centered, healthcare model.

Keywords: Artificial intelligence, Adverse drug reaction, Clinical decision support systems, Drug discovery, Drug development, Electronic health records, Genomics, Healthcare, Internet of things, Medication, Management, Precision medicine, Personalized, Prediction, Repurposing, Wearables.

***** **Corresponding author Shaweta Sharma:** School of Medical and Allied Sciences, Galgotias University Plot No. 2, Yamuna Expy, Opposite Buddha International Circuit, Sector 17A, Greater Noida, Uttar Pradesh, India; E-mail: shawetasharma@galgotiasuniversity.edu.in

INTRODUCTION

Precision medicine, also called personalized medicine or individualized medicine, is a healing technique that acknowledges the dissimilarity among persons and aims at adjusting medical care and interventions to suit individual peculiarities. In contrast to the customary "one-size-fits-all" approach to health care that depends on standardized protocols and therapies, precision medicine considers different genetic, environmental as well as lifestyle factors associated with an individual's health and disease propensity [1].

The basic idea behind precision medicine is the use of genomics, molecular biology, data science, and related technologies to understand the molecular basis of diseases and develop personal treatment options. The field has grown and changed significantly during the past years due to fast developments in genomic sequencing technology, bioinformatics tools, and computational analytics [2].

One of the major principles of precision medicine embraces genomic data for diagnosis, treatment selection, and therapeutic decision-making. Researchers and medical practitioners analyze the patient's genetic makeup using genome sequencing in order to find out genetic variations that are associated with specific diseases or drug responses among mutations and biomarkers. By understanding the genetic basis of ailments, doctors can produce individualized curatives that suit each patient's genetic blueprint [3].

Precision medicine is more than genomics. It also involves a range of other omics technologies, such as transcriptomics, proteomics, and metabolomics, that shed light on the molecular pathways and mechanisms of diseases. By combining data from various omics platforms, scientists can obtain a more comprehensive understanding of how diseases develop and even discover new drug targets [4].

Precision medicine is not confined to molecular data only; it also includes other sources of information such as Electronic Health Records (EHRs), imaging studies, and patient-reported outcomes. By integrating different datasets, healthcare providers can have a holistic view of each patient's health status and develop appropriate treatment plans [5].

The main objective of precision medicine is to go beyond a reactive, one-size-fits-all approach to healthcare and towards a more proactive and preventive model. Precision medicine enables early detection, risk stratification, and implementation of preventive interventions by identifying high-risk individuals for some diseases based on their genetic predisposition, lifestyle choices, and exposures to environmental elements [6].

Precision medicine also involves pharmacogenomics, which uses genetic information to predict how a person reacts to drugs. By determining gene variants that alter drug metabolism, efficacy, or toxicity, doctors can choose the right medication and dosage for optimum therapy results and reduced side effects [7].

Evolution and Importance

Table **1** summarizes the evolutionary milestones and the significance of precision medicine in transforming healthcare delivery and improving patient outcomes.

Table 1. The evolution and importance of precision medicine.

Evolution	Importance
Emergence of Genomic Technologies	- The emergence of genomic sequencing technologies, such as Next-Generation Sequencing (NGS), has made it possible to examine genetic information quickly and inexpensively. - Facilitates identification of genetic variants, mutations, and biomarkers linked to diseases, leading to personalized treatment decisions [8].
Advancements in Omics Technologies	- Integrating the use of transcriptomics, proteomics, metabolomics, and other 'omics' data for a more comprehensive understanding of disease mechanisms and pathways. - Provides a holistic understanding of the molecular signatures underlying diseases, helping in the identification of novel therapeutic targets [9].
Integration of Electronic Health Records	- EHRs are used to capture clinical data, imaging studies, and patient-reported outcomes to develop a complete patient profile. - Enables healthcare providers to create personalized treatment plans for each patient based on a holistic view of health status and medical history [10].
Advancements in Pharmacogenomics	- Develop pharmacogenomics testing that provides personalized prescription and dosage guidance by utilizing genomic information on drug efficacy and metabolism. Optimizes medication selection, dosing, and management to increase therapeutic results and decrease side effects [11].
Shift towards Preventive and Predictive Medicine	It is important to focus on early detection, risk stratification, and prevention strategies based on an individual's genetic predisposition, environmental exposure, and lifestyle. - Enables proactive disease management, decreases disease burden, and improves long-term health outcomes [12].
Ethical, Legal, and Social Implications	- Recognition of ethical considerations about privacy, informed consent, genetic discrimination, and equity in access to genomic technologies. - Ensures responsible and equitable implementation of precision medicine, safeguarding individual rights, autonomy, and privacy [13].

Challenges in Conventional Medication Management

One-Size-Fits-All Approach

Conventional medication management often relies on an established treatment paradigm that prescribes drugs and doses as per common guidelines or population averages. Still, this approach ignores the inherent heterogeneity in individuals with regard to genetics, physiology, and lifestyle issues. Therefore, patients with the same diagnosis may react differently to the same medicine or treatment, which can result in less-than-optimal treatment outcomes. For instance, a dosage that is effective for one patient might be too little for another due to differences in drug metabolism or genetic variations affecting drug response [14].

Moreover, some populations of patients like children, elderly persons, or the ones having certain clinical conditions, can need customized treatment approaches that deviate from the one-size-fits-all model. Addressing this challenge demands a focus on personalized medicine options like precision medicine that take into account the patient's genetic makeup, biomarkers, and other factors in order to create customized treatment plans for patients based on their unique characteristics [15].

Adverse Drug Reactions

Adverse Drug Reactions (ADRs) are unintended and harmful reactions to medications that can range from mild side effects to severe allergic reactions or organ damage. It is difficult for conventional medicine to predict or prevent ADRs since there are many factors affecting an individual's drug metabolism and response that are not easy to predict. Genetic variations in drug-metabolizing enzymes, drug-drug interactions, and patient-specific factors like age, comorbidities, and concurrent medications contribute to the risk of ADRs [16, 17].

Furthermore, ADRs can be extremely unpredictable in their occurrence, and patients may differ, making it difficult to foresee and control them. For instance, a patient could experience an upset stomach, skin inflammation, or liver damage owing to harmful reactions to a prescribed drug. To prevent and minimize ADRs, comprehensive assessment of the patient is necessary, as well as close monitoring along with personalized medication management approaches that are inclusive of individual patient characteristics and risk factors [17].

Limited Efficacy in Diverse Populations

Conventional medications are often developed and tested in relatively homogenous populations, which may not adequately represent the diversity of real-world patients. Consequently, the efficiency of drugs among mixed populations such as different ethnicities, ages, and sexes may be limited or variable. Medication response in diverse patient populations may be influenced by factors such as genetic dissimilarities in drug metabolism, divergences in the course of disease pathogenesis, and socio-cultural considerations. For instance, some ethnic groups may have their drug metabolism rates or drug-receptor interactions differently affected by specific genetic polymorphisms, which can result in changed treatment efficiency and tolerability [18, 19].

Likewise, changes in pharmacokinetics and pharmacodynamics due to age could affect medication response among children, adults, and the elderly. In dealing with this problem, research should focus on the inclusion and diversity of clinical trials as well as drug development programs so that drugs can be effective for all patients. Furthermore, personalized medicine techniques such as pharmacogenomics can also help to individualize drug regimens based on patient-specific factors, thereby optimizing treatment outcomes and reducing disparities in healthcare delivery [20].

ARTIFICIAL INTELLIGENCE (AI) IN HEALTHCARE: REVOLUTIONIZING PERSONALIZED MEDICINE

AI Technologies

AI is a broad term that covers many technologies that allow machines to imitate human-like intelligence, utilize data to learn, and make decisions or predictions by themselves. In healthcare, AI technologies are the subject of much hope and interest for their capacity to transform different parts of medical practice, research, and delivery of healthcare. AI technologies and techniques utilized in healthcare are described below and also summarized in Fig. (1).

Machine Learning (ML)

Machine learning algorithms allow computers to learn from enormous datasets and make forecasts or decisions without being explicitly programmed. In healthcare, ML techniques such as supervised learning, unsupervised learning, and reinforcement learning are utilized for disease prediction, medical image analysis, drug discovery, and personalized treatment recommendation tasks [21].

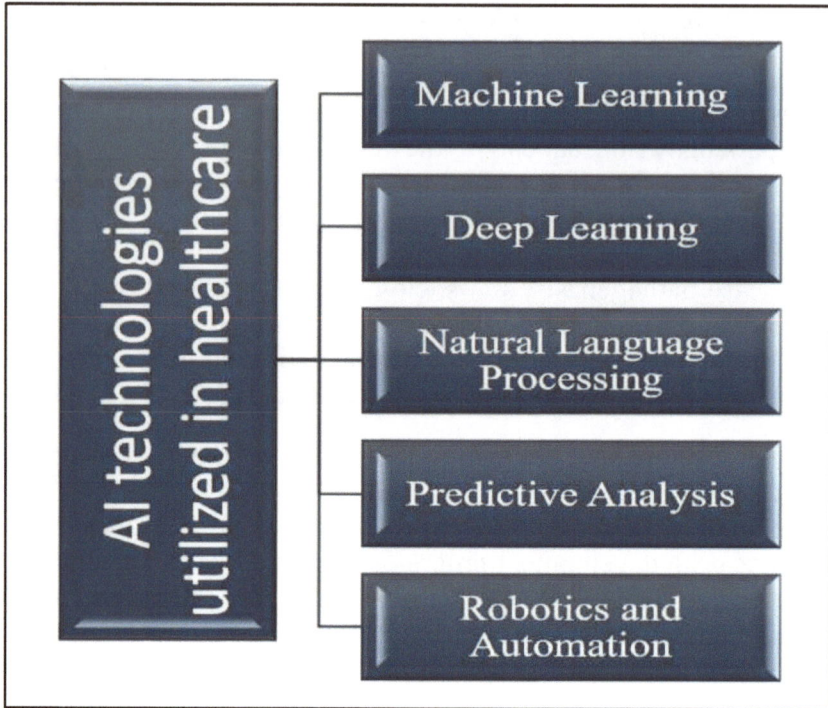

Fig. (1). AI technologies and techniques utilized in healthcare.

Deep Learning (DL)

Deep learning is a subfield of machine learning that uses neural networks with multiple layers. This ensures that DL algorithms can automatically identify hierarchical features from raw data, making them very effective for tasks like image recognition, natural language processing, and voice recognition. In healthcare, deep learning has shown promise in medical imaging analysis, diagnostic decision support, and genomics research [22].

Natural Language Processing (NLP)

Computers can understand and analyze human language using natural language processing techniques. These NLP algorithms help to extract information from clinical notes, medical literature, and patient records, which facilitate activities such as clinical documentation, information retrieval, and sentiment analysis. In addition, NLP is applied to virtual assistants, chatbots, and clinical decision support systems to enhance communication and information access in healthcare settings [23].

Predictive Analytics

Using statistical models and machine learning algorithms, predictive analytics entails analyzing historical data and predicting the future. It is used in healthcare to perform tasks such as patient risk stratification, hospital readmission prediction, early disease detection, and personalized treatment planning. It looks through patients' data from Electronic Health Records (EHRs), wearable devices as well as genetic testing to identify the most vulnerable people who may experience adverse health events that are preventable with timely interventions [24].

Robotics and Automation

Robotics and automation technologies involve the use of robotic systems and autonomous machines to perform tasks usually executed by humans. In healthcare, robotics is used for surgical procedures, rehabilitation therapy, medication dispensing, and telemedicine applications. Examples of this are robotic surgery systems that allow doctors to carry out minimally invasive surgeries with improved precision and skillfulness, leading to quicker recuperation times and better patient results [25].

Applications in Healthcare

In healthcare, numerous applications of AI technologies have the potential to change how medicine is practiced completely and how healthcare is delivered. One such application that has had the greatest effect is medical imaging analysis, where AI algorithms can help radiologists and pathologists identify any abnormalities, diagnose diseases, or predict treatment outcomes from images such as X-rays, CT scans, MRI scans, and pathology slides. These algorithms are usually based on deep learning techniques and exhibit excellent performance in tasks like tumor detection, identification of fractures, and disease classification, thereby improving diagnostic accuracy and patient outcomes [26 - 28].

Utilizing machine learning models to predict patient responses to drugs, identify genetic risk factors for diseases, or stratify patient populations based on treatment efficacy and safety profiles will improve patient outcomes and healthcare efficiency [29, 30].

In addition, AI technologies are used in healthcare management and operations to simplify administrative processes, improve resource allocation, and make workflow more effective. Predictive analytics models forecast patient volumes and hospital readmission rates and automate clinical documentation and billing procedures to reduce administrative duties, particularly in revenue cycle management. The use of AI in healthcare can revolutionize the delivery of health services by improving diagnostic accuracy, individualizing treatment plans, and streamlining healthcare operations [31].

Advantages in Personalized Medication Management

There are several benefits of individualized medical care compared to traditional approaches. AI technology and personalized patient data can be used to improve the outcome of treatments administered and enhance patient well-being. Advantages in personalized medication management are described below and also summarized in Fig. (**2**).

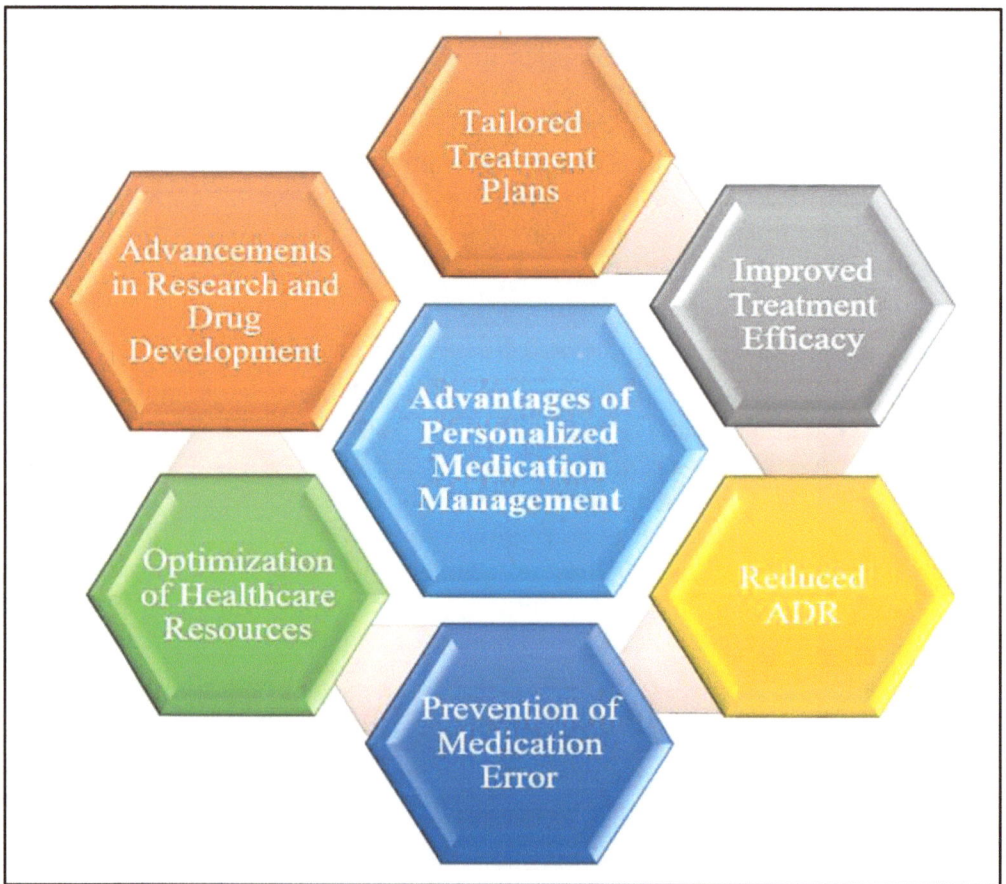

Fig. (2). Advantages in personalized medication management.

Personalized medication management takes into account various properties of each patient, such as genetics, metabolism, disease severity, and lifestyle, to generate customized treatment plans. AI algorithms can predict how patients are likely to respond to specific medications by analyzing genetic variations and biomarkers, thus enabling healthcare providers to adjust their treatment regimens. This personalized method increases the chances of successful treatment and reduces drug reactions [32].

Personalized medication management improves treatment efficacy by optimizing medication selection, dosing, and administration based on individual patient factors. When patients are prescribed medications tailored to their unique biological makeup and clinical profiles, positive outcomes and symptom relief are more likely. This also increases patient satisfaction and decreases the need for trial-and-error approaches to finding effective treatments [33].

The problem of adverse drug reactions is very important in the healthcare industry. Many times, they may result in pain and discomfort to the patient, discontinuation of treatment, or high costs of care. Personalized medication management minimizes ADR risks by identifying factors such as genetic predispositions, drug interactions, and other factors that can increase sensitivity to drug side effects. It also improves patients' safety and tolerability by avoiding drugs with several chances of causing adverse reactions and selecting alternatives that have a better safety profile [34].

The most common causes of harm to patients in healthcare environments are medication errors, such as giving an incorrect dose, combining incompatible drugs, and prescribing the wrong medication. AI-based decision support systems for personalized medication management employ real-time patient-specific data to minimize the potential errors that may arise while using medications. They also help prevent adverse events and promote adherence to medication by ensuring that they are prescribed, dispensed, and administered safely [35].

Through personalized medicine, medical resources are optimized because they focus on treatments that would benefit patients the most and reduce unnecessary healthcare use and expenses. Identifying those patients in greater danger of treatment failure or adverse outcomes helps healthcare providers to better direct interventions and allocate health services. By doing this, it is possible to improve the outcomes of patients while also decreasing the costs associated with ineffective treatments, hospitalizations, and emergency room visits in terms of healthcare spending across the country [36].

Personalized medication management produces essential insights into drug reactions, disease processes, and therapy outcomes that can guide future research and development of drugs. Researchers can discover new therapeutic targets, confirm existing drug candidates, and improve therapeutic strategies for specific populations of patients by analyzing actual patient data as well as biomarker associations. It is the process of learning and optimizing that drives healthcare innovation and paves the way for the development of better treatments that are more efficient and aimed at particular diseases [37].

DATA INTEGRATION AND ANALYSIS

Personalized medicine can be achieved by using data integration and analysis, which allows care providers to harness the potential of different sources of patient data for optimum treatment outcomes. By integrating and analyzing EHRs, genomics, wearables, and IoT devices together, healthcare teams can gain essential insights into patient health, medication reactions, and disease progression.

Electronic Health Records

EHRs revolutionize how healthcare data is collected, stored, and used by offering a fully comprehensive digital patient medical information repository. EHRs are at their heart, containing patients' demographic information, medical records including history, diagnoses, treatments, drugs they took, and imaging results, among others, from labs. Such detailed information gives the healthcare provider an overall view of the patient's status in terms of health and past medical record thus helping them to make informed choices concerning treatment options for individual patients [38].

Furthermore, EHRs enhance the accessibility and portability of medical information since healthcare providers can access patient information securely from any place with internet connectivity. Consequently, this enhances care coordination between various providers and settings to ensure continuity of care and better outcomes for patients. EHR systems incorporate interoperability as one of their key features, enabling the smooth transfer of patient data across different health systems and organizations. By promoting communication among healthcare stakeholders, EHRs that can interoperate reduce redundant testing and procedures while improving efficiency [39].

Clinical decision-support tools in the EHR provide evidence-based reminders to healthcare providers at the point of care, thereby enhancing medication safety, adherence to guidelines, and overall quality of care. EHRs also facilitate clinical documentation processes by improving accuracy and effectiveness in capturing patient encounters while also supporting automated coding and billing. Additionally, EHR data can be a valuable resource for healthcare analytics and health management efforts that help shape public health interventions and undergird data-driven decision-making [40, 41].

Genomic Data

The collection of genomic data, or the complete DNA sequences of an individual, is a critical aspect of modern healthcare that can guide personalized medication, disease risk assessments, drug development, and clinical decision-making. The advent of advanced genomic sequencing technologies, particularly Next-Generation Sequencing (NGS), has led to a significant increase in the accuracy and scale of genomic analysis, which ensures an inclusive examination of genetic variations as well as biomarkers. Within healthcare settings, genomic data is subjected to bioinformatics tools for variant identification and interpretation of their clinical significance [42, 43].

Further, these insights help inform disease risk assessments, and as a result, clinicians are able to come up with prevention tactics that are personalized to the genetic tendencies of each individual. Additionally, precision medicine initiatives that utilize genomic data enable the optimization of healthcare treatments for patients based on their genetic profiles. Pharmacogenomic testing is a process of using genomic information to predict responses to drugs, selecting appropriate medications, and minimizing adverse drug reactions. Also, profiling the genomic of tumors helps in the choice of therapy for cancer patients that is individualized, thereby improving treatment results [44].

Genetic counseling services use genomic data to evaluate hereditary conditions, direct decision-making, and enable patients as well as families to understand the consequences of genetic information. Additionally, genomics data, in conjunction with biomedical research, helps in developing drugs that identify disease-causing genes, biomarkers, and medication targets. Studies in population genomics utilize genome-level data to examine genetic diversity, evolutionary relationships, and population structures that inform public health planning as well as anthropological research. However, despite its potential impact on societal transformation, a number of problems, such as privacy issues surrounding genetic information, ethical considerations, and challenges in interpreting personal genomic data, need to be addressed for maximum utilization of genomic data in improving healthcare [45, 46].

Wearables and IoT Devices

The advent of wearables and Internet of Things (IoT) devices has opened up new horizons in healthcare technology, with significant implications for remote patient monitoring, personalized health management, and data-driven interventions. Fitness trackers, smartwatches, and biosensors are all types of wearable devices that monitor real-time health information from people as they go about their daily lives in order to determine things like pulse, strain levels, sleep patterns, or glucose concentration. These instruments use sensors as well as accelerometers together with other built-in tools to capture physiological signals and lifestyle behaviors for patients' continuous health monitoring [47].

Connected medical devices, home monitoring systems, and ambient sensors are among the IoT devices that extend wearables by integrating with healthcare ecosystems and transmitting data to those in need. This promotes proactive healthcare delivery through wearables and IoT devices which enable early recognition of health changes, timely interventions, and preventive measures. Through an analysis of wearable data, medical practitioners are able to discover disease exacerbations, medication responses, and adverse events trends and patterns, which allow them to make personalized treatment adjustments and care plans [48].

Additionally, wearables and IoT devices can facilitate active participation by people in their health management, thereby enhancing self-awareness, engagement, and adherence to healthy habits. However, to achieve the actual potential of wearables and IoT devices in healthcare, there are challenges related to data security, privacy, interoperability, and data integration that must be solved. Nonetheless, wearables and IoT devices hold a promise of being valuable tools for improving healthcare delivery, and enhancing patient outcomes while advancing the connected patient-centered care vision [49].

PREDICTIVE ANALYTICS AND PATIENT PROFILING

Anticipatory data analysis on patient profiling and predictive analytics is a powerful method of personalized medicine to predict drug responses, identify possible side effects, and modify treatment strategies according to personal characteristics. These approaches exploit patient data from numerous sources, including EHRs, genomic information, wearable devices, and clinical trials, to generate insights into action that inform clinical decision-making and optimize patient care.

Predicting Drug Responses

Personalized medicine is a critical aspect of personalized medicine that uses sophisticated data analytics to anticipate how patients will respond to a given medication. It is based on various forms of patient integration with the model for predictive modeling which include: genomics, omics, clinical history, biomarkers, and phenotypic information as well as demographic characteristics. Predictive models can be used to estimate the probability of successful treatment, side effects, and drug tolerance in medical practice by analyzing genetic variations, pharmacokinetic parameters, and disease characteristics [50, 51].

Factors such as age, gender, weight, comorbidities, concomitant medications, and lifestyle are included in predictive models to determine the effect of drugs on patients besides genetic causes. Patient data that is comprehensive can be integrated into predictive analytic models to generate individualized risk profiles and treatment recommendations that will optimize therapeutic outcomes while minimizing the risk of adverse events [52].

Clinical decision-making can be improved, medical safety can be enhanced and healthcare treatment efficiency increased by predicting drug responses. Predictive models identify those patients who are most likely to respond to specific medications and those at higher risk of adverse reactions, thus enabling clinicians to develop personalized treatment plans and dosing regimens that bring better patient outcomes and improved quality of care. However, there are still challenges in operationalizing the integration of predictive models into routine clinical practice. These include conducting robust validation studies, establishing standardized data collection methods, and interfacing with electronic medical record systems. Nevertheless, despite these challenges, the future potential of predictive analytics in predicting drug responses is a promising avenue for more individualized and efficient healthcare delivery [53, 54].

Identifying Potential Adverse Reactions

Healthcare should include the identification of potentially harmful outcomes to enhance patient safety and better treatment results. Clinicians can easily examine patients' data using advanced techniques of analytics to be ready for ADRs. In this light, a proactive approach considers several patient information sources, such as electronic health records, genomic data, medication history, and clinical observations, to identify individuals who have higher chances of experiencing adverse events [55].

Pharmacovigilance is one strategy that can be used to identify possible side effects. It is a method of tracking and analyzing data on drug safety and adverse events in the real world. In pharmacovigilance, data from healthcare databases, clinical trials, spontaneous reporting systems, post-marketing surveillance programs, and other sources are collected together and analyzed systematically to detect signals for emerging safety issues and adverse reactions related to individual medicines. Unexpected patterns of adverse events may be reflected in these signals, including disproportionate reporting of certain reactions or identification of recently reported risk factors that need to be explored further [56].

Predictive analytics models can also help identify patients who are at greater risk of experiencing negative side effects through the examination of patient-specific variables such as genetic predisposition, comorbidities, medication history, and demographic factors in addition to pharmacovigilance. Clinicians may thus incorporate these variables within their predictive models so that they produce customized risk profiles concerning specific adverse events for any given patient. Early identification of high-risk patients allows clinicians to implement preventive measures, such as dose adjustments, medication substitutions, or close monitoring, to minimize the likelihood of adverse events and enhance patient safety [57, 58].

Additionally, incorporating genomics in predicting adverse reactions can provide useful information about genetic variation that may affect a drug's metabolism, pharmacokinetics, and how it responds to drugs. Pharmacogenomic testing allows clinicians to tailor treatment plans and medication regimens because it helps them identify genetic variants that increase the chances of certain adverse reactions [59].

Tailoring Treatment Plans

The personalization of medicine, which uses sophisticated data analytics and patient-specific information to tailor therapeutic regimens according to individual needs and characteristics, is founded on the customization of treatment plans for patients. The personalized approach to health care acknowledges that people differ in the way they respond to treatments due to reasons such as genetics, severity of disease, presence of other ailments, lifestyle choices, and treatment objectives. The inclusion of different kinds of medical records like EHRs, gene data, biomarkers, and wearables information, together with other patient health details, will enable doctors to come up with custom-built treatment plans that are aimed at enhancing therapy results while reducing hazards and side effects [60, 61].

Pharmacogenomics is one of the main ways to customize treatment strategies, which assesses genetic differences to predict responses patients may have towards particular drugs. Pharmacogenomic testing detects genomic variations related to drug metabolism, efficacy, and toxicity, thus assisting in choosing medicines and dosage regimens that are most likely to be useful and well-tolerated by individual patients. Clinicians can also avoid drugs with known genetic contraindications or adjust doses based on differences in metabolic rates by taking into consideration patients' genetic profiles [62].

Apart from pharmacogenomics, patient-specific elements like age, sex, Body Mass Index (BMI), renal function, and concomitant medications are taken into account when customizing treatment protocols. Physicians take into consideration patients' medical records, clinical signs and symptoms, and treatment options to tailor healthcare plans that correspond to their specific requirements and aims in life. For example, long-term disease patients may require a combination of lifestyle changes, a team-based approach in their care plan as well as a supportive intervention to promote optimal management of the condition for improved quality of life [63].

In addition, clinicians can improve healthcare plans by using continuous monitoring systems and feedback mechanisms, including wearable devices and remote patient monitoring technologies to observe patients' response to treatment in real-time. When relied on such insights from data-driven approaches that enable doctors to get optimal treatment results for their patients, they make them stick to their prescriptions, and not expose them to high risks of negative side effects [64].

DRUG DISCOVERY AND DEVELOPMENT

Crucial steps in the process of introducing new drugs to the market include discovering and developing them to bridge therapeutic gaps and enhance patient satisfaction. With advancements in science and technology, this process has embraced new methods that speed up the identification and validation of drug candidates. These include speeding up drug discovery time frames, target identification and validation, and drug repurposing. All these are important strategies that drive innovation as well as revolutionize the healthcare landscape [65].

Accelerating Drug Discovery

The main goal of contemporary pharmaceutical research is to accelerate drug discovery, which is necessitated by the urgent need to address unmet medical needs and provide innovative therapies to patients as fast as possible. This effort involves bringing together different types of new technologies, computer methods, and cooperation arrangements in order to facilitate the identification and proofing of potential drug candidates through a range of activities. An increase in the pace of drug discovery can be attributed to computational biology and bioinformatics, which employ computational modeling, machine learning algorithms, and big data analytics to speed up the examination and analysis of large chemical libraries as well as biological datasets [66, 67].

It is also possible to use in silico docking approaches to anticipate the binding affinities of small molecule ligands towards target proteins, hence leading to the identification of drug lead compounds. There have been tremendous improvements in structural biology, *e.g.* X-ray crystallography or cryo-electron microscopy techniques, which can be used to understand how drug molecules interact with their target protein at atomic level and thus inform rational drug design and optimization. Additionally, high-throughput screening (HTS) platforms have automated the testing of thousands of compounds targeted against disease-relevant proteins, thus rapidly identifying hits for further optimization [68].

Public-private partnerships and open innovation models are some of the initiatives that encourage collaboration among higher education, industry, and government institutions; they also facilitate the translation of basic research findings into clinical applications. Integrating multidisciplinary knowledge like medicinal chemistry, pharmacology, and computational sciences, among others, can further improve the efficiency and success of drug discovery. As a result, speeding up drug discovery could potentially revolutionize the pharmaceutical industry, leading to new therapeutics for prevalent medical problems and improving patients' lives [69].

Target Identification and Validation

The drug discovery process needs target identification and validation, which are highly important in the development of effective therapeutics. Consequently, these steps necessitate the identification of specific molecules or biological pathways involved in disease pathogenesis and confirm their relevance and druggability by robust experimental validation. The process of target identification starts with a thorough understanding of the disease biology; this includes knowing about the molecular basis for its occurrence, development, and manifestation. Advances in genomics, proteomics, and systems biology have transformed target identification by offering researchers powerful tools that can be used to study biological systems at the level of molecules [70, 71].

Genome-Wide Association Studies (GWAS), for example, identify genetic variants that are associated with susceptibility to diseases and phenotype, indicating the possible therapeutic targets. Also, proteomic profiling techniques such as mass spectrometry and protein microarrays enable the identification of abnormally expressed proteins or dysregulated signaling pathways in disease tissues. Furthermore, functional genomics techniques such as RNA interference (RNAi) and CRISPR-Cas9 gene editing are used to selectively silence or edit gene expression for novel drug target discovery [72].

When potential drug targets are found, they have to be validated rigorously to confirm their significance and drugability. Target validation refers to a range of experiments conducted to show the target's relevance in disease pathogenesis and its possible therapeutic applications. *in vitro* assays judge a particular target's functionality by looking at how it interacts with others through measuring expression or activity [73].

For example, enzyme assays evaluate the catalytic activity of target proteins, while binding assays determine the affinity and specificity of potential drug candidates for the target. In addition, cellular assays use cell-based models to assess the effects of targets on phenotypes, disease pathways, and endpoints that are significant in diseases. Animal models of disease are further used to validate the target by assessing its impact on therapeutic efficacy, disease progression, and safety [74].

During target validation, several criteria must be met to establish the feasibility of targeting the molecule for therapeutic intervention. These include evidence of target engagement, modulation of disease-relevant pathways, correlation with disease phenotype, and potential for therapeutic intervention. Furthermore, considerations such as target specificity, druggability, and safety profile are critical in assessing whether or not the proposed drug is suitable [75].

Drug Repurposing

Drug repurposing is a medical technique that seeks to identify new therapeutic indications for existing drugs. This approach leverages the extensive safety and pharmacologic data available for approved drugs or compounds undergoing clinical development instead of trying to synthesize completely new molecules from scratch to hasten the process of introducing novel therapies into the market. In fact, it offers several benefits compared to traditional drug discovery methods, such as reduced development timelines, reduced costs, and decreased risks [76].

Different methods and strategies used in drug repurposing include bioinformatics analysis, data mining, network pharmacology, and other computational techniques. These techniques analyze big data to find possible drug candidates that could be repurposed. Drug-protein interaction networks, molecular pathways, and phenotypic data are the subjects of these studies, which aim to establish relationships between drugs and diseases [77].

Phenotypic screening involves testing approved drugs or investigational compounds in cell-based or animal models of disease to detect unforeseen therapeutic effects or off-target activities, hence allowing for the exploration of wider pharmacological implications of drug use beyond their original prescriptions. In this regard, even deconvoluting existing drugs could result in new and alternative cure targets or pathways that may be targeted for other diseases. Analysis of drug-target interactions through techniques such as proteomics, structural biology, and computational modeling offers insights into the mechanisms of action and potential applications of drugs in alternate disease contexts [78]. Drug repurposing offers several advantages over traditional drug discovery approaches, which are described below and shown in Fig. (3).

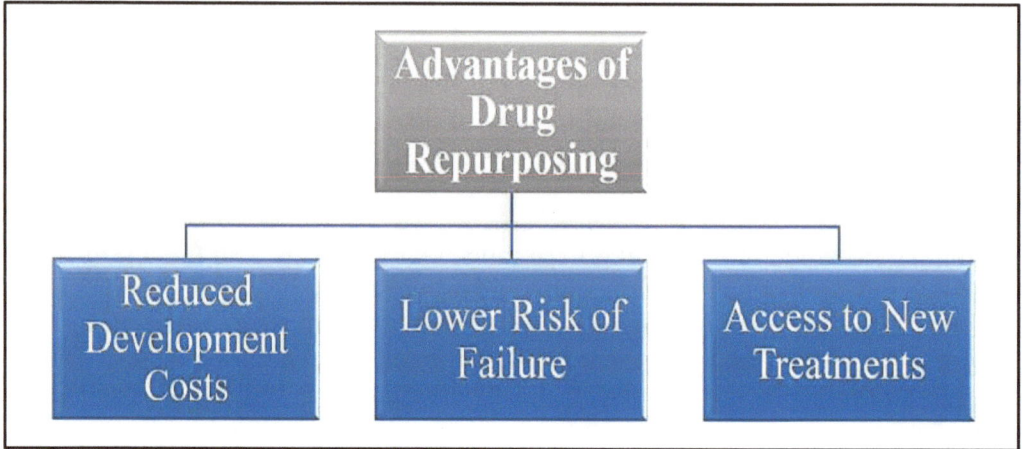

Fig. (3). Advantages of drug repurposing.

Drug repurposing is a process through which already approved drugs can be used for other medical purposes. This saves time and several resources due to the reliance on existing safety and pharmacokinetic data. Development costs can be significantly reduced, and the time required to develop new treatment options before commercialization can be shortened. Due to their known safety profiles in humans, there is a lower risk of unexpected toxicity or adverse effects compared to novel molecules. As a result, fewer late-stage clinical trial failures and regulatory setbacks are possible. Drug repurposing can lead to new therapeutic uses for currently approved drugs, thus increasing treatment choices available for patients with unmet medical needs. This method could reveal untapped indications for discontinued or overlooked drugs [79, 80].

CLINICAL DECISION SUPPORT SYSTEMS (CDSS)

CDSS plays a vital part in improving clinical decision-making by affording healthcare providers with real-time insights, evidence-based advice, and patient-specific data at the point of care. They combine clinical knowledge, patient information, and best practices to help physicians make informed choices about diagnosis, treatment, and patient management.

Enhancing Clinical Decision-Making

In healthcare, the major goal is to improve clinical decision-making in order to increase health outcomes for patients and improve quality healthcare. CDSS has a huge role to play in this by integrating advanced technology with patient data, which offers useful insights and clinical recommendations backed by evidence at the point of care delivery. These systems blend clinical guidelines, best practices, and relevant patient information from EHRs, diagnostic tests, and medical literature to assist clinicians in making decisions on diagnosis, treatment, and managing the patients. CDSS can analyze data from patients in real-time, thereby offering alerts that may help clinicians avoid possible risks of drug interaction or deviation from practice standards, thus enabling timely interventions that may prevent errors from occurring [81, 82].

In addition, CDSS can aid healthcare providers in reading intricate medical information, detecting trends, and making predictions that will result in more precise diagnoses and treatment planning. Moreover, it can promote teamwork among interdisciplinary teams, facilitating patient data sharing and care coordination. Through personalized recommendations and decision support tools, CDSS enables clinicians to work smarter, faster, and patient-focused for better clinical outcomes and reduce healthcare costs with improved satisfaction among patients. It is anticipated that as technology continues to develop and data analytics capabilities progress further, the scope of CDSS will broaden, thereby revolutionizing health systems while enhancing care across diverse clinical settings [83, 84].

Real-time Insights for Healthcare Professionals

Modern healthcare delivery is complete with real-time insights for healthcare professionals, facilitated by advanced technologies and data analytics capabilities. As a result of the wider adoption of EHRs, wearables, and interconnected health systems, clinicians can now rely on a lot of real-time patient data as well as analytical tools to make timely decisions and act proactively. Clinicians get these real-time insights, which give them current information about patients' health status, response to treatment, and the progression of diseases, thereby empowering them toward informed decision-making at the point of care [85].

For example, real-time monitoring of vital signs, lab results, and medication adherence data allows clinicians to promptly identify and respond to changes in patients' conditions, facilitating early intervention and preventing adverse outcomes. At the same time, real-time analytics platforms make use of machine learning algorithms and predictive modeling techniques to examine vast quantities of data and supply active insights on an immediate basis. These platforms make it possible for healthcare providers to predict potential risks, anticipate outcomes, and personalize treatment plans to fit individual patient's needs by allowing them to see patterns, trends, or irregularities in patient data [86].

Also, real-time insights encourage interdisciplinary collaboration and care coordination by creating a universal platform for exchanging patient information and interacting with other members of the healthcare team. Real-time insights can also be used to optimize clinical workflows, improve resource allocation, and enhance patient outcomes, thereby leading to better caregiving that is more effective, efficient, and centered on the patient. With advancing data analytics capabilities and continuous development in technology, real-time insights are expected to play an increasing role in healthcare, thus fostering innovation and driving change throughout the continuum of healthcare [87].

IMPLEMENTATION CHALLENGES AND ADOPTION BARRIER

The widespread integration of AI technologies in healthcare poses significant challenges due to obstacles to implementation and adoption. Such obstacles include three key challenges: the integration of AI with current healthcare systems, training and education for healthcare professionals, and resistance to change.

Integration with Existing Healthcare Systems

A significant challenge is that AI technologies are difficult to integrate with existing healthcare systems because of the complicated and often irregular natures of these systems. Different types of healthcare organizations have many systems, including EHRs, PACS, and LIS, as well as administrative software that support various functions while processing voluminous information about patients. Technical challenges, interoperability obstacles, and workflow problems must be overcome in order to integrate AI solutions into these systems and ensure smooth data exchange and compatibility with existing processes [88].

For AI systems to integrate into healthcare, interoperability is a key technical challenge. This is because healthcare systems usually employ different formats for data, standards, and protocols. The incompatibility of such formats can make it hard to share information and facilitate effective communication among different systems. Besides interconnection standards such as Health Level Seven International (HL7) and Fast Healthcare Interoperability Resources (FHIR), smart solutions should also be designed in a manner that enables them to interact with other EHRs seamlessly. The inclusion of Application Programming Interfaces (APIs) and the adoption of standardized data models can also help in integration by providing common platforms for exchanging or communicating data [89].

In addition, introducing AI solutions to the existing workflows comes with workflow obstacles. The medical staff are used to the already established processes and workflows, and any changes or departures that the application of AI technologies can introduce can hamper its acceptance and usage. Hence, AI solutions must be designed in a way that they can fit into existing workflows with minimal disturbances, harmonizing them into clinical processes. These could involve tailoring AI algorithms for particular clinical workflows, user-friendly interfaces, and decision support tools, as well as training and supporting healthcare professionals to adopt new technologies [90].

For healthcare IT professionals to overcome the hurdles of interoperability, workflow, and technical issues, they must work together with AI developers and clinical stakeholders. This will enable them to integrate artificial intelligence technology into existing systems and workflows so as to unlock its full potential of improving patient care and outcomes *via* customization, interoperability, and user-centered design in healthcare organizations [105].

Training and Education for Healthcare Professionals

AI adoption in healthcare hinges on effective training and education programs aimed at healthcare professionals. The nature of healthcare delivery is changing as AI technology is integrated, making it crucial for medical practitioners to develop the competencies that will enable them to use such tools in real-life situations. The key areas for training and educational interventions must cover several things to ensure that clinicians are ready to exploit the total benefits of AI technology's potential [91].

Healthcare practitioners should have a basic understanding of AI concepts such as machine learning, natural language processing, and data analytics. This means that educational programs should provide basic concepts of AI, its use in healthcare, and the possible advantages and limitations of an AI-driven decision support system. To bridge this knowledge gap and foster a culture of AI literacy within healthcare organizations, they need to be trained on terminologies and methodologies used in AI [92].

In clinical settings, healthcare practitioners require specialized training in the application of AI tools and techniques. This will involve practical experience in using AI-enabled diagnostic and decision support systems, as well as understanding the results and recommendations provided by AI programs. Clinicians need to be trained to use AI interfaces, feed patient data into algorithms, and make medical judgments based on their outputs. Moreover, it is important to have continuous training sessions or other continuing education options for healthcare professionals who want to stay updated with innovations in AI technology or best practices pertaining to AI-driven healthcare delivery [93].

In addition, training and education programs should cover the ethical, legal, and regulatory aspects related to the adoption of AI in healthcare. Doctors have to see the moral implications of artificial intelligence algorithms, such as privacy for patients, data protection, and algorithmic bias. Training programs should also make clinicians aware of appropriate regulatory frameworks such as HIPAA and GDPR, thus enabling them to adhere to data protection legislation and follow ethical dimensions [94].

Overcoming Resistance to Change

It is crucial to overcome opposition when introducing AI technologies into medical settings. Healthcare providers may exhibit reluctance towards new technologies such as AI for various reasons, including the fear of job displacement, loss of autonomy, or uncertainty about the benefits of AI. Dealing with resistance to change calls for a broad strategy that includes promoting an innovation culture, teaching and development programs, and stakeholder engagement during implementation [95].

Healthcare organizations must foster an innovative and open-minded culture to facilitate the adoption of AI. This means ensuring a common vision toward integrating AI technologies and encouraging dialogue and cooperation between stakeholders. By iterating on the good outcomes of employing AI in patient care, clinical workflow optimization, and efficiency promotion, healthcare managers can reduce concerns about and doubts about it [96].

In order to overcome the resistance to change that prevails among healthcare practitioners, it is indispensable that they receive education and training. Offering full-fledged programs on AI concepts, applications, and best practices can equip clinicians with the capacity required to make effective use of AI technologies in their everyday professional activities. Hands-on training sessions, workshops, and continuous learning options would be helpful in demystifying AI as well as boosting the confidence of healthcare providers utilizing AI-supported decision-making tools [97].

Also, the process of involving stakeholders in implementation is necessary for overcoming resistance to change and gaining acceptance from front-line personnel. This means that organizations in the health sector should actively engage physicians, administrators, IT specialists, and other important players at all stages of AI activities, including planning, designing, and implementing it. Inviting contributions, reacting to worries, and involving people who have a stake in what gets decided to provide leadership in healthcare with opportunities to harmonize AI solutions with corporate objectives and user requirements [98].

In addition, it is crucial to offer ongoing support and resources to help caregivers transition into AI-driven care delivery. Otherwise, there might be resistance to change. This may involve things such as giving technical aid, problem-solving services, or even opportunities for feedback and contemplation. Consequently, if healthcare organizations show dedication to backing their staff in the implementation process of this innovation, they will create a foundation of trust and confidence in artificial intelligence tools that can promote successful implementation [99].

FUTURE DIRECTIONS AND OPPORTUNITIES

Future strides hold enormous opportunities for personalizing medicine and changing healthcare results in AI-driven advances. By using AI, health institutions can draw on immense amounts of patient details to come up with more specific individual-oriented treatments that are fit to every person's differences in needs and attributes. The overlap between genomic data, other omics data, and artificial intelligence has the potential to fundamentally change how medicine is practiced by enabling an improved understanding of how diseases work, predicting how patients will react to treatments, and discovering drugs that act selectively on disease targets [100].

Innovations in personalized medicine powered by AI offer multiple chances to enhance the outcomes of health care. Foremost, AI algorithms can scrutinize genomic data on a large scale and clinical information to find out trends, biomarkers, and genetic variations linked to disease vulnerability, evolution, and responsiveness to therapy. The integration of genomic information into the clinical data allows AI-supported decision systems that can help physicians make better diagnoses and treatment determinations, resulting in improved patient outcomes and enhanced disease management [101].

Additionally, the use of AI technology enables the formation of predictive models and risk stratification tools that can identify high-risk individuals for diseases or events. By employing machine learning algorithms, healthcare providers can take preventive measures against sickness; this helps to prevent disease progression, improve treatment strategies, and enhance patient outcomes. For instance, AI-powered predictive analytics can help identify patients at a high risk of hospital readmission and adverse drug reactions, hence enabling interventions that would reduce health care costs and enhance patient safety [102].

Healthcare providers, AI developers, and regulators must work together to exploit AI-driven personalized medicine fully. By sharing clinical data with domain knowledge and real-world experience, clinicians play an important role in shaping the development and validation of AI algorithms. When they partner with AI developers and researchers, healthcare companies can develop ground-breaking solutions to unaddressed clinical issues and ensure practical results for patients and healthcare professionals [103].

Further, regulatory agencies should collaborate with them to ensure that AI-driven innovations meet strict safety standards and are effective and of good quality. Regulatory frameworks and guidelines play a vital role in overseeing and directing the development, validation, and deployment of artificial intelligence-based medical devices and software. By engaging regulators closely, AI developers and healthcare providers can negotiate complicated regulatory pathways to hasten the adoption of AI technologies into clinical settings, ensuring patient safety and confidence [104, 105].

CONCLUSION

In conclusion, the promise of transforming patient care, enhancing results, and promoting medical standards exists with the integration of AI technologies in healthcare. While personalized medication management to clinical decision support systems, AI-driven innovations provide unprecedented avenues for improving diagnostic accuracy, optimizing treatment strategies, and delivering more patient-focused care. The AI algorithms analyze massive amounts of patients' data and are able to extract valuable insights, identify trends, and predict outcomes better than ever before. Healthcare providers can individualize their treatments toward patients by using genomic data, wearable devices, and digital health records. The final result is improved quality of life and better health outcomes as the medications that are prescribed to individuals are optimized, hence making them adhere to medical instructions. However, implementing AI technologies in healthcare faces a number of challenges. For AI-driven solutions to be successful, integration with existing systems, training/education for healthcare professionals, and overcoming resistance to change must be addressed. Furthermore, ethical and regulatory concerns such as privacy of information, algorithmic favoritism, and meeting the requirements for healthcare are key to ensuring the safety of patients and trust in AI-based healthcare services. Notwithstanding these obstacles, joint efforts among AI developers, health providers, and regulators can be a good starting point for exploiting the full potential of AI in the medical sector. Through collaboration aimed at tackling technical, organizational, and ethical issues, stakeholders can overcome the barriers that hinder innovation, thus causing positive changes in healthcare service delivery. In conclusion, artificial intelligence technology will be vital in shaping the future of healthcare. Continual investment, cooperation, and adherence to moral values can enable AI to turn around patient handling, improve health outcomes, and transform medicine as a profession for good. While we explore this new field, we must be aware of how AI supports us as patients, medical practitioners, and society at large.

ACKNOWLEDGEMENTS

Authors are highly thankful to their Universities/Colleges for providing library facilities for the literature survey.

REFERENCES

[1]   O. Strianese, F. Rizzo, M. Ciccarelli, G. Galasso, Y. D'Agostino, A. Salvati, C. Del Giudice, P. Tesorio, and M.R. Rusciano, "Precision and personalized medicine: How genomic approach improves the management of cardiovascular and neurodegenerative disease", *Genes (Basel),* vol. 11, no. 7, p. 747, 2020.
[http://dx.doi.org/10.3390/genes11070747] [PMID: 32640513]

[2]   S. Green, A. Carusi, and K. Hoeyer, "Plastic diagnostics: The remaking of disease and evidence in personalized medicine", *Soc. Sci. Med.,* vol. 304, p. 112318, 2022.
[http://dx.doi.org/10.1016/j.socscimed.2019.05.023] [PMID: 31130237]

[3]   S. Mathur and J. Sutton, "Personalized medicine could transform healthcare (Review)," *Biomedical Reports*, vol. 7, no. 1. pp. 3-5, 2017.
[http://dx.doi.org/10.3892/br.2017.922]

[4]   L. H. Goetz and N. J. Schork, "Personalized medicine: motivation, challenges, and progress," *Fertility and Sterility*, vol. 109, no. 6. pp. 952-963, 2018.
[http://dx.doi.org/10.1016/j.fertnstert.2018.05.006]

[5]   T. Nilchaikovit, J. M. Hill and J. C. Holland, "The effects of culture on illness behavior and medical care. Asian and American differences," *Gen. Hosp. Psychiatry*, vol. 15, no. 1, pp. 41–50, Jan. 1993.

[6]   J. Hartog and E. A. Hartog, "Cultural aspects of health and illness behavior in hospitals," *West. J. Med.*, vol. 139, no. 6, pp. 910–916, Dec. 1983

[7]   F. J. Bekker, U. Hentschel, and M. Fujita, "Basic cultural values and differences in attitudes towards health, illness and treatment preferences within a psychosomatic frame of reference," *Psychother. Psychosom.*, vol. 65, no. 4, pp. 191–198, 1996.
[http://dx.doi.org/10.1159/000289074]

[8]   A. Cunha, "Genomic technologies-from tools to therapies," *Genome Medicine,* vol. 9, no. 1. 2017.
[http://dx.doi.org/10.1186/s13073-017-0462-9]

[9]   X. Dai and L. Shen, "Advances and Trends in Omics Technology Development," *Frontiers in Medicine*, vol. 9. 2022.
[http://dx.doi.org/10.3389/fmed.2022.911861]

[10]   P. Duke, R.M. Frankel, and S. Reis, "How to integrate the electronic health record and patient-centered communication into the medical visit: a skills-based approach", *Teach. Learn. Med.,* vol. 25, no. 4, pp. 358-365, 2013.
[http://dx.doi.org/10.1080/10401334.2013.827981] [PMID: 24112206]

[11]   C.R. Bhasker, and G. Hardiman, "Advances in pharmacogenomics technologies", *Pharmacogenomics,* vol. 11, no. 4, pp. 481-485, 2010.
[http://dx.doi.org/10.2217/pgs.10.10] [PMID: 20350126]

[12]   O. Golubnitschaja, "Paradigm change from curative to predictive medicine: novel strategic trends in Europe", *Croat. Med. J.,* vol. 50, no. 6, pp. 596-597, 2009.
[http://dx.doi.org/10.3325/cmj.2009.50.596] [PMID: 20017229]

[13]   C.J. Guerrini, A.L. McGuire, and G. Lazaro-Munoz, "Ethical, Legal, and Social Implications", In: *Handbook of Clinical Adult Genetics and Genomics: A Practice-Based Approach.* Elsevier, 2020, pp. 431-442.
[http://dx.doi.org/10.1016/B978-0-12-817344-2.00027-7]

[14]   M. Kapalla, J. Kubáň, V. Costigliola, and O. Golubnitschaja, "Vision of the first EPMA center for predictive, preventive and personalized medicine in Europe", *EPMA Journal,* vol. Feb;5, no. Suppl 1, pp. A153-, 2014.

[15]   L. H. Goetz and N. J. Schork, "Personalized medicine: motivation, challenges, and progress," *Fertility and Sterility, vol. 109, no. 6. pp. 952-963,* 2018.
[http://dx.doi.org/10.1016/j.fertnstert.2018.05.006]

[16]   Pourpak Z, Fazlollahi MR, Fattahi F. "Understanding adverse drug reactions and drug allergies: principles, diagnosis and treatment aspects". *Recent patents on inflammation & allergy drug discovery.* 2008 Jan 1;2(1):24-46
[http://dx.doi.org/10.2174/187221308783399289]

[17]   Marzano AV, Borghi A, Cugno M. "Adverse drug reactions and organ damage: the skin". *European journal of internal medicine.* 2016 Mar 1;28:17-24.
[http://dx.doi.org/10.1016/j.ejim.2015.11.017]

[18]   A. S. Gross, A. C. Harry, C. S. Clifton, and O. Della Pasqua, "Clinical trial diversity: An opportunity for improved insight into the determinants of variability in drug response," *Br. J. Clin. Pharmacol.,* vol. 88, no. 6. pp. 2700-2717, 2022.
[http://dx.doi.org/10.1111/bcp.15242]

[19]   A. Sharma and L. Palaniappan, "Improving diversity in medical research," *Nature Reviews Disease Primers, Nature Research,* vol. 7, no. 1, 2021.
[http://dx.doi.org/10.1038/s41572-021-00316-8]

[20]   L.D. Lindley, "The paradox of self-efficacy: Research with diverse populations", *J. Career Assess.,* vol. 14, no. 1, pp. 143-160, 2006.
[http://dx.doi.org/10.1177/1069072705281371]

[21]   I. H. Sarker, "Machine Learning: Algorithms, Real-World Applications and Research Directions," *SN Computer Science,* vol. 2, no. 3. 2021
[http://dx.doi.org/10.1007/s42979-021-00592-x]

[22]   I. H. Sarker, "Deep Learning: A Comprehensive Overview on Techniques, Taxonomy, Applications and Research Directions," *SN Computer Science,* vol. 2, no. 6. 2021.
[http://dx.doi.org/10.1007/s42979-021-00815-1]

[23]   D. Khurana, A. Koli, K. Khatter, and S. Singh, "Natural language processing: state of the art, current trends and challenges", *Multimedia Tools Appl.,* vol. 82, no. 3, pp. 3713-3744, 2023.
[http://dx.doi.org/10.1007/s11042-022-13428-4] [PMID: 35855771]

[24]   M. Rustagi and N. Goel, "Predictive Analytics: A study of its Advantages and Applications," 2022. Available from: https://www.redalyc.org/journal/6638/663872727008/html/1/4
[http://dx.doi.org/10.51611/iars.irj.v12i01.2022.192]

[25]   R. D. S. G. Campilho and F. J. G. Silva, "Industrial Process Improvement by Automation and Robotics," *Machines.,* vol. 11, 2023.
[http://dx.doi.org/10.3390/machines11111011]

[26]   C. Lee Ventola, "Medical applications for 3D printing: Current and projected uses," *P&T,* vol. 39, no. 10, pp. 704-711, Oct. 2014.
[http://dx.doi.org/10.1016/j.ijpharm.2020.119732]

[27]   B. Pradhan, S. Bhattacharyya, and K. Pal, "IoT-Based Applications in Healthcare Devices", *J. Healthc. Eng.,* vol. 2021, pp. 1-18, 2021.
[http://dx.doi.org/10.1155/2021/6632599] [PMID: 33791084]

[28]   L. Lämmermann, P. Hofmann, and N. Urbach, "Managing artificial intelligence applications in healthcare: Promoting information processing among stakeholders", *Int. J. Inf. Manage.,* vol. 75, p. 102728, 2024.
[http://dx.doi.org/10.1016/j.ijinfomgt.2023.102728]

[29]   M. Yamin, "IT applications in healthcare management: a survey", *Int. J. Inf. Technol.,* vol. 10, no. 4, pp. 503-509, 2018.
[http://dx.doi.org/10.1007/s41870-018-0203-3] [PMID: 32289102]

[30]   A. Haleem, M. Javaid, R. P. Singh, R. Suman, and S. Rab, "Blockchain technology applications in healthcare: An overview," *International Journal of Intelligent Networks*, vol. 2. pp. 130-139, 2021.
[http://dx.doi.org/10.1016/j.ijin.2021.09.005]

[31]   A. S. M. Mosa, I. Yoo, and L. Sheets, "A systematic review of healthcare applications for smartphones," *BMC Medical Informatics and Decision Making,* vol. 12, no. 1. 2012.
[http://dx.doi.org/10.1186/1472-6947-12-67]

[32]   G. Luo, *Proceedings of the 2nd ACM SIGHIT International Health Informatics Symposium*, ACM, 2012. https://dl.acm.org/doi/proceedings/10.1145/2110363

[33]   D. Primorac *et al.*, "Pharmacogenomics at the center of precision medicine: Challenges and perspective in an era of Big Data," *Pharmacogenomics*, vol. 21, no. 2. pp. 141-156, 2020.
[http://dx.doi.org/10.2217/pgs-2019-0134]

[34]   M. M. Ghassemi, T. Alhanai, M. B. Westover, R. G. Mark, and S. Nemati, "Personalized medication dosing using volatile data streams," In: *Proc. Workshops of the Thirty-Second AAAI Conf. Artif. Intell.*, 2018. Available from: www.aaai.org

[35]   J.P. Jarvis, A.P. Peter, M. Keogh, V. Baldasare, G.M. Beanland, Z.T. Wilkerson, S. Kradel, and J.A. Shaman, "Real-World Impact of a Pharmacogenomics-Enriched Comprehensive Medication Management Program", *J. Pers. Med.,* vol. 12, no. 3, p. 421, 2022.
[http://dx.doi.org/10.3390/jpm12030421] [PMID: 35330421]

[36]   R.P. Aquino, S. Barile, A. Grasso, and M. Saviano, "Envisioning smart and sustainable healthcare: 3D Printing technologies for personalized medication", *Futures,* vol. 103, pp. 35-50, 2018.
[http://dx.doi.org/10.1016/j.futures.2018.03.002]

[37]   F.N.U. Sugandh, M. Chandio, F.N.U. Raveena, L. Kumar, F.N.U. Karishma, S. Khuwaja, U.A. Memon, K. Bai, M. Kashif, G. Varrassi, M. Khatri, and S. Kumar, "Advances in the Management of Diabetes Mellitus: A Focus on Personalized Medicine", *Cureus,* vol. 15, no. 8, p. e43697, 2023.
[http://dx.doi.org/10.7759/cureus.43697] [PMID: 37724233]

[38]   P.B. Jensen, L.J. Jensen, and S. Brunak, "Mining electronic health records: towards better research applications and clinical care", *Nat. Rev. Genet.,* vol. 13, no. 6, pp. 395-405, 2012.
[http://dx.doi.org/10.1038/nrg3208] [PMID: 22549152]

[39]   E. Ammenwerth, and A. Hoerbst, "Electronic health records. A systematic review on quality requirements", *Methods Inf. Med.,* vol. 49, no. 4, pp. 320-336, 2010.
[http://dx.doi.org/10.3414/ME10-01-0038] [PMID: 20603687]

[40]   M. R. Cowie *et al.*, "Electronic health records to facilitate clinical research," *Clinical Research in Cardiology*, vol. 106, no. 1. 2017.
[http://dx.doi.org/10.1007/s00392-016-1025-6]

[41]   R.S. Evans, "Electronic Health Records: Then, Now, and in the Future", *Yearb. Med. Inform.,* vol. 25, no. S 01, suppl. Suppl. 1, pp. S48-S61, 2016.
[http://dx.doi.org/10.15265/IYS-2016-s006] [PMID: 27199197]

[42]   G.R.G. Lanckriet, T. De Bie, N. Cristianini, M.I. Jordan, and W.S. Noble, "A statistical framework for genomic data fusion", *Bioinformatics,* vol. 20, no. 16, pp. 2626-2635, 2004.
[http://dx.doi.org/10.1093/bioinformatics/bth294] [PMID: 15130933]

[43]   L. Chin, W.C. Hahn, G. Getz, and M. Meyerson, "Making sense of cancer genomic data", *Genes Dev.,* vol. 25, no. 6, pp. 534-555, 2011.
[http://dx.doi.org/10.1101/gad.2017311] [PMID: 21406553]

[44]   F. Hahne and R. Ivanek, "Visualizing genomic data using Gviz and Bioconductor," In: *E. Mathé and S. Davis, Eds. Statistical Genomics. Methods in Molecular Biology*, vol. 1418, New York, NY: Humana Press, 2016, pp. 335–351.
[http://dx.doi.org/10.1007/978-1-4939-3578-9_16]

[45]   M. Manni, M.R. Berkeley, M. Seppey, and E.M. Zdobnov, "BUSCO: Assessing Genomic Data Quality and Beyond", *Curr. Protoc.,* vol. 1, no. 12, p. e323, 2021.
[http://dx.doi.org/10.1002/cpz1.323] [PMID: 34936221]

[46]   S.D. Kahn, "On the future of genomic data", *Science,* vol. 331, no. 6018, pp. 728-729, 2011.
[http://dx.doi.org/10.1126/science.1197891] [PMID: 21311016]

[47]   F. John Dian, R. Vahidnia, and A. Rahmati, *"Wearables and the Internet of Things (IoT), Applications, Opportunities, and Challenges: A Survey," IEEE Access.* vol. 8. Institute of Electrical and Electronics Engineers Inc., 2020, pp. 69200-69211.
[http://dx.doi.org/10.1109/ACCESS.2020.2986329]

[48]   J. Passos *et al.*, "Wearables and internet of things (Iot) technologies for fitness assessment: A systematic review," *Sensors*, vol. 21, no. 16. MDPI AG, Aug. 02, 2021.
[http://dx.doi.org/10.37766/inplasy2021.6.0041]

[49]   J. Hajny, P. Dzurenda, and L. Malina, "Multi-device authentication using wearables and IoT," in *ICETE 2016 - Proceedings of the 13th International Joint Conference on e-Business and Telecommunications, SciTePress*, pp. 483-488, 2016.
[http://dx.doi.org/10.5220/0006000004830488]

[50]   Y.C. Chiu, H.I.H. Chen, T. Zhang, S. Zhang, A. Gorthi, L.J. Wang, Y. Huang, and Y. Chen, "Predicting drug response of tumors from integrated genomic profiles by deep neural networks", *BMC Med. Genomics,* vol. 12, no. S1, suppl. Suppl. 1, p. 18, 2019.
[http://dx.doi.org/10.1186/s12920-018-0460-9] [PMID: 30704458]

[51]   G. Adam, L. Rampášek, Z. Safikhani, P. Smirnov, B. Haibe-Kains, and A. Goldenberg, "Machine learning approaches to drug response prediction: challenges and recent progress," *Npj Precision Oncology*, vol. 4, no. 1. 01, 2020.
[http://dx.doi.org/10.1038/s41698-020-0122-1]

[52]   B.M. Kuenzi, J. Park, S.H. Fong, K.S. Sanchez, J. Lee, J.F. Kreisberg, J. Ma, and T. Ideker, "Predicting Drug Response and Synergy Using a Deep Learning Model of Human Cancer Cells", *Cancer Cell,* vol. 38, no. 5, pp. 672-684.e6, 2020.
[http://dx.doi.org/10.1016/j.ccell.2020.09.014] [PMID: 33096023]

[53]   J. Robert, V.L. Morvan, D. Smith, P. Pourquier, and J. Bonnet, "Predicting drug response and toxicity based on gene polymorphisms", *Crit. Rev. Oncol. Hematol.,* vol. 54, no. 3, pp. 171-196, 2005.
[http://dx.doi.org/10.1016/j.critrevonc.2005.01.005] [PMID: 15890268]

[54]   F. Azuaje, "Computational models for predicting drug responses in cancer research", *Brief. Bioinform.,* vol. 18, no. 5, p. bbw065, 2016.
[http://dx.doi.org/10.1093/bib/bbw065] [PMID: 27444372]

[55]   I. Sushko, E. Salmina, V.A. Potemkin, G. Poda, and I.V. Tetko, "ToxAlerts: a Web server of structural alerts for toxic chemicals and compounds with potential adverse reactions", *J. Chem. Inf. Model.,* vol. 52, no. 8, pp. 2310-2316, 2012.
[http://dx.doi.org/10.1021/ci300245q] [PMID: 22876798]

[56]   Available from: https://www.nccmerp.org/about-medication-errors

[57]   R. Leone, L. Magro, U. Moretti, P. M. Cutroneo, M. Moschini, D. Motola, and A. Conforti, "Identifying adverse drug reactions associated with drug-drug interactions: Data mining of a spontaneous reporting database in Italy," *Drug Safety*, vol. 33, no. 8, pp. 667-675, Aug. 2010. [http://dx.doi.org/10.2165/11534400-000000000-00000]

[58]   E.C.C. Lai, C.Y. Hsieh, Y.H. Kao Yang, and S.J. Lin, "Detecting potential adverse reactions of sulpiride in schizophrenic patients by prescription sequence symmetry analysis", *PLoS One,* vol. 9, no. 2, p. e89795, 2014. [http://dx.doi.org/10.1371/journal.pone.0089795] [PMID: 24587038]

[59]   K. Patton and D. C. Borshoff, "Adverse drug reactions," Anaesthesia, vol. 73. Blackwell Publishing Ltd, pp. 76-84, 2018. [http://dx.doi.org/10.1111/anae.14143]

[60]   E. Aakhus, I. Granlund, A.D. Oxman, and S.A. Flottorp, "Tailoring interventions to implement recommendations for the treatment of elderly patients with depression: a qualitative study", *Int. J. Ment. Health Syst.,* vol. 9, no. 1, p. 36, 2015. [http://dx.doi.org/10.1186/s13033-015-0027-5] [PMID: 26366193]

[61]   S. Zilcha-Mano, M.J. Constantino, and C.F. Eubanks, "Evidence-based tailoring of treatment to patients, providers, and processes: Introduction to the special issue", *J. Consult. Clin. Psychol.,* vol. 90, no. 1, pp. 1-4, 2022. [http://dx.doi.org/10.1037/ccp0000694] [PMID: 35225633]

[62]   K.G. Thompson, M. Shuster, B.C. Ly, C. Antonescu, L. Florea, A.L. Chien, and S. Kang, "Variability in skin microbiota between smokers, former smokers, and nonsmokers", *J. Am. Acad. Dermatol.,* vol. 83, no. 3, pp. 942-944, 2020. [http://dx.doi.org/10.1016/j.jaad.2020.01.042] [PMID: 32004647]

[63]   K. Matchett, N. Lynam-Lennon, R. Watson, and J. Brown, "Advances in precision medicine: Tailoring individualized therapies", *Cancers (Basel),* vol. 9, no. 11, p. 146, 2017. [http://dx.doi.org/10.3390/cancers9110146] [PMID: 29068364]

[64]   D.M. Hilty, C.M. Armstrong, A. Edwards-Stewart, *et al.* "Sensor, Wearable, and Remote Patient Monitoring Competencies for Clinical Care and Training: Scoping Review". *J. technol. behav. sci.,* vol. 6, pp. 252–277, 2021. [http://dx.doi.org/10.1007/s41347-020-00190-3]

[65]   K.C. Nicolaou, "Advancing the drug discovery and development process", *Angew. Chem. Int. Ed.,* vol. 53, no. 35, pp. 9128-9140, 2014. [http://dx.doi.org/10.1002/anie.201404761] [PMID: 25045053]

[66]   A. Tripathi, K. Misra, R. Dhanuka, and J.P. Singh, "Artificial Intelligence in Accelerating Drug Discovery and Development", *Recent Pat. Biotechnol.,* vol. 17, no. 1, pp. 9-23, 2023. [http://dx.doi.org/10.2174/1872208316666220802151129] [PMID: 35927896]

[67]   Z. Liu, J. Du, J. Fang, Y. Yin, G. Xu, and L. Xie, "DeepScreening: a deep learning-based screening web server for accelerating drug discovery", *Database (Oxford),* vol. 2019, no. 1, p. baz104, 2019. [http://dx.doi.org/10.1093/database/baz104] [PMID: 31608949]

[68]   S. Kraljević, P. J. Stambrook, and K. Pavelić, "Accelerating drug discovery," *EMBO Reports*, vol. 5, no. 9, pp. 837-842, 2004. [http://dx.doi.org/10.1038/sj.embor.7400236]

[69]   D. W. Shineman, G. S. Basi, J. L. Bizon, C. A. Colton, B. D. Greenberg, B. A. Hollister, J. Lincecum, G. G. Leblanc, L. H. Lee, F. Luo, D. Morgan, I. Morse, L. M. Refolo, D. R. Riddell, K. Scearce-Levie, P. Sweeney, J. Yrjänheikki, and H. M. Fillit, "Accelerating drug discovery for Alzheimer's disease: Best practices for preclinical animal studies," *Alzheimers Res. Ther.*, vol. 3, no. 5, p. 28, 2011. Available: https://alzres.biomedcentral.com/articles/10.1186/ar343

[70]   J. Moll, and S. Carotta, *Target Identii cation and Validation in Drug Discovery Methods and Protocols.* 2nd ed. Methods in Molecular Biology, 1953. Available from: http://www.springer.com/series/7651

[71]   C. McNamara, and E.A. Winzeler, "Target identification and validation of novel antimalarials", *Future Microbiol.,* vol. 6, no. 6, pp. 693-704, 2011.
[http://dx.doi.org/10.2217/fmb.11.45] [PMID: 21707315]

[72]   C. Finan, S. L. S. P. Overington, A. L. C. Hopkins, E. J. Schreiber, A. B. B. Smith, P. R. Green, and D. R. E. L. Houghton, "The druggable genome and support for target identification and validation in drug development," *Sci. Transl. Med.,* vol. 9, no. 380, 2017, Art. no. eaag1166. https://www.science.org
[http://dx.doi.org/10.1126/scitranslmed.aag1166]

[73]   J. D. Moore, "The impact of CRISPR-Cas9 on target identification and validation," *Drug Discovery Today,* vol. 20, no. 4. pp. 450-457, 2015.
[http://dx.doi.org/10.1016/j.drudis.2014.12.016]

[74]   M. Jayapal and A. J. Melendez, "Dna microarray technology for target identification and validation," 2006. Available from: http://www.affymetrix.com
[http://dx.doi.org/10.1111/j.1440-1681.2006.04398.x]

[75]   G. Koscielny, P. An, D. Carvalho-Silva, J.A. Cham, L. Fumis, R. Gasparyan, S. Hasan, N. Karamanis, M. Maguire, E. Papa, A. Pierleoni, M. Pignatelli, T. Platt, F. Rowland, P. Wankar, A.P. Bento, T. Burdett, A. Fabregat, S. Forbes, A. Gaulton, C.Y. Gonzalez, H. Hermjakob, A. Hersey, S. Jupe, Ş. Kafkas, M. Keays, C. Leroy, F.J. Lopez, M.P. Magarinos, J. Malone, J. McEntyre, A. Munoz-Pomer Fuentes, C. O'Donovan, I. Papatheodorou, H. Parkinson, B. Palka, J. Paschall, R. Petryszak, N. Pratanwanich, S. Sarntivijal, G. Saunders, K. Sidiropoulos, T. Smith, Z. Sondka, O. Stegle, Y.A. Tang, E. Turner, B. Vaughan, O. Vrousgou, X. Watkins, M.J. Martin, P. Sanseau, J. Vamathevan, E. Birney, J. Barrett, and I. Dunham, "Open Targets: a platform for therapeutic target identification and validation", *Nucleic Acids Res.,* vol. 45, no. D1, pp. D985-D994, 2017.
[http://dx.doi.org/10.1093/nar/gkw1055] [PMID: 27899665]

[76]   T. U. Singh, S. Parida, M. C. Lingaraju, M. Kesavan, D. Kumar, and R. K. Singh, "Drug repurposing approach to fight COVID-19," *Pharmacological Reports,* vol. 72, no. 6. pp. 1479-1508, 2020.
[http://dx.doi.org/10.1007/s43440-020-00155-6]

[77]   Pushpakom *et al.,* "Drug repurposing: Progress, challenges and recommendations," *Nature Reviews Drug Discovery,* vol. 18, no. 1. pp. 41-58, 2018.
[http://dx.doi.org/10.1038/nrd.2018.168]

[78]   C. Daphna Laifenfeld, "Themed Section: Inventing New Therapies Without Reinventing the Wheel: The Power of Drug Repurposing Drug repurposing from the perspective of pharmaceutical companies LINKED ARTICLES", *Br. J. Pharmacol.,* vol. 175, p. 168, 2018.
[http://dx.doi.org/10.1111/bph.v175.2/issuetoc]

[79]   P. P. Sharma, S. K. Yadav, A. K. Dubey, N. K. Sharma, S. K. Soni, A. M. Z. Altwaijry, and A. P. Ghosh, "Computational methods directed towards drug repurposing for COVID-19: Advantages and limitations," *RSC Adv.,* vol. 11, no. 57, pp. 36181-36198, 2021.
[http://dx.doi.org/10.1039/D1RA05320E]

[80]   V. Parvathaneni and V. Gupta, "Utilizing drug repurposing against COVID-19 - Efficacy, limitations, and challenges," *Life Sciences,* vol. 259. 2020.
[http://dx.doi.org/10.1016/j.lfs.2020.118275]

[81]   S. Powell-Laney, S. Powell-Laney, C. Keen, and K. Hall, *The Use of Human Patient Simulators to Enhance Clinical Decision-making of Nursing Students,* 2012. Available from: http://journals.lww.com/edhe
[http://dx.doi.org/10.4103/1357-6283.99201]

[82]   A. Masood, U. Naseem, J. Rashid, J. Kim, and I. Razzak, "Review on enhancing clinical decision support system using machine learning", In: *CAAI Transactions on Intelligence Technology.* John

Wiley and Sons Inc, 2024.
[http://dx.doi.org/10.1049/cit2.12286]

[83] P. J. Scott, P. A. Altenburger, and J. Kean, "A collaborative teaching strategy for enhancing learning of evidence-based clinical decision-making," *J. Allied Health*, vol. 40, no. 3, pp. 120–127, Sep. 2011.

[84] E. Nango and Y. Tanaka, "Problem-based learning in a multidisciplinary group enhances clinical decision making by medical students: a randomized controlled trial," *J. Med. Dent. Sci.*, vol. 57, no. 1, pp. 109–118, Mar. 2010.

[85] R. Miranda, C. Alves, A. Abelha, and J. Machado, "Data Platforms for Real-time Insights in Healthcare: Systematic Review," in *Procedia Computer Science*, Elsevier B.V., 2023, pp. 826-831.
[http://dx.doi.org/10.1016/j.procs.2023.03.110]

[86] P. J. Scott, P. A. Altenburger, and J. Kean, "A collaborative teaching strategy for enhancing learning of evidence-based clinical decision-making," *J. Allied Health*, vol. 40, no. 3, pp. 120–127, 2011.

[87] S. Shukla, "Real-time Monitoring and Predictive Analytics in Healthcare: Harnessing the Power of Data Streaming", *Int. J. Comput. Appl.*, vol. 185, no. 8, pp. 32-37, 2023.
[http://dx.doi.org/10.5120/ijca2023922738]

[88] E. Tensen, J.P. van der Heijden, M.W.M. Jaspers, and L. Witkamp, "Two Decades of Teledermatology: Current Status and Integration in National Healthcare Systems", *Curr. Dermatol. Rep.*, vol. 5, no. 2, pp. 96-104, 2016.
[http://dx.doi.org/10.1007/s13671-016-0136-7] [PMID: 27182461]

[89] R. Atun, T. de Jongh, F. Secci, K. Ohiri, and O. Adeyi, "Integration of targeted health interventions into health systems: a conceptual framework for analysis", *Health Policy Plan.*, vol. 25, no. 2, pp. 104-111, 2010.
[http://dx.doi.org/10.1093/heapol/czp055] [PMID: 19917651]

[90] M. Breton, R. Pineault, J.F. Levesque, D. Roberge, R.B. Da Silva, and A. Prud'homme, "Reforming healthcare systems on a locally integrated basis: is there a potential for increasing collaborations in primary healthcare?", *BMC Health Serv. Res.*, vol. 13, no. 1, p. 262, 2013.
[http://dx.doi.org/10.1186/1472-6963-13-262] [PMID: 23835105]

[91] M. Li, Y. Fan, X. Zhang, W. Hou, and Z. Tang, "Fruit and vegetable intake and risk of type 2 diabetes mellitus: meta-analysis of prospective cohort studies", *BMJ Open*, vol. 4, no. 11, p. e005497, 2014.
[http://dx.doi.org/10.1136/bmjopen-2014-005497] [PMID: 25377009]

[92] L.J. Nayahangan, L. Konge, L. Russell, and S. Andersen, "Training and education of healthcare workers during viral epidemics: a systematic review", *BMJ Open*, vol. 11, no. 5, p. e044111, 2021.
[http://dx.doi.org/10.1136/bmjopen-2020-044111] [PMID: 34049907]

[93] L. Hecht, S. Buhse, and G. Meyer, "Effectiveness of training in evidence-based medicine skills for healthcare professionals: A systematic review", *BMC Med Educ*, vol. 16, p. 103, 2016.
[http://dx.doi.org/10.1186/s12909-016-0616-2]

[94] M. Peduzzi, I.J. Norman, A.C.C.G. Germani, J.A.M. da Silva, and G.C. de Souza, "Interprofessional education: Training for healthcare professionals for teamwork focusing on users", *Rev. Esc. Enferm.*, vol. 47, no. 4, 2013.

[95] J. Repper, and J. Breeze, "User and carer involvement in the training and education of health professionals: A review of the literature", *Int. J. Nurs. Stud.*, vol. 44, no. 3, pp. 511-519, 2007.
[http://dx.doi.org/10.1016/j.ijnurstu.2006.05.013] [PMID: 16842793]

[96] R. J. Recardo, "Overcoming resistance to change," *Natl. Product. Rev.*, vol. 14, no. 2, pp. 5–12, Spring 1995.

[97] Hon AH, Bloom M, Crant JM. Overcoming resistance to change and enhancing creative performance. Journal of management. 2014 Mar;40(3):919-41.
[http://dx.doi.org/10.1177/0149206311415418]

[98]   M.M. Kan, and K.W. Parry, "Identifying paradox: A grounded theory of leadership in overcoming resistance to change", *Leadersh. Q.*, vol. 15, no. 4, pp. 467-491, 2004.
[http://dx.doi.org/10.1016/j.leaqua.2004.05.003]

[99]   S. Murrar, and M. Brauer, "Overcoming Resistance to Change: Using Narratives to Create More Positive Intergroup Attitudes", *Curr. Dir. Psychol. Sci.,* vol. 28, no. 2, pp. 164-169, 2019.
[http://dx.doi.org/10.1177/0963721418818552]

[100] D. R. Self, "Overcoming resistance to change by managing readiness for change," 2008.

[101] A. Singam, "Revolutionizing Patient Care: A Comprehensive Review of Artificial Intelligence Applications in Anesthesia", *Cureus,* vol. 15, no. 12, p. e49887, 2023.
[http://dx.doi.org/10.7759/cureus.49887] [PMID: 38174199]

[102] K. B. Johnson *et al.*, "Precision Medicine, AI, and the Future of Personalized Health Care," *Clinical and Translational Science*, vol. 14, no. 1. pp. 86-93, 2021.
[http://dx.doi.org/10.1111/cts.12884]

[103] S. Verma, R. Sharma, S. Deb, and D. Maitra, "Artificial intelligence in marketing: Systematic review and future research direction", *Int. J. Inf. Manag. Data Insights,* vol. 1, no. 1, p. 100002, 2021.
[http://dx.doi.org/10.1016/j.jjimei.2020.100002]

[104] T. T. Nguyen, A. N. Pham, H. M. Nguyen, S. H. Nguyen, and L. T. Hoang, "Artificial Intelligence in the Battle against Coronavirus (COVID-19): A Survey and Future Research Directions," 2020. Available: http://arxiv.org/abs/2008.07343

[105] A. F. S. Borges, F. J. B. Laurindo, M. M. Spínola, R. F. Gonçalves, and C. A. Mattos, "The strategic use of artificial intelligence in the digital era: Systematic literature review and future research directions," *International Journal of Information Management*, vol. 57. 2021.
[http://dx.doi.org/10.1016/j.ijinfomgt.2020.102225]

CHAPTER 3

IoT Integration: Tracking Medication Intake

Shekhar Singh[1], Akhil Sharma[2], Sunita[3], P. Ravi Kishore[4] and Shaweta Sharma[5,*]

[1] *Faculty of Pharmacy, Babu Banarasi Das Northern India Institute of Technology, Lucknow, Uttar Pradesh, India*

[2] *R.J. College of Pharmacy, Raipur, Gharbara, Tappal, Khair, Uttar Pradesh, India*

[3] *Metro College of Health Sciences and Research, Greater Noida, Uttar Pradesh, India*

[4] *Department of Civil Engineering, Aditya University, Surampalem, India*

[5] *School of Medical and Allied Sciences, Galgotias University Plot No. 2, Yamuna Expy, Opposite Buddha International Circuit, Sector 17A, Greater Noida, Uttar Pradesh, India*

Abstract: Non-adherence occurs when patients do not take their medications as prescribed. This is a major challenge in healthcare that has detrimental consequences on the health outcomes of patients and health systems. An emerging solution to this problem has been identified by using Internet of Things (IoT) capabilities. This chapter investigates the use of IoT for medication intake tracking, giving a detailed account of its advantages, mechanisms, limitations, and prospects. The IoT's role in healthcare and medication non-adherence are examined at the beginning of the discussion. The chapter explores various IoT solutions for medication management, including smart pill boxes, wearables, and apps, their functions, and real-time monitoring abilities. The chapter highlights the key benefits of integrating IoT into healthcare for patients and care providers, such as better compliance rates, greater patient involvement, and the availability of immediate adherence data to enhance decision-making. Additionally, the chapter examines the practicality of IoT in medication tracking by looking at how it works technically and how sensors, connectivity, and data analytics are used to collect and analyze adherence data. Also, privacy concerns, as well as integration with existing healthcare systems, are some of the possible challenges that are discussed. The chapter also outlines forthcoming trends such as an improvement in IoT technology, possibilities for AI and machine learning incorporation within it, and a wider use of IoT solutions in other healthcare sectors. This chapter takes insights from different fields to give an all-inclusive understanding of how IoT integration can disrupt medication management, leading to better patient outcomes and healthcare delivery.

---

[*] **Corresponding author Shaweta Sharma:** School of Medical and Allied Sciences, Galgotias University Plot No. 2, Yamuna Expy, Opposite Buddha International Circuit, Sector 17A, Greater Noida, Uttar Pradesh, India; E-mail: shawetasharma@galgotiasuniversity.edu.in

Akhil Sharma, Neeraj Kumar Fuloria, Pankaj Kumar Singh & Shaweta Sharma (Eds.)

Keywords: Adherence, Data analytics, Health, Healthcare, Internet of things, Medication, Mobile applications, Non-adherence, Patient, Real-time, Sensors, Smart pill dispensers, Wearable devices.

INTRODUCTION

Adhering to prescribed medication is a major problem in health care, comprising many complex difficulties that highly affect the health of patients and the efficiency of healthcare systems in general. One of the main challenges in this case is the intricacy associated with prescription regimens, whereby patients have to deal with multiple drugs, each having different doses, timing, and administration requirements. The complicated balancing involved can be too much for patients, resulting in perplexity, mistakes, and finally noncompliance with prescribed schedules [1].

Furthermore, forgetfulness is a common problem, with patients finding it hard to stick to their medication schedules because of momentary memory lapses or inability to sustain regular routines in the middle of day-to-day commitments. Financial obstacles also make the situation worse by imposing a huge financial burden on patients because of the high cost of prescription drugs, thereby forcing them to choose between life-saving drugs and food, shelter, and other basic requirements. Additionally, there is looming dread about possible side effects or any other unwanted reactions that stop individuals from adhering to what has been prescribed for the fear of their own lives and health [2].

Furthermore, adherence difficulties are worsened by inadequate health literacy since patients without enough knowledge of how to take medicines or doses can mistakenly move away from their prescriptions, bringing ineffective treatment results or effects on them. Another thing that hampers adherence attempts is social factors such as stigma towards some medical conditions or lack of support system; in this regard, patients may feel guilty and be unwilling to express themselves through discussing openly their medication use and asking for help with their treatment [3].

The importance of medication adherence for achieving positive health outcomes must be emphasized in this labyrinthine landscape of challenges. As the cornerstone to effective disease management and control, adhering to prescribed medications is especially critical in cases of chronic illnesses such as diabetes, hypertension, and HIV/AIDS. For instance, optimal adherence can enable patients to achieve and maintain optimum disease control, which reduces the risk of disease exacerbation and complications while enhancing overall well-being [4].

When patients follow their recommended medication plan, they can cut down considerably on the probability of hospitalizations or ER visits, easing pressure from healthcare providers and reducing health care costs. More so, constant adherence is vital in blocking diseases from spreading further, enabling individuals to maintain their capability status, improve their life standards, and reduce the long-term effects of untreated or inadequately treated cases. From an economic perspective, adherence to medications leads to significant savings through a reduction in healthcare utilization, prevention of expensive complications, and a decrease in the need for costly medical interventions or procedures [5].

At the population level, public health implications of adherence improvement are extensive and include disease prevention, mitigation of healthcare disparities, and community health promotion and well-being. Consequently, addressing the multiple challenges around medication adherence is essential in order to achieve optimal health outcomes, enhance patient care, and ensure the viability of healthcare delivery systems. By using individualized procedures, inventing new technologies, and encouraging interaction among healthcare givers, policymakers, and other parties concerned, we can attempt to overcome these hurdles and support the use of drugs as an important building block in health service provision. The importance of medication adherence for health outcomes is shown in Fig. (**1**) [6, 7].

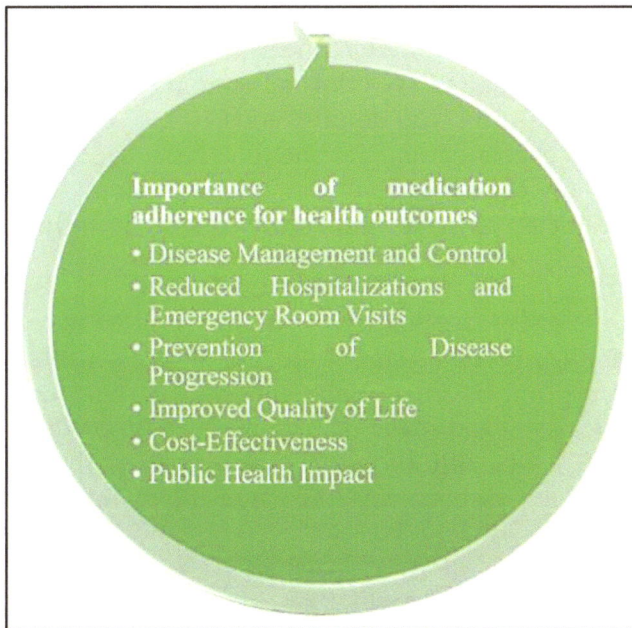

Fig. (1). Importance of medication adherence for health outcomes.

Prescribed medicines need to be taken as directed if chronic diseases such as diabetes, hypertension, and HIV/AIDS are to be adequately managed, as this helps patients gain the best disease control and avoid complications. Strictly following medication prescriptions can greatly reduce the chances of having a flare-up of a condition that would lead to hospitalization or emergency room visits, which puts an enormous strain on healthcare facilities. In specific diseases like mental health disorders and cardiovascular conditions, among others where early intervention is key in their management, adherence to drugs has been identified as the most important factor in preventing their progression [8].

Patients who follow the doctor's orders with regard to taking their medication can get a better quality of life in general by reducing symptoms, improving functional capacity, and promoting well-being thereby enabling individuals to live rewarding and productive lives. Optimal adherence to medications will result in significant financial gains, including decreased healthcare utilization, prevention of costly complications, and reduction in expensive medical interventions or procedures. A population-level increase in drug therapy adherence could lead to a major public health impact, such as disease prevention, reduction in disparities in the healthcare system, and improvement in community health outcomes [9].

IOT IN HEALTHCARE

The Internet of Things (IoT) is an innovative technological framework that makes it possible to link up normal things to the internet so that they can collect, share, and analyze data by themselves. At its heart, IoT encompasses a collection of connected devices, sensors, and systems that communicate with one another and with cloud-based platforms or applications, thus creating an integrated environment of data exchange and interaction. Such gadgets may involve cell phones, wearable devices, household machines, among others right up to industrial machinery cars as well as medical equipment [10].

The essence of IoT is its transformative potential, which can turn passive objects into smart, proactive ones that sense, process, and respond to real-time data. This transformative ability involves the embedding of sensors, actuators, and communication technologies in physical objects that help them monitor their environment, collect data, and make decisions based on predefined rules or user inputs. For example, a wearable fitness band has trackers that capture heart rate, activity level, and sleep patterns and then transmit it for further analysis in a mobile application or cloud platform [11].

In the healthcare context, the IoT is highly likely to transform patient care, clinical workflows, and healthcare delivery. Healthcare service providers can capture real-time patient data, monitor vital signs, track medication adherence, and remotely manage chronic conditions by integrating IoT devices and sensors into medical devices, diagnostic equipment, and healthcare facilities. For example, IoT wearables will be able to continually monitor a patient's blood glucose levels, heart rate, and physical activity, thereby giving timely interventions or adjustments to treatment plans based on their health status with regard to that particular point in time [12].

Additionally, IoT allows for the easy sharing of data relating to healthcare among various concerned parties such as patients, providers, insurance companies, and teachers. This facilitates teamwork, makes communication easier, and improves the quality of decisions made by different individuals involved. For instance, EHR systems that IoT enables can interchangeably send patient information from one doctor to another without putting the information at risk or duplicating it. Such platforms also enable e-consultation through telemedicine, that is remote monitoring and telehealth services, thereby expanding the coverage of health care access and improving patient outcomes, especially in underprivileged areas [13].

IoT is a transformative factor in healthcare as it gives room for novel ways of enhancing service provision to patients, improving clinical outcomes, and streamlining healthcare delivery. With the help of data analytics and AI by connecting medical devices, sensors, and systems to the internet, this will enable healthcare providers to develop an interconnected ecosystem of care that is patient-centered, cost-effective, and sustainable. Nevertheless, like every other technology, IoT in healthcare has its share of difficulties, which include security issues on data privacy, interoperability as well and regulatory compliance that need to be tackled so as to maximize its full potential in reshaping how healthcare is delivered [14, 15].

The IoT has a great impact on healthcare and medication management by providing creative propositions that change how healthcare is given, regulated, and arranged. Through IoT technology, it is possible to smoothly incorporate linked devices, sensors, and systems that allow real-time data acquisition, processing, and exchange for better patient outcomes, more efficient operations, and innovative healthcare delivery [16]. The roles of IoT in healthcare and medication management are described below and shown in Fig. (**2**).

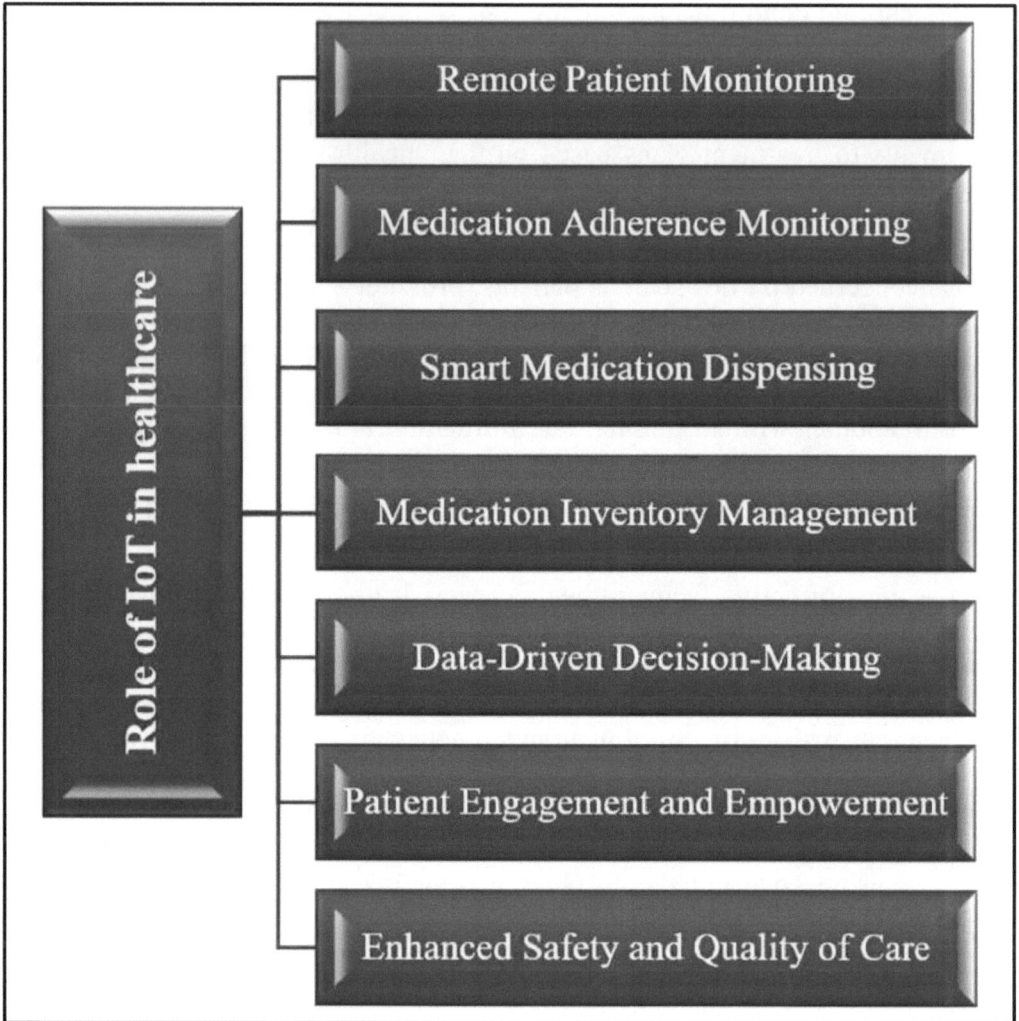

Fig. (2). Role of IoT in healthcare.

Remote Patient Monitoring

The IoT plays a critical role in Remote Patient Monitoring (RPM), transforming the provision and management of healthcare away from conventional clinical settings. To provide information on patient's health, vital signs, and symptoms in real-time, it combines connected devices, sensors, and telecommunication technologies. For example, wearable sensors, smartwatches, and medical-grade wearables are examples of IoT devices through which patient information is collected securely for proactive intervention by doctors as well as a timely adjustment of treatment plans [17].

Telecommunication systems help facilitate smooth communication between patients and providers, thus allowing remote consultations, virtual visits, and data access. Advanced analytics alongside artificial intelligence analyze the IoT collected information identifying trends and abnormalities as well as forecasting potential health risks, making it possible for healthcare givers to monitor their patients' health from miles away and intervene whenever a need arises. When IoT systems trigger alerts and notifications, they allow timely interventions and coordination of care by informing healthcare providers about notable variations in the health status of patients [18-20].

Smart Medication Dispensing

In smart medication dispensing, the IoT is transformative as it revolutionizes how medication is managed and enhances patient adherence to prescribed treatment regimens. Thus, when IoT technology is integrated into medication dispensing systems, healthcare providers can make sure that patients get their drugs accurately, on time, and in a personalized manner. Smart medication dispensers are equipped with sensors, connectivity features, and intelligent algorithms that automate the process of medication dispensing and boost security and effectiveness. They can be set to dispense drugs at particular times, dosages, and intervals as indicated by patient treatment plans, thereby lowering cases of incorrect dosages, side effects, or noncompliance [21].

IoT-enabled smart dispensers monitor medication usage in real time, track adherence behaviors, and provide patients with timely reminders and alerts to take their medications as prescribed. Healthcare providers can remotely monitor patients' medication adherence, review adherence data, and intervene promptly when adherence issues arise. By promoting medication adherence through personalized reminders, dosage tracking, and feedback, IoT-enabled smart medication dispensers improve patient outcomes, enhance medication management, and optimize healthcare delivery [22].

Medication Inventory Management

Pharmaceutical usage is monitored by smart dispensers enabled by the IoT in real-time, adherence behavior is tracked, and patients are reminded at the right time. Doctors can follow up on their patient's adherence to medication remotely and examine this information before intervening. By providing personalized reminders, dosage tracking, and feedback, IoT-enabled smart medication dispensers enhance patient outcomes, improve medication management, and optimize healthcare delivery [23].

These are some of the ways that these systems enabled by IoT help automate inventory replenishment processes in order to have enough medications when needed and avoid stockouts or overstocking. They also provide useful information for medication usage trends, demand forecasting, and inventory optimization through IoT-driven data analytics and predictive modeling. Through this, the healthcare system will be able to achieve efficiencies in medication procurement, thus lowering costs associated with carrying an inventory while at the same time increasing the availability of medicines, hence enhancing patient safety as well as care quality [24].

Data-Driven Decision-Making

The significance of IoT in data-driven decision-making is essential, as it provides healthcare providers with an invaluable understanding of patient health, treatment outcomes, and operational efficiency. Health organizations can collate extensive real-time information related to patients' medication compliance records, health status, healthcare utilization, or treatment effectiveness through the use of IoT-enabled devices, sensors, and systems. Advanced analytics tools are used to process the information into meaningful patterns for better decisions on clinical practice and quality improvement projects (Artificial Intelligence (AI) & Machine Learning (ML) algorithms) [25].

Health experts can examine patient data, create personalized wellness plans, and anticipate health risks using the Internet of Things. Besides, IoT enables seamless data sharing among various stakeholders in the healthcare sector, thereby ensuring ease of communication and knowledge sharing among healthcare providers. By utilizing IoT for decision-making through data management, healthcare organizations are able to improve patient outcomes, enhance operational efficiency, and drive innovation in healthcare delivery [26].

Patient Engagement and Empowerment

The role of the IoT in patient engagement and empowerment is transformative, making it possible to empower people in order for them to control their health and well-being. The application of IoT-enabled devices, applications, and platforms allows patients to have real-time health data, personalized feedback as well as educational materials that enhance self-identity and self-control. Patients are able to monitor vital signs, track symptoms, and manage chronic conditions with wearable sensors, smart devices, and mobile health apps from home; this results in a feeling of independence concerning their wellness [27].

Additionally, IoT-enabled patient commitment platforms are tools that encourage patients and health providers to be able to discuss problems related to treatment remotely, find support in virtual groups, or come to common decisions. Through individualized interactions, education, and support that increases user engagement, IoT enables people to take responsibility for their health through making informed choices on their healthcare options, adopting healthier lifestyles, and actively engaging in their care, which will ultimately result in improved health outcomes as well as better quality of life [28].

Enhanced Safety and Quality of Care

IoT plays a crucial role in reinforcing the safety and quality of healthcare and transforming healthcare delivery in general by reducing mistakes, improving patient outcomes, and optimizing operational efficiency. By integrating IoT-enabled devices, sensors, and systems, healthcare providers can monitor patients' health conditions in real-time and also keep track of their medication adherence as well as environmental conditions so that they can intervene proactively before things go wrong. Smart medical devices fitted with IoT sensors enable correct drug administration, monitor the vital signs of a patient, and detect early signs of complications, thus minimizing dispensing errors or other problems that may arise from their use [29].

Additionally, healthcare providers can identify trends, predict patient needs, and personalize treatment plans through IoT-driven analytics and predictive modeling, enhancing clinical decision-making as well as care delivery. Moreover, improving communication and coordination among healthcare teams, promoting infection control measures, and reducing the risk of hospital-acquired infections and medical errors are all benefits of IoT to patients' safety. This can be achieved through leveraging the use of IoT technology in healthcare organizations in an effort to enhance safety and quality of care, which can make a positive difference in patient outcomes by lowering health costs besides increasing continuous improvement culture [30].

MEDICATION ADHERENCE PROBLEM

Medication non-adherence poses a significant challenge in healthcare, leading to adverse health outcomes, increased healthcare costs, and decreased quality of life for patients. Some statistics, consequences, and common reasons associated with medication non-adherence are described below.

Statistics on Medication Non-adherence

In healthcare, medication non-adherence is very common, and it becomes a huge obstacle to effective disease management and its impact on the patients. According to the World Health Organization (WHO), about half of all patients with chronic diseases in developed countries fail to comply with the drugs that have been prescribed for their treatment. This trend cuts across different types of medical conditions and patient populations. For example, research showed that among cardiovascular disease patients, adherence ranged from 40% up to 60%, while diabetes cases had adherence rates as low as 50%. Even psychiatric disorders are associated with difficulties in adhering; hence prevalence rates are reported between 20% and 60% [31, 32].

Chemotherapy and oral medication usage is not adhered to by 25% of patients who have cancer. There are also instances where the non-adherence rates range between 30-50% in relation to the pediatric population. The elderly who live with multiple chronic diseases at the same face adherence rates below 50%, indicating how difficult it is for them to manage their medications. All these statistics prove that the problem of non-compliance with treatment is so widespread among various medical conditions and different groups of patients [33].

Non-compliance imperils personal health and escalates medical care, admissions, and death costs. Solving a medication non-adherence issue requires many-sided interventions tailored to fit individual patients' needs, such as education, patient involvement tactics, and technology-based supports for adherence to drugs and overall well-being improvement [34].

Consequences of Non-adherence

There are far-reaching consequences on personal health outcomes, healthcare systems, and society as a whole when drug prescription instructions are violated. Firstly, non-adherence leads to suboptimal treatment outcomes and disease progression. Patients who fail to comply with their prescribed medications run the risk of developing complications, worsening their chronic conditions, and having worse general health outcomes. This can lead to exacerbation of symptoms leading to decreased quality of life, morbidity, and mortality rates, among other things [35].

Non-adherence also increases the cost of healthcare and its resource utilization. Patients who fail to adhere to their medications are more prone to requiring further medical interventions, hospitalizations, emergency room visits, and protracted health care. These enhanced rates of healthcare utilization impose a significant economic burden on healthcare systems and can stretch scarce resources, resulting in increased overall healthcare costs [36].

Moreover, medication non-compliance compromises the success of public health efforts as well as disease control programs. It then becomes difficult to control infectious diseases' spread, prevent their complications, or even achieve public health goals due to the fact that patients who are not compliant with their medication may fail to get the desired therapeutic results. As a result, this has huge implications for public health and welfare by undermining population-based strategies to reduce chronic illness burden and improve overall well-being [37].

Furthermore, failure to adhere contributes to the resistance of drugs and treatment failures, in particular for antibiotics and long-term therapies for chronic conditions. In addition to that, if patients do not complete their prescribed courses of medication or take them inconsistently, this can lead to the emergence of bacteria or viruses resistant to drugs, which make treatment ineffective and significantly impede public health measures [38].

Drug non-compliance has far-reaching implications for people, healthcare systems, and public health efforts. Dealing with non-adherence demands holistic approaches that encompass patient education, provider-patient communication, medication management support, and the integration of innovative technologies to promote adherence and improve health outcomes for all [39].

Common Reasons for Non-adherence

Non-compliance with medication routines stems from diverse sources that are influenced by factors such as distinct characteristics of the patients, dynamics within healthcare systems, and socioeconomic determinants. An example of this is forgetfulness, where patients might just ignore their doses or even fail to take them when they should be, especially those with complex dose schedules or cognitive decline. Furthermore, lack of knowledge or misinformation about the significance of drugs, dosages required, possible side effects, and long-term outcomes can also result in non-compliance [40].

Medications can cause patients to change their treatment or discontinue it altogether if they suffer from unwanted side effects. Compliance is a major issue for underserved communities owing to financial constraints, such as the cost of medication, the absence of insurance coverage, and the affordability of medications. Patients may feel overwhelmed by the complexity of medication regimens, which might include multiple medicines, dosing times, and ways of administering them, leading to non-adherence [41].

However, patients' medications can be effectively managed only if they have social support or good communication channels with healthcare providers. The use of certain drugs and having some medical conditions may attract reproach; hence; the patient opts to hide their medication. For that reason, interventions intended to address these common causes of non-adherence require appropriate actions according to individual patient's needs, provision of information and assistance, overcoming financial obstacles, enhancing the flow of communication, and employing technology for tracking adherence and managing drug prescriptions [42, 43].

IOT SOLUTIONS FOR MEDICATION INTAKE TRACKING

IoT solutions for medication intake tracking offer innovative ways to improve medication adherence and enhance patient outcomes. Below, we discuss IoT-enabled technologies and solutions for medication intake tracking.

Wearable Devices for Medication Reminders

Wearable medication reminder devices are an advanced application of wearable technology in healthcare designed to provide patients with a convenient and personalized way to enhance treatment outcomes through improved drug adherence. These novel devices use wearable sensors, connectivity features, and smart algorithms that ensure the timely administration of medications while assisting patients in adhering to their prescribed medicine schedules [44, 45].

The chief characteristic of wearable devices for medication reminders is that they can transmit personalized reminiscences and warnings to the user's wrist or smartphone. Such appliances usually come as smartwatches, fitness bracelets, or other wearable gadgets that have embedded sensors as well as such connectivity options as Bluetooth or Wi-Fi. When linked with accompanying mobile apps, wearables can auto-sync medication schedules, set up reminder alerts, and notify patients according to personal preferences and drug doses [46, 47].

Wearable devices have some advantages over other medication reminders, one of them is their ability to give secret nudges. Unlike usual alarm clocks or smartphone alerts, wearables bring it right on the user's wrist making sure that patients get notified of their consumption without disturbing what they are doing throughout the day or drawing much attention to their regular medications. The discreetness of this approach assists patients in integrating taking drugs into their routines and reducing cases when doses are missed [48, 49].

Furthermore, medication reminder wearable devices are very much customizable and adaptable to suit specific patient requirements. For instance, patients can easily tune reminder timing, frequency as well as types to fit into their medication schedule and lifestyle; this may include vibrations, alarms or visual cues among others. These include additional features like snooze options, tracking of medications taken, and logging doses in a way that enables the patients to actively participate in the self-management process and observe their adherence levels over time [50, 51].

Furthermore, an additional benefit of wearable devices for medication reminders is their capability to give reminders based on real-time data and user activities. For instance, by employing sensors like accelerometers, gyroscopes, and heart rate monitors, these devices may determine when levels of user activity are high or low, and identify sleep patterns and physiological signals so as to send out prompts at the most favorable times. In some situations, notifications can be inhibited during strenuous exercises or reminder timing can be adjusted by following the cycle of sleep-wake of a patient with a view to best adherence while also avoiding chaos [52, 53].

Moreover, wearable medication reminder devices may also make it easy for medical professionals to check on the patient remotely. As a result of such connections like Bluetooth or cellular networks, such devices can send to healthcare teams any information about adherence to medication that is usually stored in the cloud. Thus, healthcare providers are able to oversee drug-taking practices from their respective places of work and promptly apply proactive measures when problems arise. Additionally, wearables can be used by patients to establish personalized feedback channels with their doctors; they can also use them as platforms for receiving reminder messages on drugs and educational materials [54, 55].

Wearable devices that remind one to take medication may allow for the compliance of medicine while empowering patients to become more health-conscious, and thus improve treatment. This integration is done by the use of personalized alerts, customization features, as well as real-time information analysis providing individuals with the ability to incorporate adherence into their everyday routines and this helps them develop good habits. These reminders could become a vital part of supporting patient-responsive care and bettering drug management in the modern wearable technology era [56, 57].

Mobile Applications for Medication Tracking

Healthcare has found valuable aids in medication tracking on mobile applications. These tools help patients manage their drug-taking regimens more efficiently by increasing adherence to prescription treatments. Innovative apps make the most out of smartphones' popularity and mobility to offer user-friendly platforms for planning their pill intake, receiving reminder messages, monitoring compliance, as well as accessing other health-related data. Mobile medication tracking applications have extensive characteristics and utilities that provide a holistic approach to improving medicine management and perfecting treatment results [58, 59].

In addition, personalized medication schedules are one of the key features of mobile applications for medication tracking, which can be tailored according to each user's specific treatment schedule. A user can enter information about their medications such as drug names, dosages, frequencies, and routes of administration into the application. From this data, the app creates an individualized medication timetable that tells when exactly each drug should be taken thereby aiding patients in getting organized and sticking to their treatment program [60, 61].

Mobile tracking apps also offer reminder functions to alert users when it is time for them to take their drugs. One can therefore program these reminders according to his/her own liking, allowing one to decide about the timing, frequency, and even the type of alarm; could be a sound, shaking or push notification, *etc*. If mobile apps send timely reminders straight to users' smartphones, they make it possible for patients to develop the right medication habits and reduce the risks of dose omission [62, 63].

Moreover, these mobile medication monitoring apps for example assist with adherence monitoring and tracking by allowing patients to log their everyday medication intake and keep track of their adherence to treatment over time. This helps them to remember all the drugs they take hence promoting better patient adherence. It may provide users with graphs that display various aspects of medication-taking behaviors, like the number of pills taken, or displayed as a line graph, which depicts the number of days per week that people took no medicine in a given time period [64, 65].

Additionally, mobile medication tracking apps often have extra characteristics that can help users manage their general health and wellness. Such characteristics might include medication refilling reminders, medication interaction checkers, side effects tracking, and integration with wearable devices or health tracking platforms. Mobile apps offer patients a comprehensive approach to drug management, empowering them to take charge of their own care and treatment [66, 67].

Furthermore, there is another important advantage of mobile medication tracking applications that they allow for communication and collaboration between patients and healthcare providers. A few apps make it possible for individuals to share their medication adherence information with their medical team, hence making it possible for the doctors to monitor adherence from a distance, locate any instances of non-adherence that may be present, and respond before such happenings have occurred. Mobile apps can also offer educational resources, medicine details, or service links that assist users in taking informed choices about their health [68, 69].

Medication monitoring mobile applications provide a strong way of promoting adherence to medication, enhancing treatment results, and improving patients' involvement in healthcare systems. These applications have user-friendly interfaces, personalized options, and connection abilities that give power to users on how they manage their medicine timetables, keep order and understand everything concerning their health. The emerging healthcare field will see the widespread use of these apps with regard to patient-centered care taking into account the optimization of medication control [70].

HOW IOT WORKS IN MEDICATION TRACKING

IoT technology revolutionizes medication tracking by incorporating sensors, connectivity features, and advanced data analytics to provide real-time monitoring capabilities. How IoT works in medication tracking is described below.

Sensors and Connectivity in IoT Devices

IoT gadgets rely on sensors and connectivity as key pillars; the very tenets that allow for interaction, data gathering, and communication with the physical environment to occur. In terms of drug monitoring, it is important to have in place sensors as well as connectivity features that would help in monitoring medication intake and tracking compliance as well as facilitate communication among devices and health systems.

Sensors in IoT Devices

Sensors used in IoT devices are described below and shown in Fig. (**3**).

Presence Sensors

Presence sensors can be used to detect the presence or absence of things or people within a given area. When it comes to medication tracking, presence sensors are applied in smart pill dispensers to detect pills removed from them, which means that medication has been taken. These sensors may employ infrared (IR) sensors, motion sensors, or proximity sensors as technology to identify environmental changes [71].

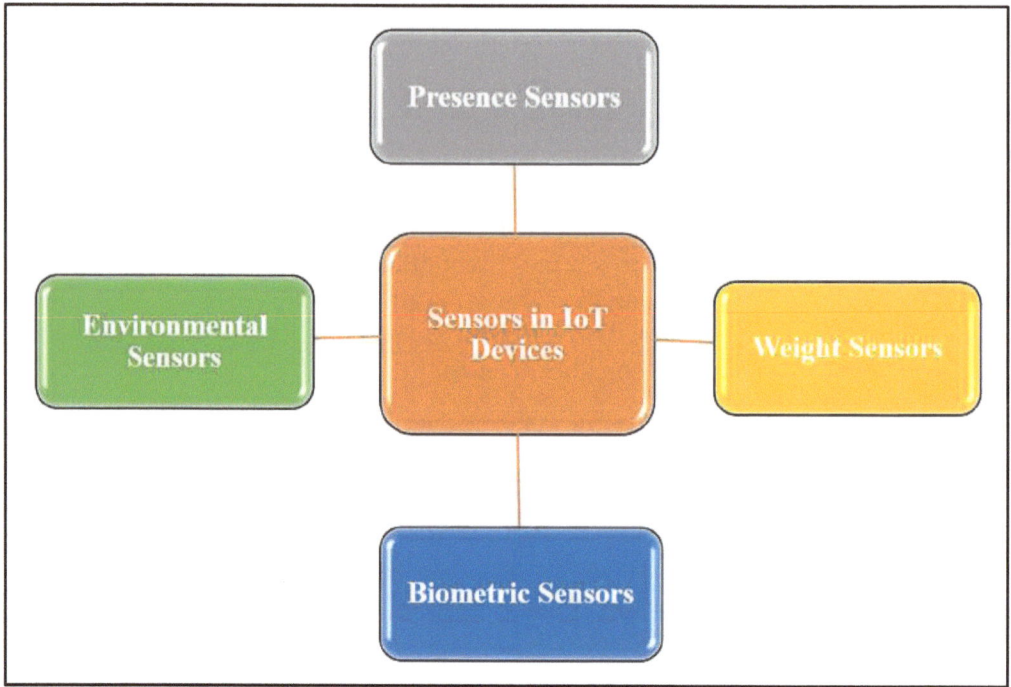

Fig. (3). Sensors used in IoT devices.

Weight Sensors

Weight sensors are capable of measuring the weight or mass of anything placed close to them. In smart pill dispensers, weight sensors can be deployed to check the amount of medicine and detect any changes in pill count that show the need for refilling medications. They give live updates about drug quantities and use, ensuring timely management of stock levels [72].

Biometric Sensors

Biometric sensors measure physiological parameters or characteristics of individuals, like pulse rate, blood pressure, or temperature. For instance, in the technology of medicine, tracking wearable devices with biometric sensors assists in monitoring relevant vital signs that are related to medication adherence. For example, heart rate variability and activity levels can be monitored by wearable devices to determine whether a patient adheres to a given medication regimen [73].

Environmental Sensors

Environmental sensors measure all parameters in the environment like temperature, humidity, and light intensity. For example, these sensors can help in knowing how medication should be stored as well as monitoring patients' adherence to medication. To illustrate, environmental sensors identify variations from perfect storage conditions like temperature changes or levels of humidity that could affect the efficiency of medicines [74].

Connectivity Features in IoT Devices

Wi-Fi

IoT devices can connect to local wireless networks through Wi-Fi connectivity hence they are able to communicate with other devices, the internet or cloud-based platforms. Medication tracking, on the other hand, uses Wi-Fi to facilitate data transmission, remote monitoring, and software updates for IoT-enabled devices. For instance, smart pill dispensers with Wi-Fi capabilities can send real-time information about drug adherence to healthcare providers [75].

Bluetooth

IoT devices and nearby smartphones, tablets, or Bluetooth-enabled devices are connected by Bluetooth technology to facilitate short-range wireless communication. Mediation tracking involves the use of Bluetooth connectivity in wearable devices to synchronize data with mobile applications or transmit alerts and notifications to user's smartphones. For instance, using a wearable device *via* Bluetooth connectivity; one can receive drug reminders plus adherence alerts [76].

Cellular Connectivity

4G or 5G cellular networks and other forms of cellular connectivity connect IoT devices to such networks for the transmission of data over long distances. The medication tracking feature in which remote monitoring and communication are made possible through cellular connectivity, allows IoT devices to have access to different locations like patients' homes or healthcare facilities . For instance, smart pill dispensers with cellular connectivity can send medication adherence statistics to a central monitoring system regardless of where these devices are physically located [77].

Data Collection and Analysis

For medication monitoring IoT, data collection and analysis are a must-have. They provide information on patient behavior, drug usage patterns, treatment outcomes, and compliance records. Data collection in medication management encompasses gathering information about medication intake, adherence behaviors, and relevant environmental factors while data analysis involves the processing of such information for extracting useful insights as well as determining trends to guide decision-making [78].

Data Collection

To monitor medication intake and adherence behaviors, data collection in medication tracking is mainly centered. IoT devices like intelligent pill dispensers or wearable devices gather information on the time when medicines are given, taken off, or consumed by patients. This data provides real-time knowledge about medication adherence thus helping healthcare providers gauge patient compliance with prescribed regimens and identify issues of adherence [79].

Apart from tracking medication intake, the Internet of Things may also gather environmental data concerning drug management. The IoT gadgets possess environmental sensors that can monitor temperature, humidity, and light among other things which affect the efficacy of drugs and their storage conditions. Thus, through monitoring these parameters, IoT systems help to ascertain that medicines are adequately stored as well as maintain their original shelf-life [80, 81].

For instance, wearable technology with biometric sensors may collect information on either physiological parameters or activities that are relevant to drug compliance. Biometric sensors can check vital signs like pulse rate, blood pressure, and activity levels, which give clues regarding the patient's medical condition and his willingness to take drugs as required. It is possible for healthcare providers to use biometric data in order to determine how drugs affect people's health as well as note down the side effects that may appear during treatment [82, 83].

The IoT systems may also take note of how their users interact with medication-tracking apparatuses or applications. This encompasses the time when the user will work with a device, see medication reminders, and log manually for medication intake. Data concerning user interactions allows us to gain insights into engagement, barriers to compliance, and preferences thereof ; this enables personalized interventions and support strategies [84, 85].

Data Analysis

The application of data analysis methods to medication intake data helps identify adherence patterns, trends, and deviations from prescribed regimens. By analyzing medication intake timestamps and dosage information, healthcare providers can assess the consistency of medication adherence, identify missed doses or irregularities, and evaluate overall adherence levels over time [86, 87].

Predictive models exploit prior medication adherence details for future forecasts of conformity behaviors and apprehend looming adherence difficulties. They also describe high-risk patients by analyzing previous patterns and patient features to indicate those who are prone to non-adherence and then treat them in a special way. This kind of modelling allows an early response to any threats or breaches of medication compliance [88, 89].

Data analysis helps healthcare providers determine the efficacy of medication adherence on treatment results and patients' well-being. By relating medicine taking to health outcomes like a worsening condition, symptom control or re-hospitalization, doctors can measure the adequacy of therapies and identify ways to improve them. Assessment of outcomes supports the delivery of quality care and attainment of appropriate therapeutic goals by patients [90, 91].

Healthcare providers can access actionable insights and decision support tools in data analysis to inform clinical decisions as well as help in treatment planning. Other clinical information such as patient demographics, medical history, and laboratory data are synthesized with medication adherence data to enable healthcare providers make decisions on medication adjustments based on evidence-based therapy modification or patient intervention. With the aid of decision support tools, the quality of care is enhanced, patient outcomes improve and medication management strategies are optimized [92, 93].

BENEFITS OF IOT INTEGRATION FOR PATIENTS

Table **1** describes the benefits of IoT integration, which enhances medication management, improves patient outcomes, and promotes patient-centered care by leveraging technology to support patients in adhering to their prescribed treatment regimens.

Table 1. Benefits of IoT integration for patients.

Benefit	Description
Improved Medication Adherence	With IoT integration, medication reminders can be automated, medication intake can be monitored in real-time, and personalized adherence supports can be provided, leading to improved adherence to prescribed treatment plans [94].
Enhanced Convenience and Accessibility	Patients can access opportunities to be reminded about medicine, adherence data, and educational materials through mobile apps or wearable devices, which makes it easy for them to manage medication tools anytime from anywhere [95].

Benefit	Description
Personalized Treatment Plans	IoT devices gather real-time data on medication intake, physiological parameters, and behavioral patterns, making it easier for healthcare providers to craft treatment plans that fit individual patient's needs and adherence behaviors [96].
Remote Monitoring and Support	Healthcare providers can remotely monitor patient medication adherence, intervene in case of non-adherence on time, and provide personalized support and assistance that will promote patient engagement and boost treatment outcomes [97].
Increased Patient Engagement	Patient participation in medication management is improved through interactive apps, educational resources, and feedback mechanisms. These allow patients to assume responsibility for their health and contribute to shared decision-making concerning their care [98].
Enhanced Safety and Medication Management	Features of smart pill dispensers equipped with IoT include medication verification, dose monitoring, and safety alarms that ensure correct medication administration, minimize the possibility of drug errors, and enhance patient safety [99].

BENEFITS FOR HEALTHCARE PROVIDERS

The integration of IoT greatly facilitates healthcare providers in acquiring real-time data regarding the extent to which patients comply with or adhere to medication. This capability enables them to track continuous adherence levels, helping them intervene faster if the need arises. Healthcare service providers may be able to identify adherence problems that emerge as they occur through accessing real-time adherence data, enabling them to intervene in non-adherence and prevent complications. In case patients miss doses of medication or deviate from their prescribed treatment regimens, doctors can instantly receive alerts or notifications prompting immediate action [100, 101].

Providers can use IoT technology to obtain timely and correct information on adherence, hence improving patient outcomes, preventing adverse events, and optimizing healthcare delivery. Real-time adherence data is a key component in proactive medication management strategies that enable healthcare providers to deliver quality, personalized patient care [102, 103].

IoT technology enables healthcare providers to check remotely if patients have taken their medicine, regardless of where they are. *via* connected devices and platforms, providers can view adherence data in real time and avoid having patients go to healthcare facilities for adherence assessment purposes. This feature makes it easier for both patients and doctors to adhere to medication regularly without interruptions in daily routines through remote monitoring [104, 105].

Integration of IoT enables healthcare providers to deliver individualized interventions based on the specific needs and patterns of adherence of each patient. By analyzing real-time data for adherence, practitioners can become aware of patients' preferences and behaviors about medication intake. This information helps them come up with personalized approaches such as customized reminders, educational materials, or counseling sessions aimed at helping patients adhere to their prescribed treatment protocols more effectively [106, 107].

With improved patient monitoring and intervention using IoT technology, healthcare providers can more efficiently allocate resources. Remotely monitoring medication adherence and intervening proactively assist in pinpointing the focus on patients who may need more support or interventions, enabling healthcare providers to concentrate their efforts and resources on them. This approach reduces wasted healthcare resources by allocating them specifically where they are needed the most [108].

Healthcare providers benefit from the integration of the IoT into medication management through improved patient outcomes and reduced costs, which are two major benefits. It improves patient care delivery, encourages medication adherence, and hence leads to better health outcomes and cost savings. IoT-enabled medication tracking and adherence monitoring help to improve patient outcomes by ensuring that patients follow their prescribed treatment regimen. Real-time monitoring enables healthcare providers to promptly identify medication non-adherence problems and intervene in a pre-emptive manner [109].

Promoting the integration of IoT in medicine and encouraging adherence to medication can aid in stopping diseases from getting worse, thereby lowering complications and improving the general health of a patient. The success of treatment depends upon adhering to prescribed medications, leading to better management of symptoms, reduced hospitalizations, and improved quality of life for patients. Furthermore, incorporating the IoT into medication administration decreases medical costs by decreasing the number of preventable adverse events and healthcare utilization that are due to non-adherence to medications. By improving patients' adherence to prescribed therapies, IoT can decrease complications, hospital readmissions, and emergency department visits [110].

Healthcare providers and payers can save a lot by avoiding unwanted incidents as a result of non-compliant medication consumption. This is also facilitated by the Internet of Things (IoT) supported medication monitoring, which enables better allocation of resources, thereby helping healthcare providers to efficiently use their available healthcare stocks so as to minimize unnecessary expenses. To summarize, the benefits associated with IoT adoption in pharmaceutical management include improved patient outcomes and lower healthcare costs, illustrating the importance of IoT-driven medication management solutions in enhancing patient care delivery systems, optimizing healthcare resource usage rates, and ensuring the long-term functionality of healthcare services [111].

CHALLENGES AND LIMITATIONS

Several problems and constraints must be addressed by healthcare providers concerning the incorporation of IoT technology into medication management so as to make the implementation and adoption of these solutions successful. Among the major challenges are the privacy and security matters associated with gathering and transmitting sensitive patient information *via* IoT devices. Concerns may arise from patients about the possibility of their health information being misused or accessed by unauthorized persons, which in turn can lead to the fear of data leakage and violation of privacy. To reduce these risks, healthcare providers need to ensure that strong security measures such as encryption, access controls, and secure data storage practices are put in place to protect patient data while maintaining its confidentiality [112].

Additionally, there are also challenges with accessibility, particularly for specific groups such as senior citizens and those with disabilities. Poor digital skills, physical handicaps, or social obstacles may hamper the effectiveness of these IoT devices among these populations. For this reason, health providers have to cater to this issue by designing inclusive IoT solutions that can be accessed by all patients irrespective of their age, abilities, or income level. This can include the provision of training and support resources designed to meet different patient populations as well as IoT devices that have interfaces that are simple to use and accessibility features for users with varying degrees of technological literacy [113].

Furthermore, integration into the existing healthcare systems presents technical difficulties for healthcare providers to navigate in order to guarantee seamless interoperability and compatibility and successful integration of IoT-enabled medication management solutions into EHRs, medication management systems, and other relevant existing healthcare IT infrastructure. However, the goal of achieving this level of integration can be a complex issue due to data integration complexities, interoperability issues, and compatibility with legacy systems. Healthcare providers should work together with IT experts as well as technology vendors to surmount such challenges, hence allowing IoT solutions to align properly with existing workflows and systems and enhance their usability and effectiveness [114].

In order to achieve maximum benefits while at the same time minimizing the risks and setbacks related to Internet of Things (IoT) integration in medication management, healthcare providers should consider dealing with these challenges and limitations. Healthcare providers must remember that IoT technology can be instrumental in enhancing medication management as well as improving patient care delivery *via* addressing patients' accessibility issues, overcoming technical difficulties connected with system integration, and focusing on patient privacy and security [115].

FUTURE TRENDS AND OPPORTUNITIES

Healthcare delivery will be revolutionized, and patient outcomes will be improved by future trends and opportunities in medicine management exploiting IoT technology. One of the dominant trends is the persistent advancements in IoT technology, which are specifically designed for medication management. We should expect to see more advanced and user-friendly features, such as smart pill dispensers, wearable sensors, and mobile applications that can keep track of medication adherence seamlessly and provide real-time data to healthcare providers as IoT technology advances. These technological developments will make medication management solutions more accurate, dependable, and efficient, enabling closer monitoring of patients taking their drugs properly as well as customized responses to help optimize treatment results [116].

Additionally, IoT-enabled medication management systems can be enhanced through the integration of AI as well as machine learning algorithms. Through the utilization of AI-driven algorithms, patterns may be identified by analyzing a great deal of data that comes from IoT devices and even anticipate patient adherence behaviors to result in recommendations for healthcare providers. Healthcare providers can use AI and machine learning to build predictive models for anticipated non-adherence, individualized interventions in accordance with patient's needs, and effective medication arrangements that maximize the benefits and minimize the side effects. The conjunction of AI and machine learning has the potential to improve the efficiency, effectiveness, and personalization of medication management strategies [117].

Furthermore, we expect the growth of IoT solutions beyond medication management to other healthcare offerings in various patient care facilities. Patient monitoring, disease management, and healthcare delivery across different healthcare settings can also be revolutionized by using the Internet of Things technology. For instance, the Internet of Things provided systems for remote monitoring of patients, which will enable proactive management of chronic diseases, early detection of deteriorating health conditions, and timely interferences to prevent hospitalization. IoT solutions can support telehealth in addition to enabling virtual consultations, telemedicine services, and remote patient monitoring, thereby improving access to care as well as enhancing the engagement of patients. Healthcare providers are offered a unique prospect to transform healthcare delivery and enhance the overall quality of care while using the innovative potential of IoT to revolutionize healthcare outcomes [118].

CONCLUSION

In conclusion, IoT technology implementation for medication schedule observance is a milestone in healthcare delivery as far as patient care and treatment outcomes are concerned. For instance, with the help of IoT-based drug management systems, medical practitioners would have real-time adherence information to enable proactive surveillance, personalized assistance, and better involvement by patients in their treatment. Advances in medicinal adherence can be beneficial to clients, which results in improved treatment results, lessened expenses related to healthcare, and increased standard of life. This is only achievable if the challenges, including accessibility, privacy, and system integration, are resolved for effective IoT use. The forthcoming future presents several exciting trends, such as IoT technology developments, integration with AI and machine learning, and expansion into other areas of healthcare. These offer opportunities to enhance medication management further so as to revolutionize healthcare delivery. Through the transformative power of IoT integration, healthcare providers can optimize their strategies for managing medications; this will help improve patient outcomes and eventually advance global care quality for all patients.

ACKNOWLEDGEMENTS

Authors are highly thankful to their Universities/Colleges for providing library facilities for the literature survey.

REFERENCES

[1]   K. Kvarnström, A. Westerholm, M. Airaksinen, and H. Liira, "Factors contributing to medication adherence in patients with a chronic condition: A scoping review of qualitative research", *Pharmaceutics,* vol. 13, no. 7, p. 1100, 2021.
[http://dx.doi.org/10.3390/pharmaceutics13071100] [PMID: 34371791]

[2]   K. Souliotis, T.V. Giannouchos, C. Golna, and E. Liberopoulos, "Assessing forgetfulness and polypharmacy and their impact on health-related quality of life among patients with hypertension and dyslipidemia in Greece during the COVID-19 pandemic", *Qual. Life Res.,* vol. 31, no. 1, pp. 193-204, 2022.
[http://dx.doi.org/10.1007/s11136-021-02917-y] [PMID: 34156596]

[3]   F. I. Rahman, F. Aziz, S. Huque, and S. A. Ether, "Medication understanding and health literacy among patients with multiple chronic conditions: A study conducted in Bangladesh," *J. Pub. Heal. Res.,* vol. 9, no. 1, p. 1792, Jun. 2020.

[4]   B. Jimmy and J. Jose, "Patient medication adherence: Measures in daily practice," O. M. J, vol. 26, no. 3, pp. 155–159, Mar. 2011.
[http://dx.doi.org/10.5001/omj.2011.38]

[5]   T.H. Baryakova, B.H. Pogostin, R. Langer, and K.J. McHugh, "Overcoming barriers to patient adherence: the case for developing innovative drug delivery systems", *Nat. Rev. Drug Discov.*, vol. 22, no. 5, pp. 387-409, 2023.
[http://dx.doi.org/10.1038/s41573-023-00670-0] [PMID: 36973491]

[6]   S.H. Ihm, K.I. Kim, K.J. Lee, J.W. Won, J.O. Na, S.W. Rha, H.L. Kim, S.H. Kim, and J. Shin, "Interventions for Adherence Improvement in the Primary Prevention of Cardiovascular Diseases: Expert Consensus Statement", *Korean Circ. J.*, vol. 52, no. 1, pp. 1-33, 2022.
[http://dx.doi.org/10.4070/kcj.2021.0226] [PMID: 34989192]

[7]   Religioni U, Barrios-Rodríguez R, Requena P, Borowska M, Ostrowski J. Enhancing therapy adherence: impact on clinical outcomes, healthcare costs, and patient quality of life. Medicina. 2025 Jan 17;61(1):153.
[http://dx.doi.org/10.3390/medicina61010153]

[8]   H.B. Bosworth, B.B. Granger, P. Mendys, R. Brindis, R. Burkholder, S.M. Czajkowski, J.G. Daniel, I. Ekman, M. Ho, M. Johnson, S.E. Kimmel, L.Z. Liu, J. Musaus, W.H. Shrank, E.W. Buono, K. Weiss, and C.B. Granger, "Medication adherence: A call for action", *Am. Heart J.*, vol. 162, no. 3, pp. 412-424, 2011.
[http://dx.doi.org/10.1016/j.ahj.2011.06.007] [PMID: 21884856]

[9]   R. Nieuwlaat, N. Wilczynski, T. Navarro, N. Hobson, R. Jeffery, A. Keepanasseril, T. Agoritsas, N. Mistry, A. Iorio, S. Jack, B. Sivaramalingam, E. Iserman, R. A. Mustafa, D. Jedraszewski, C. Cotoi, and R. B. Haynes, "Interventions for enhancing medication adherence," *Cochrane Database, Sys. Rev.*, vol. 2014, no. 11, Nov, 2014.

[10]   M.A. Azzawi, R. Hassan, K. Azmi, and A. Bakar, *A Review on Internet of Things (IoT) in Healthcare*, 2016. Available from: https://www.researchgate.net/publication/309718253

[11]   S. Selvaraj, and S. Sundaravaradhan, "Challenges and opportunities in IoT healthcare systems: a systematic review", *SN Applied Sciences*, vol. 2, no. 1, p. 139, 2020.
[http://dx.doi.org/10.1007/s42452-019-1925-y]

[12]   A. Chacko, and T. Hayajneh, "Security and Privacy Issues with IoT in Healthcare", *EAI Endorsed Trans. Pervasive Health Technol.*, vol. 4, no. 14, p. e2, 2018.
[http://dx.doi.org/10.4108/eai.13-7-2018.155079]

[13]   R. K. Kodali, G. Swamy, and B. Lakshmi, "An implementation of IoT for healthcare," *In: Proc. 2015 IEEE Recent Advances in Intelligent Computational Systems (RAICS)*, Trivandrum, India, 2015, pp. 411–416.

[14]   Y. Yin, Y. Zeng, X. Chen, and Y. Fan, "The internet of things in healthcare: An overview", *J. Ind. Inf. Integr.*, vol. 1, pp. 3-13, 2016.
[http://dx.doi.org/10.1016/j.jii.2016.03.004]

[15]   B. Sobhan Babu, K. Srikanth, T. Ramanjaneyulu, and I. Lakshmi, "IoT for Healthcare," *Int. J. Sci. Res. (IJSR)*, vol. 5, no. 2, pp. 2319–7064, 2016.

[16]   M.A. Khan, "Challenges Facing the Application of IoT in Medicine and Healthcare", *International Journal of Computations, Information and Manufacturing (IJCIM)*, vol. 1, no. 1, 2021. [IJCIM].
[http://dx.doi.org/10.54489/ijcim.v1i1.32]

[17]   F.A.C. Farias, C.M. Dagostini, Y.A. Bicca, V.F. Falavigna, and A. Falavigna, "Remote patient monitoring: A systematic review", *Telemed. J. E Health*, vol. 26, no. 5, pp. 576-583, 2020.
[http://dx.doi.org/10.1089/tmj.2019.0066] [PMID: 31314689]

[18]   M.J. Field, and J. Grigsby, *Telemedicine and Remote Patient Monitoring*, 2008. Available from: http://www.hcfa.gov/pubforms/transmit/AB0169

[19]   M. Aldeer, M. Javanmard, and R. Martin, "A review of medication adherence monitoring technologies", *Applied System Innovation,* vol. 1, no. 2, p. 14, 2018.
[http://dx.doi.org/10.3390/asi1020014]

[20]   W. Y. Lam and P. Fresco, "Medication adherence measures: An overview," *Biomed. Res. Int.,* vol. 2015, Art. no. 217047, 2015.

[21]   P.H. Tsai, T.Y. Chen, C.R. Yu, C.S. Shih, and J.W.S. Liu, "Smart medication dispenser: Design, architecture and implementation", *IEEE Syst. J.,* vol. 5, no. 1, pp. 99-110, 2011.
[http://dx.doi.org/10.1109/JSYST.2010.2070970]

[22]   A. Kassem, W. Antoun, M. Hamad, and C. El-Moucary, "A comprehensive approach for a smart medication dispenser", In: *International Journal of Computing and Digital Systems.* University of Bahrain, 2019, pp. 131-141.
[http://dx.doi.org/10.12785/ijcds/080205]

[23]   Y. Yin, Y. Zeng, X. Chen, and Y. Fan, "The internet of things in healthcare: An overview", *J. Ind. Inf. Integr.,* vol. 1, pp. 3-13, 2016.
[http://dx.doi.org/10.1016/j.jii.2016.03.004]

[24]   M.R. Holm, M.I. Rudis, and J.W. Wilson, "Medication supply chain management through implementation of a hospital pharmacy computerized inventory program in Haiti", *Glob. Health Action,* vol. 8, no. 1, p. 26546, 2015.
[http://dx.doi.org/10.3402/gha.v8.26546] [PMID: 25623613]

[25]   E. B. Mandinach, M. Honey, and D. Light, "A theoretical framework for data-driven decision making," In: *Annual Meeting of the American Educational Research Association (AERA)*, San Francisco, CA, Apr. 9, 2006.

[26]   N. C. Farah, Medication inventory optimization and oral solution workflow implementation and integration into pharmacy inventory management system, Essay, University of Pittsburgh, Pittsburgh, PA, USA. 2021.

[27]   J. Khuntia, D. Yim, M. Tanniru, and S. Lim, "Patient empowerment and engagement with a health infomediary", *Health Policy Technol.,* vol. 6, no. 1, pp. 40-50, 2017.
[http://dx.doi.org/10.1016/j.hlpt.2016.11.003]

[28]   A. Pekonen, S. Eloranta, M. Stolt, P. Virolainen, and H. Leino-Kilpi, "Measuring patient empowerment – A systematic review", *Patient Educ. Couns.,* vol. 103, no. 4, pp. 777-787, 2020.
[http://dx.doi.org/10.1016/j.pec.2019.10.019] [PMID: 31767243]

[29]   C.W. Hicks, M. Rosen, D.B. Hobson, C. Ko, and E.C. Wick, "Improving safety and quality of care with enhanced teamwork through operating room briefings", *JAMA Surg.,* vol. 149, no. 8, pp. 863-868, 2014.
[http://dx.doi.org/10.1001/jamasurg.2014.172] [PMID: 25006700]

[30]   B. Middleton, M. Bloomrosen, M.A. Dente, B. Hashmat, R. Koppel, J.M. Overhage, T.H. Payne, S.T. Rosenbloom, C. Weaver, and J. Zhang, "Enhancing patient safety and quality of care by improving the usability of electronic health record systems: recommendations from AMIA", *J. Am. Med. Inform. Assoc.,* vol. 20, no. e1, pp. e2-e8, 2013.
[http://dx.doi.org/10.1136/amiajnl-2012-001458] [PMID: 23355463]

[31]   D. Russell, Y.K. Cho, and E. Cylwik, "Learning Opportunities and Career Implications of Experience with BIM/VDC", *Pract. Period. Struct. Des. Constr.,* vol. 19, no. 1, pp. 111-121, 2014.
[http://dx.doi.org/10.1061/(ASCE)SC.1943-5576.0000191]

[32]   M. Amorim-Lopes, W. Fu, K. Papp, and H. Lang, "Role of patient safety attitudes between career identity and turnover intentions of new nurses in China: A cross-sectional study."

[33]   Almendra Mattos RM, de Mendonça RM, dos Santos Aguiar S. Adherence to dental treatment reduces oral complications related to cancer treatment in pediatric and adolescent patients. Supportive Care in Cancer. 2020 Feb;28(2):661-70.

[http://dx.doi.org/10.1007/s00520-019-04857-3]

[34]   R.K. Adeniran, A. Bhattacharya, and A.A. Adeniran, "Professional excellence and career advancement in nursing: a conceptual framework for clinical leadership development", *Nurs. Adm. Q.,* vol. 36, no. 1, pp. 41-51, 2012.
[http://dx.doi.org/10.1097/NAQ.0b013e31823b0fec] [PMID: 22157789]

[35]   M.V. Lenti, and C.P. Selinger, "Medication non-adherence in adult patients affected by inflammatory bowel disease: a critical review and update of the determining factors, consequences and possible interventions", *Expert Rev. Gastroenterol. Hepatol.,* vol. 11, no. 3, pp. 1-12, 2017.
[http://dx.doi.org/10.1080/17474124.2017.1284587] [PMID: 28099821]

[36]   D. Novick, J.M. Haro, D. Suarez, V. Perez, R.W. Dittmann, and P.M. Haddad, "Predictors and clinical consequences of non-adherence with antipsychotic medication in the outpatient treatment of schizophrenia", *Psychiatry Res.,* vol. 176, no. 2-3, pp. 109-113, 2010.
[http://dx.doi.org/10.1016/j.psychres.2009.05.004] [PMID: 20185182]

[37]   K. Denhaerynck, F. Burkhalter, P. Schäfer-Keller, J. Steiger, A. Bock, and S. De Geest, "Clinical consequences of non adherence to immunosuppressive medication in kidney transplant patients", *Transpl. Int.,* vol. 22, no. 4, pp. 441-446, 2009.
[http://dx.doi.org/10.1111/j.1432-2277.2008.00820.x] [PMID: 19144090]

[38]   R.L. Cutler, F. Fernandez-Llimos, M. Frommer, C. Benrimoj, and V. Garcia-Cardenas, "Economic impact of medication non-adherence by disease groups: a systematic review", *BMJ Open,* vol. 8, no. 1, p. e016982, 2018.
[http://dx.doi.org/10.1136/bmjopen-2017-016982] [PMID: 29358417]

[39]   J. Hong, C. Reed, D. Novick, J.M. Haro, and J. Aguado, "Clinical and economic consequences of medication non-adherence in the treatment of patients with a manic/mixed episode of bipolar disorder: Results from the European Mania in Bipolar Longitudinal Evaluation of Medication (EMBLEM) Study", *Psychiatry Res.,* vol. 190, no. 1, pp. 110-114, 2011.
[http://dx.doi.org/10.1016/j.psychres.2011.04.016] [PMID: 21571375]

[40]   Y. Wang, H. Chen, Z. Huang, E.B. McNeil, X. Lu, and V. Chongsuvivatwong, "Drug non-adherence and reasons among multidrug-resistant tuberculosis patients in Guizhou, China: A cross-sectional study", *Patient Prefer. Adherence,* vol. 13, pp. 1641-1653, 2019.
[http://dx.doi.org/10.2147/PPA.S219920] [PMID: 31686790]

[41]   P. Kardas, "Prevalence and reasons for non-adherence to hyperlipidemia treatment", *Open Med. (Wars.),* vol. 8, no. 5, pp. 539-547, 2013.
[http://dx.doi.org/10.2478/s11536-013-0198-x]

[42]   E. Unni, N. Sternbach, and A. Goren, "Using the Medication Adherence Reasons Scale (MAR-Scale) to identify the reasons for non-adherence across multiple disease conditions", *Patient Prefer. Adherence,* vol. 13, pp. 993-1004, 2019.
[http://dx.doi.org/10.2147/PPA.S205359] [PMID: 31308635]

[43]   R. Lingam, and J. Scott, "Treatment non-adherence in affective disorders", *Acta Psychiatr. Scand.,* vol. 105, no. 3, pp. 164-172, 2002.
[http://dx.doi.org/10.1034/j.1600-0447.2002.1r084.x] [PMID: 11939969]

[44]   T. Zijp, D. Touw, and J. van Boven, "User acceptability and technical robustness evaluation of a novel smart pill bottle prototype designed to support medication adherence", *Patient Prefer. Adherence,* vol. 14, pp. 625-634, 2020.
[http://dx.doi.org/10.2147/PPA.S240443] [PMID: 32256053]

[45]   X. Toh, H.X. Tan, H. Liang, and H.P. Tan, "Elderly medication adherence monitoring with the Internet of Things", In: *2016 IEEE International Conference on Pervasive Computing and Communication Workshops, PerCom Workshops 2016* Institute of Electrical and Electronics Engineers Inc., 2016.
[http://dx.doi.org/10.1109/PERCOMW.2016.7457133]

[46]   G. Latif, A. Shankar, J.M. Alghazo, V. Kalyanasundaram, C.S. Boopathi, and M. Arfan Jaffar, "I-CARES: advancing health diagnosis and medication through IoT", *Wirel. Netw.*, vol. 26, no. 4, pp. 2375-2389, 2020.
[http://dx.doi.org/10.1007/s11276-019-02165-6]

[47]   W. Antoun, A. Abdo, S. Al-Yaman, A. Kassem, M. Hamad, and C. El-Moucary, "Smart Medicine Dispenser (SMD", *Middle East Conference on Biomedical Engineering, MECBME,* IEEE Computer Society, pp. 20-23, 2018.
[http://dx.doi.org/10.1109/MECBME.2018.8402399]

[48]   Arora K, Singh U. Smart pill dispenser using internet of things. International Journal of Engineering Research and Technology (IJERT). 2018 Jul;7(07). Available from: https://d1wqtxts1xzle7.cloudfront.net/59350817/smart-pill-dispenser-using-internet-of-things-IJERTV7IS07015520190522-80692-gbsghw-libre.pdf?1558508975=&response-content-disposition=inline%3B+filename%3DIJERT_Smart_pill_dispenser_using_interne.pdf&Expires=1756146615&Signature=eRUetXPG9-RzC-aM0xrGlh4fKtaOhqYe0Ik7kAXxkjxLpbE0nzxi-hGo8VLCs3eKrXGm0HGAuOjBsi4wAWk3aGsDMHyLbi6bEfnwstfwYtuXZ-5DLrbbR0MLDFYCsD9s2GVsVq5qAtDiQWOKXe3rdsfkH~GZGdKPIXbgBRajf5MYosyuo0y81i1jU4qhvvSI3W26yk3Fhnxt9tMs06HVeG57Zp06ZMx0XILIZQtj8h8gY~q67hiwcbHA-tfZKe7Bf-jQHlRQhCp5aRdPseSMPIrisb2Ob60yWe0PFZy6EdE6ch1Ec7XY-k-Myzg9TtU7JukTLRjZTglVv9IozA3OGg__&Key-Pair-Id=APKAJLOHF5GGSLRBV4ZA

[49]   V. Gawde, A. Panada, and R. Solanki, *Electronic Drug Reminder: A New Innovation in the Domain of Automatic Drug Dispensers,* 2013. Available from: www.ijsr.net

[50]   G. De, J. Grau, and D. Díaz Sánchez, "Smart pill dispenser for dependent people," 2015.

[51]   N. Singh, and U. Varshney, "Medication adherence: A method for designing context-aware reminders", *Int. J. Med. Inform.*, vol. 132, p. 103980, 2019.
[http://dx.doi.org/10.1016/j.ijmedinf.2019.103980] [PMID: 31586826]

[52]   M. Abu, S. Mondol, A. Emi, and J. A. Stankovic, "MedRem: An Interactive Medication Reminder and Tracking System on Wrist Devices." 2016.

[53]   D. Bhadauria, "Health Monitoring of Elderly, Children, and Alzheimer's Patients through Medication Reminder Apps and Wearable Sensors", *J. Algebr. Stat.*, vol. 13, no. 2, pp. 3546-3554, 2022. [Online]. [. Available: https://publishoa.com].

[54]   A. Cheon, S. Y. Jung, C. Prather, M. Sarmiento, K. Wong, and D. M.-K. Woodbridge, "A machine learning approach to detecting low medication state with wearable technologies," in *Proc. 42nd Annu. Int. Conf. IEEE Eng. Med. Biol. Soc. (EMBC)*, 2020, pp. 1–4,
[http://dx.doi.org/10.1109/EMBC44109.2020.9176310]

[55]   U. Varshney, "Smart medication management system and multiple interventions for medication adherence", *Decis. Support Syst.*, vol. 55, no. 2, pp. 538-551, 2013.
[http://dx.doi.org/10.1016/j.dss.2012.10.011]

[56]   C. Crema, A. Depari, A. Flammini, M. Lavarini, E. Sisinni and A. Vezzoli, "A smartphone-enhanced pill-dispenser providing patient identification and in-take recognition," In: *Proc. 2015 IEEE Int. Symp. Med. Meas. Appl. (MeMeA)*, Turin, Italy, 2015, pp. 484–489.
[http://dx.doi.org/10.1109/MeMeA.2015.7145252]

[57]   Greiwe and S. M. Nyenhuis, "Wearable Technology and How This Can Be Implemented into Clinical Practice," Current Allergy and Asthma Reports, vol. 20, no. 8. 2020.
[http://dx.doi.org/10.1007/s11882-020-00927-3]

[58]   R. Ng, S.R. Carter, and S. El-Den, "The impact of mobile applications on medication adherence: a systematic review", *Transl. Behav. Med.*, vol. 10, no. 6, p. ibz125, 2019.
[http://dx.doi.org/10.1093/tbm/ibz125] [PMID: 31384950]

[59]   T. Kim, and P. Müller, "Institute of Electrical and Electronics Engineers., and IEEE Communications Society", In: *2013 IEEE International Conference on Communications (ICC)*, 2013. Budapest,

Hungary

[60]   N. Díaz-Rodríguez, *Smart Dosing: A mobile application for tracking the medication tray-filling and dispensation processes in hospital wards,* 2014. Available from: https://www.researchgate.net/publication/270763222

[61]   J.C.Y. Jupp, H. Sultani, C.A. Cooper, K.A. Peterson, and T.H. Truong, "Evaluation of mobile phone applications to support medication adherence and symptom management in oncology patients", *Pediatr. Blood Cancer,* vol. 65, no. 11, p. e27278, 2018.
[http://dx.doi.org/10.1002/pbc.27278] [PMID: 29943893]

[62]   J. Rajj, *EAI/Springer Innovations in Communication and Computing International Conference onnMobile Computing and Sustainable Informatics ICMCSI 2020,* 2020. Available from: http://www.springer.com/series/15427

[63]   J.C.Y. Jupp, H. Sultani, C.A. Cooper, K.A. Peterson, and T.H. Truong, "Evaluation of mobile phone applications to support medication adherence and symptom management in oncology patients", *Pediatr. Blood Cancer,* vol. 65, no. 11, p. e27278, 2018.
[http://dx.doi.org/10.1002/pbc.27278] [PMID: 29943893]

[64]   B. Spiller, M. Bpharm, A.B. Btech, D. Biduski Bsc, A. Carolina, and B. De Marchi Bsc, *Mobile Health Applications and Medication Adherence of Patients With Hypertension: A Systematic Review and Meta-Analysis-S.....* Available from: https://www.sciencedirect.com/science/article/abs/pii/S0749379721005948

[65]   C.H. Patil, N. Lightwala, M Sherdiwala, A.D. Vibhute, S.A. Naik, and S.M. Mali, "An IoT based smart medicine dispenser model for healthcare", In: *2022 IEEE World Conference on Applied Intelligence and Computing (AIC)* vol. 17. IEEE, 2022, pp. 391-395.

[66]   K.M. Cresswell, A. Worth, and A. Sheikh, "Integration of a nationally procured electronic health record system into user work practices", *BMC Med. Inform. Decis. Mak.,* vol. 12, no. 1, p. 15, 2012.
[http://dx.doi.org/10.1186/1472-6947-12-15] [PMID: 22400978]

[67]   K.K. Jetelina, T.T. Woodson, R. Gunn, B. Muller, K.D. Clark, J.E. DeVoe, B.A. Balasubramanian, and D.J. Cohen, "Evaluation of an electronic health record (EHR) tool for integrated behavioral health in primary care", *J. Am. Board Fam. Med.,* vol. 31, no. 5, pp. 712-723, 2018.
[http://dx.doi.org/10.3122/jabfm.2018.05.180041] [PMID: 30201667]

[68]   S. Al-Arkee, J. Mason, D.A. Lane, L. Fabritz, W. Chua, M.S. Haque, and Z. Jalal, "Mobile apps to improve medication adherence in cardiovascular disease: Systematic review and meta-analysis", *J. Med. Internet Res.,* vol. 23, no. 5, p. e24190, 2021.
[http://dx.doi.org/10.2196/24190] [PMID: 34032583]

[69]   A. Koren, M. Jurcevic, and D. Huljenic, "Requirements and challenges in the integration of aggregated personal health data for inclusion into formal electronic health records (EHR)," in *2019 2nd Int. Colloquium Smart Grid Metrol., SMAGRIMET 2019 - Proc.,* Institute of Electrical and Electronics Engineers Inc., 2019
[http://dx.doi.org/10.23919/SMAGRIMET.2019.8720389]

[70]   M.P. Gagnon, E.K. Ghandour, P.K. Talla, D. Simonyan, G. Godin, M. Labrecque, M. Ouimet, and M. Rousseau, "Electronic health record acceptance by physicians: Testing an integrated theoretical model", *J. Biomed. Inform.,* vol. 48, pp. 17-27, 2014.
[http://dx.doi.org/10.1016/j.jbi.2013.10.010] [PMID: 24184678]

[71]   T. A. Nguyen and M. Aiello, "Beyond indoor presence monitoring with simple sensors," in *PECCS 2012 - Proc. 2nd Int. Conf. Pervasive Embedded Comput. Commun. Syst.,* 2012, pp. 5–14.
[http://dx.doi.org/10.5220/0003801300050014]

[72]   W.J. Fleming, "New automotive sensors - A review", *IEEE Sens. J.,* vol. 8, no. 11, pp. 1900-1921, 2008.
[http://dx.doi.org/10.1109/JSEN.2008.2006452]

[73]   C. Conati, R. Chabbal, and H. Maclaren, "A Study on Using Biometric Sensors for Monitoring User Emotions in Educational Games." 2004.

[74]   Duk-Dong Lee, and Dae-Sik Lee, 2014. "Environmental gas sensors", *IEEE Sens. J.,* vol. 1, no. 3, pp. 214-224, 2001.
[http://dx.doi.org/10.1109/JSEN.2001.954834]

[75]   E.J. Oughton, W. Lehr, K. Katsaros, I. Selinis, D. Bubley, and J. Kusuma, "Revisiting Wireless Internet Connectivity: 5G vs Wi-Fi 6", *Telecomm. Policy,* vol. 45, no. 5, p. 102127, 2021.
[http://dx.doi.org/10.1016/j.telpol.2021.102127]

[76]   S. Raza, P. Misra, Z. He, and T. Voigt, "Building the Internet of Things with bluetooth smart", *Ad Hoc Netw.,* vol. 57, pp. 19-31, 2017.
[http://dx.doi.org/10.1016/j.adhoc.2016.08.012]

[77]   J. Ding, M. Nemati, C. Ranaweera, and J. Choi, "IoT connectivity technologies and applications: A survey", *IEEE Access,* vol. 8, pp. 67646-67673, 2020.
[http://dx.doi.org/10.1109/ACCESS.2020.2985932]

[78]   R. Sapsford and V. Jupp, *Data Collection and Analysis,* 2nd ed., London, UK: SAGE Publications Ltd, 2006.

[79]   M.P. Couper, "Technology trends in survey data collection", *Soc. Sci. Comput. Rev.,* vol. 23, no. 4, pp. 486-501, 2005.
[http://dx.doi.org/10.1177/0894439305278972]

[80]   Z. R. Steelman, B. I. Hammer, and M. Limayem, "Increasing the Willingness to Collaborate Online: An Analysis of Sentiment-Driven Interactions in Peer Content Production," 2010.

[81]   O.P. Aborisade, "Data collection and new technology", *Int. J. Emerg. Technol. Learn.,* vol. 8, no. 2, pp. 48-52, 2013.
[http://dx.doi.org/10.3991/ijet.v8i2.2157]

[82]   M. I. Broese van Groenou, T. G. van Tilburg, E. de Leeuw, and A. C. Liefbroer, "Appendix Data Collection," in *Sourcebook of Living Arrangements and Social Networks of Older Adults in the Netherlands,* NESTOR-LSN Program, Vrije Universiteit Amsterdam, 2003.

[83]   S. Brandt, *Data Analysis: Statistical and Computational Methods for Scientists and Engineers,* 4th ed. Cham, Switzerland: Springer International Publishing, 2014.

[84]   Santos A, Macedo J, Costa A, Nicolau MJ. Internet of things and smart objects for M-health monitoring and control. Procedia Technology. 2014 Jan 1;16:1351-60.
[http://dx.doi.org/10.1016/j.protcy.2014.10.152]

[85]   J. W. Tukey, *Exploratory Data Analysis.* Reading, MA: Addison-Wesley, 1977.

[86]   F. Rabiee, "Focus-group interview and data analysis", *Proc. Nutr. Soc.,* vol. 63, no. 4, pp. 655-660, 2004.
[http://dx.doi.org/10.1079/PNS2004399] [PMID: 15831139]

[87]   P. García, P. Arboleya, B. Mohamed, A.A.C. Vega, and M.C. Vega, "Implementation of a Hybrid Distributed/Centralized Real-Time Monitoring System for a DC/AC Microgrid With Energy Storage Capabilities", *IEEE Trans. Industr. Inform.,* vol. 12, no. 5, pp. 1900-1909, 2016.
[http://dx.doi.org/10.1109/TII.2016.2574999]

[88]   T. Paiva, and J.P. Reiter, "Stop or continue data collection: A nonignorable missing data approach for continuous variables", *J. Off. Stat.,* vol. 33, no. 3, pp. 579-599, 2017.
[http://dx.doi.org/10.1515/jos-2017-0028]

[89]   Shouling Ji, R. Beyah, and Zhipeng Cai, "Snapshot and continuous data collection in probabilistic wireless sensor networks", *IEEE Trans. Mobile Comput.,* vol. 13, no. 3, pp. 626-637, 2014.
[http://dx.doi.org/10.1109/TMC.2013.30]

[90]   J. Liu, A. J. Khattak, and B. Professor, "Delivering Improved Alerts, Warnings, and Control Assistance Using Basic Safety Messages Transmitted between Connected Vehicles," 2016. [http://dx.doi.org/10.1016/j.trc.2016.03.009]

[91]   E. E. Thomas, J. Haydon, A. Mehrotra, J. Caffery, D. Snoswell, C. Banbury, R. Smith, and C. Gray, "Factors influencing the effectiveness of remote patient monitoring interventions: A realist review," *BMJ Open*, vol. 11, no. 8, p. e051844, Aug. 2021. [http://dx.doi.org/10.1136/bmjopen-2021-051844]

[92]   L. Guelman, M. Guillén, and A.M. Pérez-Marín, "A decision support framework to implement optimal personalized marketing interventions", *Decis. Support Syst.*, vol. 72, pp. 24-32, 2015. [http://dx.doi.org/10.1016/j.dss.2015.01.010]

[93]   M.Y. Ng, and J.R. Weisz, "Annual Research Review: Building a science of personalized intervention for youth mental health", *J. Child Psychol. Psychiatry*, vol. 57, no. 3, pp. 216-236, 2016. [http://dx.doi.org/10.1111/jcpp.12470] [PMID: 26467325]

[94]   E. Costa, S. Pecorelli, A. Giardini, M. Savin, E. Menditto, E. Lehane, O. Laosa, A. Monaco, and A. Marengoni, "Interventional tools to improve medication adherence: review of literature", *Patient Prefer. Adherence*, vol. 9, pp. 1303-1314, 2015. [http://dx.doi.org/10.2147/PPA.S87551] [PMID: 26396502]

[95]   W. Almobaideen, M. Allan, and M. Saadeh, "Smart archaeological tourism: Contention, convenience and accessibility in the context of cloud-centric IoT", *Mediterr. Archaeol. Archaeom. Int. J.*, vol. 16, no. 1, pp. 227-236, 2016. [http://dx.doi.org/10.5281/zenodo.35535]

[96]   Z. Wen, S. Wang, D. M. Yang, and J. Liu, "Deep learning in digital pathology for personalized treatment plans of cancer patients," *Seminars in Diagnostic Pathology*, vol. 40, pp. 1–8, Apr. 2023 [http://dx.doi.org/10.1053/j.semdp.2023.02.003]

[97]   T. Grubic, "Servitization and remote monitoring technology", *J. Manuf. Tech. Manag.*, vol. 25, no. 1, pp. 100-124, 2014. [http://dx.doi.org/10.1108/JMTM-05-2012-0056]

[98]   C.M. Jenerette, and D.K. Mayer, "Patient-Provider Communication: the Rise of Patient Engagement", *Semin. Oncol. Nurs.*, vol. 32, no. 2, pp. 134-143, 2016. [http://dx.doi.org/10.1016/j.soncn.2016.02.007] [PMID: 27137470]

[99]   C.L. Lai, S.W. Chien, S.C. Chen, and K. Fang, "Enhancing Medication Safety and Reduce Adverse Drug Events on Inpatient Medication Administration using RFID," 2008.

[100]   A. Hannaford, Y. Arens, and H. Koenig, ""Real-time monitoring and point-of-care testing: A review of the current landscape of prep adherence monitoring," Patient Preference and Adherence", *Dove Medical Press Ltd*, vol. 15, pp. 259-269, 2021. [http://dx.doi.org/10.2147/PPA.S248696]

[101]   G.R. Goodman, A. Kikut, M.J. Bustamante, L. Mendez, Y. Mohamed, C. Shachar, I.G. Cohen, S. Gerke, E.W. Boyer, R.K. Rosen, K.H. Mayer, C. O'Cleirigh, and P.R. Chai, ""I'd feel like someone was watchin' me... watching for a good reason": perceptions of data privacy, access, and sharing in the context of real-time PrEP adherence monitoring among HIV-negative MSM with substance use", *AIDS Behav.*, vol. 26, no. 9, pp. 2981-2993, 2022. [http://dx.doi.org/10.1007/s10461-022-03614-8] [PMID: 35303187]

[102]   M. Vervloet, L. van Dijk, J. Santen-Reestman, B. van Vlijmen, M.L. Bouvy, and D.H. de Bakker, "Improving medication adherence in diabetes type 2 patients through Real Time Medication Monitoring: a Randomised Controlled Trial to evaluate the effect of monitoring patients' medication use combined with short message service (SMS) reminders", *BMC Health Serv. Res.*, vol. 11, no. 1, p. 5, 2011. [http://dx.doi.org/10.1186/1472-6963-11-5] [PMID: 21219596]

[103] S. Faisal, J. Ivo, S. Abu Fadaleh, and T. Patel, "Exploring the Value of Real-Time Medication Adherence Monitoring: A Qualitative Study", *Pharmacy (Basel)*, vol. 11, no. 1, p. 18, 2023. [http://dx.doi.org/10.3390/pharmacy11010018] [PMID: 36827656]

[104] M.D. Jain, and J.Y. Spiegel, "Imagining the cell therapist: Future CAR T cell monitoring and intervention strategies to improve patient outcomes", *eJHaem*, vol. 3, no. S1, suppl. Suppl. 1, pp. 46-53, 2022. [http://dx.doi.org/10.1002/jha2.357] [PMID: 35844298]

[105] L.G. Glynn, A.W. Murphy, S.M. Smith, K. Schroeder, and T. Fahey, "Self-monitoring and other non-pharmacological interventions to improve the management of hypertension in primary care: a systematic review", *Br. J. Gen. Pract.*, vol. 60, no. 581, pp. e476-e488, 2010. [http://dx.doi.org/10.3399/bjgp10X544113] [PMID: 21144192]

[106] L.G. Planas, "Intervention design, implementation, and evaluation", *Am. J. Health Syst. Pharm.*, vol. 65, no. 19, pp. 1854-1863, 2008. [http://dx.doi.org/10.2146/ajhp070366] [PMID: 18796429]

[107] Y. Hong, and S.H. Lee, "Effectiveness of tele-monitoring by patient severity and intervention type in chronic obstructive pulmonary disease patients: A systematic review and meta-analysis", *Int. J. Nurs. Stud.*, vol. 92, pp. 1-15, 2019. [http://dx.doi.org/10.1016/j.ijnurstu.2018.12.006] [PMID: 30690162]

[108] C.O. Okeke, H.A. Quigley, H.D. Jampel, G. Ying, R.J. Plyler, Y. Jiang, and D.S. Friedman, "Interventions improve poor adherence with once daily glaucoma medications in electronically monitored patients", *Ophthalmology*, vol. 116, no. 12, pp. 2286-2293, 2009. [http://dx.doi.org/10.1016/j.ophtha.2009.05.026] [PMID: 19815286]

[109] J.K. Silver, "Cancer prehabilitation and its role in improving health outcomes and reducing health care costs", *Semin. Oncol. Nurs.*, vol. 31, no. 1, pp. 13-30, 2015. [http://dx.doi.org/10.1016/j.soncn.2014.11.003] [PMID: 25636392]

[110] J.H. Hibbard, and J. Greene, "What the evidence shows about patient activation: better health outcomes and care experiences; fewer data on costs", *Health Aff. (Millwood)*, vol. 32, no. 2, pp. 207-214, 2013. [http://dx.doi.org/10.1377/hlthaff.2012.1061] [PMID: 23381511]

[111] D.M. Cosgrove, M. Fisher, P. Gabow, G. Gottlieb, G.C. Halvorson, B.C. James, G.S. Kaplan, J.B. Perlin, R. Petzel, G.D. Steele, and J.S. Toussaint, "Ten strategies to lower costs, improve quality, and engage patients: the view from leading health system CEOs", *Health Aff. (Millwood)*, vol. 32, no. 2, pp. 321-327, 2013. [http://dx.doi.org/10.1377/hlthaff.2012.1074] [PMID: 23381525]

[112] B. Fireman, J. Bartlett, and J. Selby, "Can disease management reduce health care costs by improving quality?", *Health Aff. (Millwood)*, vol. 23, no. 6, pp. 63-75, 2004. [http://dx.doi.org/10.1377/hlthaff.23.6.63] [PMID: 15584100]

[113] B.A. Bunting, D. Nayyar, and C. Lee, *Number 4 Article 227 2015 Reducing Health Care Costs and Improving Clinical Outcomes Using an Improved Asheville Project Model*, 2015. Available from: http://pubs.lib.umn.edu/innovations/vol6/iss4/9

[114] D. Dimmock, S. Caylor, B. Waldman, W. Benson, C. Ashburner, J.L. Carmichael, J. Carroll, E. Cham, S. Chowdhury, J. Cleary, A. D'Harlingue, A. Doshi, K. Ellsworth, C.I. Galarreta, C. Hobbs, K. Houtchens, J. Hunt, P. Joe, M. Joseph, R.H. Kaplan, S.F. Kingsmore, J. Knight, A. Kochhar, R.G. Kronick, J. Limon, M. Martin, K.A. Rauen, A. Schwarz, S.P. Shankar, R. Spicer, M.A. Rojas, O. Vargas-Shiraishi, K. Wigby, N. Zadeh, and L. Farnaes, "Project Baby Bear: Rapid precision care incorporating rWGS in 5 California children's hospitals demonstrates improved clinical outcomes and reduced costs of care", *Am. J. Hum. Genet.*, vol. 108, no. 7, pp. 1231-1238, 2021. [http://dx.doi.org/10.1016/j.ajhg.2021.05.008] [PMID: 34089648]

[115] J.L. Pringle, A. Boyer, M.H. Conklin, J.W. McCullough, and A. Aldridge, "The Pennsylvania Project:

pharmacist intervention improved medication adherence and reduced health care costs", *Health Aff. (Millwood)*, vol. 33, no. 8, pp. 1444-1452, 2014.
[http://dx.doi.org/10.1377/hlthaff.2013.1398] [PMID: 25092847]

[116]   M. Hassanalieragh, A. Page, T. Soyata, G. Sharma, M. Aktas, G. Mateos, B. Kantarci, and S. Andreescu, "Health Monitoring and Management Using Internet-of-Things (IoT) Sensing with Cloud-Based Processing: Opportunities and Challenges," in *Proceedings of the 2015 IEEE International Conference on Services Computing (SCC)*, New York, NY, USA, Jun. 2015, pp. 285–292.
[http://dx.doi.org/10.1109/SCC.2015.47]

[117]   A.N. Navaz, M.A. Serhani, H.T. El Kassabi, N. Al-Qirim, and H. Ismail, "Trends, Technologies, and Key Challenges in Smart and Connected Healthcare", *IEEE Access*, vol. 9, pp. 74044-74067, 2021.
[http://dx.doi.org/10.1109/ACCESS.2021.3079217] [PMID: 34812394]

[118]   M. Chan, D. Estève, J.Y. Fourniols, C. Escriba, and E. Campo, "Smart wearable systems: Current status and future challenges", *Artif. Intell. Med.*, vol. 56, no. 3, pp. 137-156, 2012.
[http://dx.doi.org/10.1016/j.artmed.2012.09.003] [PMID: 23122689]

CHAPTER 4

Remote Patient Monitoring: A Paradigm Shift

Dimple Singh Tomar¹, Shaweta Sharma², Akanksha Sharma³, Gaddam Dinesh⁴ and Akhil Sharma³,*

¹ *Kharvel Subharti College of Pharmacy, Swami Vivekanand Subharti University, Meerut, India*

² *School of Medical and Allied Sciences, Galgotias University Plot No. 2, Yamuna Expy, Opposite Buddha International Circuit, Sector 17A, Greater Noida, Uttar Pradesh, India*

³ *R.J. College of Pharmacy, Raipur, Gharbara, Tappal, Khair, Uttar Pradesh, India*

⁴ *Department of Civil Engineering, Aditya University, Surampalem, India*

Abstract: Revolutionizing the healthcare delivery process, Remote Patient Monitoring (RPM) alters the traditional way of communication between care providers and patients. It delves into the multifaceted effect of RPM that relates to its changing position in the healthcare environment. This also means that with technological advancements, like wearable techs, integrating other devices under IoT, and using AI technologies, RPM allows for healthcare parameters' tracking outside normal clinical settings. Consequently, this transition towards proactive data-enabled medical practice provides patients with a chance to take part in their treatment as well as offering doctors immediate information for making decisions. In this chapter, we explore the use of Remote Patient Monitoring (RPM) in different healthcare areas, such as long-term condition care, senior care, and post-surgery recovery, to demonstrate its capacity to enhance patients' results, cut down on health expenses, and improve the quality of care. The paper also highlights legal policies that govern RPM's implementation, putting a lot of emphasis on privacy issues, security measures, and adherence to healthcare legislation. Furthermore, it addresses ethical considerations, including patient consent, ownership of data, and fairness in reaching information. We seek for the future in aspects like predictive analytics, personalized medicine, and global expansion of RPM initiatives. But despite all these encouraging possibilities that RPM holds, there are still some challenges that must be overcome, such as lack of interoperability, reimbursement difficulties, and differences in digital health literacy. This abstract concludes by highlighting the transformative capabilities of RPM in reforming healthcare landscapes toward a more connected patient-centric model of care delivery. By promoting teamwork between stakeholders and addressing barriers that exist today, RPM could change healthcare delivery, which will enhance patient outcomes thus improving lives across the globe.

* **Corresponding author Akhil Sharma:** R.J. College of Pharmacy, Raipur, Gharbara, Tappal, Khair, Uttar Pradesh, India; E-mail: xs2akhil@gmail.com

Akhil Sharma, Neeraj Kumar Fuloria, Pankaj Kumar Singh & Shaweta Sharma (Eds.)

Keywords: Artificial intelligence, Chronic, Clinical, Compliance, Digital health, Disease, Healthcare, Internet of things, Patient, Personalized medicine, Post-operation, Privacy, Recovery, Remote patient monitoring, Security, Wearable devices.

INTRODUCTION

Remote Patient Monitoring (RPM) is a healthcare practice that uses innovative technology for monitoring as well as managing patients' health from a different location. RPM merges wearable devices, mobile apps, telecommunication platforms, and other digital tools to track patients' signs of life, symptoms, and health parameters in non-traditional healthcare settings. Thus, this method enables healthcare practitioners to get current information about the condition of their patients; they can also detect diseases at an early stage and take necessary steps before they complicate or worsen the medical status [1].

The basic principle of RPM is that it gives patients the means to monitor their health and communicate with caregivers from home, thus enabling them to play a more active role in their treatment decisions. Often, RPM focuses on people with long-term ailments, the elderly, or those convalescing from surgery; it seeks to improve their lives, reduce the number of patients returning to hospitals more frequently, and lessen expenses for healthcare in general [2].

RPM components involve wearable sensors that monitor physiological parameters like heart rate, blood pressure, and glucose levels. They also include mobile applications that enable data gathering, transmission, and analysis. Other times, it may be a remote video consultation, prescription adherence monitoring, or personalized health coaching to support patients' self-management of their condition. A brief history of RPM is presented in Table **1**.

The importance of RPM is that it allows people who live far away or in places with few services to get better access to care. For instance, RPM enables doctors to oversee patients' vital signs, signs, and adherence to medication, among others. By doing so, it helps identify complications at its earliest stages, hence reducing hospitalizations and improving long-term medical outcomes. Also, as the world's population ages rapidly, RPM meets the rising demand for health care, especially among elderly individuals suffering from multiple medical conditions [9].

RPM makes it possible to age in place and takes the burden off caregivers and health care institutions because it allows for proactive monitoring of seniors' health. Besides, RPM has been designed to facilitate preventive care and early intervention through patient empowerment for self-monitoring of vital signs as well as lifestyle choices. Prompt management is enabled by this type of surveillance, preventing further development of diseases with less risk of developing further complications. Furthermore, RPM offers cost-effective healthcare delivery by reducing costly healthcare services such as hospitalization, emergency room visits, and avoidable medical procedures [10].

Table 1. Brief history of RPM.

Year	Milestone
1950s	Early experiments with telemetry systems for monitoring cardiac patients [3].
1960s	Development of the first wearable cardiac monitors for ambulatory patients [4].
1970s	Introduction of early telemedicine systems for remote consultations [5].
1980s	Advancements in telemetry technology enable remote monitoring of vital signs [6].
1990s	Expansion of RPM into chronic disease management, focusing on diabetes care [7].
2000s	Integration of RPM with mobile technology and electronic health records [7].
2010s	The rapid growth of the RPM market is driven by advancements in sensors and connectivity [8].
Present Day	RPM has become integral to healthcare delivery, transforming patient care [8].

Further, RPM inspires interactions between patients and healthcare providers, promotes self-management actions, and improves patient satisfaction with the healthcare experience. Finally, RPM produces huge volumes of patient data that can be studied to support clinical decision-making, develop personalized therapeutic plans, estimate health outcomes, and optimize care delivery pathways. Basically, RPM is a game-changing healthcare delivery method that provides advantages like increased accessibility to treatment, better management of chronic diseases, preventive healthcare, cost-effectiveness, patient involvement, and data-driven decision-making with regard to the future of healthcare delivery [11].

TECHNOLOGICAL ADVANCEMENTS

RPM is a very dynamic and evolutional practice in healthcare that technological progress has supported. These developments include different creative solutions that boost RPM's efficiency, effectiveness, and accessibility [12 - 18]. Tech-nological advancements in RPM are shown in Fig. (**1**).

IMPACT ON HEALTHCARE DELIVERY

The impact of RPM on healthcare delivery is profound. It has reshaped traditional models of care and ushered in a new era of patient-centric and proactive healthcare. Below and in Fig. (**2**), we describe ways in which RPM has transformed healthcare delivery.

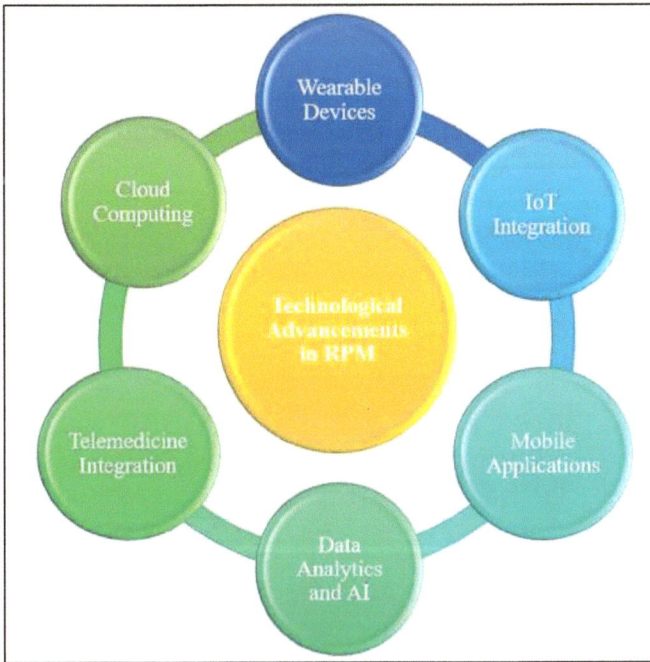

Fig. (1). Technological advancements in RPM.

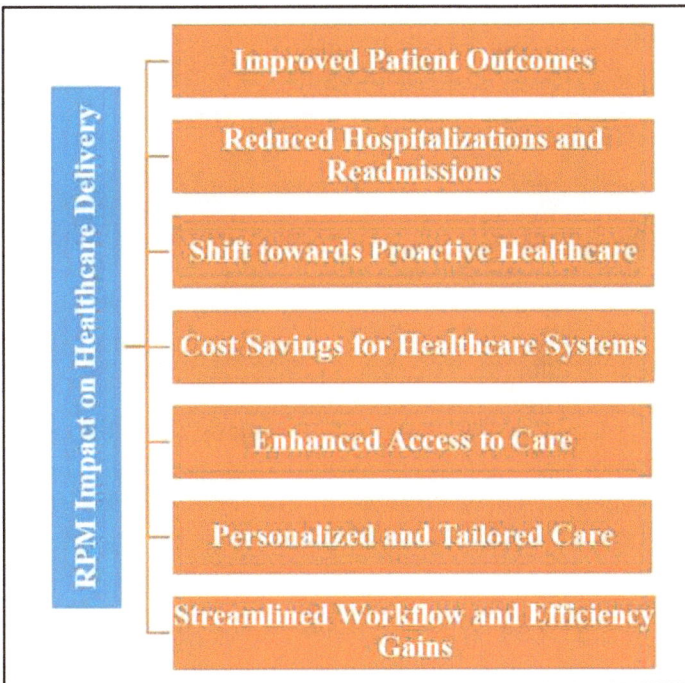

Fig. (2). RPM impact on healthcare delivery.

Improved Patient Outcomes

Early detection of health issues and timely interventions are possible through the use of RPM, which ultimately leads to improved patient outcomes. Healthcare providers can continuously monitor vital signs, symptoms, and other health metrics to safeguard against potential complications in this situation that may arise or deviations from baseline and intervene immediately to prevent any untoward happening [19].

Reduced Hospitalizations and Readmissions

RPM is helpful in preventing avoidable hospitalizations and rehospitalizations by monitoring patients' health from afar to identify the beginning of worsening. Consequently, it reduces pressure on healthcare institutions and enhances patient wellness by enabling them to access treatment within familiar locations or their homes [20].

Shift towards Proactive Healthcare

Healthcare RPM takes a proactive approach and allows patients to control their health and be involved in preventive procedures. This initiative gives them the chance to monitor their own vital signs, drug use, adherence, and lifestyles, among other factors that would require early intervention. Thus, promoting self-management reduces the need for reactive medical interventions [21].

Cost Savings for Healthcare Systems

RPM provides cost-effective solutions for managing long-term illnesses and continuously delivering patient care. By decreasing the number of unnecessary hospitalizations, emergency room visits, and medical interventions, RPM optimizes healthcare resources and lowers healthcare costs generally [22].

Enhanced Access to Care

RPM enhances the availability of medical services for individuals who live in remote, underserved regions. It breaks down geographical hindrances by facilitating telemedicine and virtual health consultations, which provide timely access to healthcare professionals, thereby enhancing equity and inclusivity in the system [23].

Personalized and Tailored Care

RPM allows personalization and tailoring of care delivery by providing health providers with real-time data insights on patient health status and trends. This makes it possible to personalize treatment plans, adjust medications, and make lifestyle recommendations based on the specific needs and preferences of each patient [24].

Streamlined Workflow and Efficiency Gains

RPM, or remote patient monitoring, reduces procedural and administrative burdens by automating processes involved in data collection, communication, and analysis. This ultimately improves efficiency and makes quality healthcare provision possible [25].

In healthcare delivery, RPM has a transformative effect by improving patient outcomes, avoiding hospitalizations, encouraging proactive care, reducing costs to access healthcare, enhancing personalized medicine, and streamlining workflow efficiency. As RPM continues evolving and integrating deeper into the healthcare systems, its impact on healthcare delivery will keep growing, thus shaping the future of healthcare into a more patient-centered and efficient care model [26].

INTEGRATION WITH TELEMEDICINE

The integration of telemedicine is a landmark in RPM that fuses two innovative healthcare delivery approaches and improves patient care [27]. The main attributes of the integration of telemedicine with RPM are discussed below.

Virtual Consultations

Telemedicine platform integration with RPM enables healthcare practitioners to provide virtual consultations remotely. The patient can interact *via* videoconferencing with his or her healthcare team and discuss any health concerns, thus receiving medical advice without physically visiting a hospital [28].

Continuous Monitoring and Follow-Up

The integration of telemedicine improves continuity of care by helping in constant monitoring and follow-up between healthcare visits. Doctors can monitor their patients' progress using RPM devices that transmit real-time health data, enabling them to adjust their treatment plans and provide timely intervention [29].

Improved Access to Specialty Care

Telemedicine and RPM can provide specialist treatment to patients in remote areas, particularly those that are underserved. This will reduce the requirement for traveling to meet the specialists and bridge the geographical barrier to healthcare access [30].

Post-Operative Care

RPM, integrated with telemedicine after surgical procedures, helps healthcare providers monitor patients' recovery progress remotely and issue post-surgical instructions. Patients can use RPM devices to report their symptoms, degree of pain, and adherence to prescribed medications, thus allowing for early detection of complications and timely interventions [31, 32].

Medication Management

The incorporation of telemedicine into RPM has made medication management more efficient by allowing remote prescription renewals and virtual medication reviews. Healthcare providers can monitor patients for drug adherence from remote locations through telemedicine and can also address any concerns or issues related to medication therapy through teleconsultations [33].

Patient Education and Engagement

Patients can communicate with their healthcare providers, track their improvement, and access relevant educational information, such as personalized lifestyle recommendations and self-management support, provided by telemedicine inclusion into remote patient monitoring [34].

RPM integration with telemedicine is a comprehensive and patient-centered approach to healthcare delivery that facilitates virtual consultations, real-time monitoring, better access to specialty care, improved management of chronic diseases, simplified medication management, and increased participation by patients. As technology advances further, this incorporation holds great potential for the improvement of health outcomes and consumer satisfaction [35].

CHRONIC DISEASE MANAGEMENT

RPM has revolutionized the management of chronic diseases such as diabetes, hypertension, and heart disease, offering innovative solutions to improve patient outcomes and quality of life [36].

Diabetes

RPM has revolutionized how diabetes is managed and provides a holistic way to improve the lives of people with this constant sickness. These wearable devices utilize advancing innovations such as mobile applications, which give patients the opportunity to monitor blood sugar levels continuously while empowering them to manage their diabetes. The technology allows patients to keep tabs on their glucose levels throughout their day, giving insights that benefit both the patient and the doctors. Continuous monitoring helps in identifying variations in blood sugar that are not within normal limits in time for corrective action to be taken, thus preventing hyperglycemia or hypoglycemia episodes and reducing the chances of diabetic complications [37].

Furthermore, RPM can increase compliance with medication among patients by reminding them about their oral drugs and insulin shots. For mobile apps to work with medication management, reminders can be tailored for each patient's dose so that they comply with the treatment plans. Remote monitoring by healthcare providers helps identify noncompliance patterns in patients and corrects them in a timely, thus optimizing medication management and improving glycemic control [38].

Apart from that, the RPM enables remote patient teaching and assistance, which assists diabetic patients in making sound decisions about eating, exercising, and changing their way of life. *via* teleconsultations and virtual coaching sessions, healthcare providers provide personalized guidance and support to address specific needs and obstacles faced by individual patients. Mobile apps provide access to educational tools such as dietary guidelines, exercise plans, or self-management habits that allow patients to adopt healthy lifestyle choices and have a better control of diabetes [39].

In addition to monitoring glucose levels and medication adherence, RPM also enables remote monitoring of other diabetes-related parameters like physical activity, sleep patterns, and stress. By integrating these lifestyle factors into the monitoring process, RPM allows for a comprehensive view of the patient's health and can enable personalized interventions aimed at addressing underlying risk factors contributing to poor glycemic control [40].

RPM changed diabetes management by providing complete care centered on patients. This has improved outcomes and the quality of life for those living with diabetes through real-time data insights, medication adherence support, remote education and support, and lifestyle issues. With the advancement in technology, RPM holds great promise to optimize the management of diabetes further, reducing the burden of this chronic condition on both patients and healthcare systems [41].

Hypertension

Hypertension, a common chronic ailment that is defined by higher levels of blood pressure, changes for the better in how it is managed through the introduction of RPM. This health technology provides a dynamic approach to checking and regulating high blood pressure, empowering people who suffer from hypertension in their role in control processes. Wearable devices and home monitors can help patients regularly keep track of their blood pressure and send it immediately to healthcare providers, which ensures constant monitoring. In this way, not only may one pick up BP fluctuations at a very early stage but also avoid hypertensive crises/complications *via* prompt interventions that mitigate cardiovascular risks and prevent damage to end organs [42, 43].

In addition to blood pressure control, RPM helps patients manage their medication by reminding them about antihypertensive pills and giving feedback. It ensures that through mobile apps with medication adherence features, patients receive personalized notifications for taking drugs, thus increasing compliance with the prescribed treatment plans. Healthcare providers may observe the trends of patient adherence remotely and act before the deviations occur, thereby optimizing medicine use and improving BP control [44].

Also, RPM promotes hypertension patient self-management and e-learning about better life choices. There are personalized recommendations and support from medical practitioners during teleconsultations with patients through virtual coaching sessions. Moreover, mobile apps available today offer a wealth of resources on dietary changes, workout routines, and stress reduction techniques for helping individuals make healthy choices that can positively affect their well-being in relation to blood pressure level control [45].

Furthermore, the remote tracking of lifestyle habits that affect blood pressure, such as diet, exercise, and stress levels, can be achieved through RPM. This allows for the integration of these factors into monitoring, hence offering a comprehensive picture of the health status of an individual, which in turn assists in tailoring strategies targeted at mitigating any hypertension triggers. Patients can track their lifestyle actions, set goals for improvement, and get feedback and motivation from medical professionals, thereby enhancing their commitment to healthier living [46].

Remote Patient Monitoring is a life-changing method of handling hypertension as it lets patients have more control over the condition, gives them custom-made help or support, and provides them with proactive interventions to secure their own bodies' optimal blood pressures. By giving real-time patient data insights to the patients, helping them take medications better, allowing remote education and support, and treating lifestyle issues, RPM ensures better outcomes while increasing the quality of life for hypertensive individuals. As technology evolves further, RPM could enhance hypertension management even further and potentially reduce its impact on patients and healthcare systems alike in this era of technological advancement [47, 48].

Heart Disease

RPM has emerged as a game-changer in the management of heart disease, offering a comprehensive approach to monitoring, managing, and preventing cardiovascular complications. By leveraging advanced technology, RPM enables continuous monitoring of cardiac parameters, facilitating early detection of abnormalities and timely interventions to prevent adverse events. Wearable devices equipped with sensors allow patients to monitor their heart rate, rhythm, and other cardiac metrics in real time, providing valuable data insights to both patients and healthcare providers. This continuous monitoring not only helps in detecting arrhythmias, heart failure exacerbations, or other cardiac events early but also supports post-operative care for patients recovering from cardiac procedures [49].

Additionally, RPM facilitates remote cardiac rehabilitation programs, where patients can carry out exercise sessions in the comfort of their homes, receive educational resources, and track their progress. The teleconsultations with cardiac rehabilitation specialists provide personalized support and guidance to patients during their recovery journey, thus enhancing adherence to rehabilitation protocols and optimizing outcomes. By incorporating these remote rehab programs into the monitoring process, RPM enhances patient engagement while reducing recurring cardiovascular events through healthier lifestyle behaviors [50].

Lastly, RPM manages medication by reminding patients of their cardiac medications and providing them with feedback. Mobile apps with drug adherence features will give prompts on when to take a pill and, therefore, boost personalized treatment. Healthcare providers should closely monitor the medication-taking habits of patients from a distance and act in anticipation of any possible non-compliance that may affect medicine administration, which is done better using mobile technology for patients suffering from heart conditions [51].

Additionally, RPM facilitates remote patient education and support, empowering heart disease patients to deliberate on their health and lifestyle. Individual needs and constraints are addressed through teleconsultations and virtual coaching sessions, where healthcare experts offer personalized advice. Dietary changes, exercise programs, and stress reduction methods can be found on mobile apps for healthy lifestyle choices by patients with heart conditions [52].

Heart disease management is improved by RPM, which empowers patients with real-time data insights, helps them to adhere to medication, and supports them remotely through education and lifestyle changes, which in turn lead to better outcomes and improved life quality. The promise of further optimizing heart disease management and reducing the burden of cardiovascular disease on patients or healthcare systems lies in the future development of technology as it continues to improve from time to time [53].

ELDERLY CARE

Addressing diverse challenges of aging, such as falls, medication management, and cognitive decline, RPM has become indispensable in providing holistic care for the elderly population [54, 55]. The following are descriptions of how RPM benefits elderly care in critical areas.

Fall Detection

In the field of elderly care, one important thing to consider is fall detection among aged individuals, and RPM seems to be a valuable method that will alleviate this problem. In real-time, RPMs utilize wearable gadgets and sensors, which are very advanced in technology, to detect falls in aged people. These devices contain accelerometers and gyroscopes that can measure changes in movement patterns or body orientation, thus distinguishing normal activities from falls. In case of a fall, an alert is activated by the RPM system, and it can be sent to caregivers, family members, or healthcare givers, facilitating prompt help and intervention [56, 57].

Its importance in RPM lies in its ability to solve fall-related risks among older people. Falls are a leading cause of injury and hospitalization of old adults, often resulting in fractures, head traumas, and other grave complications. In detecting falls as they happen, RPM ensures quick response and treatment, thus reducing the likelihood of staying on the ground for an extended time and lowering the seriousness of injuries. Such fast intervention can be life-saving, particularly for aged people who live by themselves or have immobility issues [58, 59].

Additionally, RPM's fall detection encourages self-determination and eases the minds of elderly people and their friends. Older adults can continue to live in their own houses safely yet independently, provided that they are aware that support teams will attend a fall. Furthermore, falling detection technology serves as a good anchor for family members or caregivers, knowing that their loved ones are watched over even when they are not present [60, 61].

Fall detection through RPM provides not only immediate support but also post-fall analysis and intervention. Healthcare providers can analyze the data collected by remote patient monitoring systems to uncover intrinsic risks for falls like abnormal gaits or balance problems. From here, one-on-one prevention playbooks such as exercises, home adjustments, and assistive devices can be tailored to avoid future fall episodes while improving the safety of older adults at large [62, 63].

Cognitive Decline Detection

Detecting cognitive decline is a crucial facet of elderly care, and RPM offers pioneering alternatives that help identify the early stages of cognitive impairment and dementia. RPM systems use cutting-edge technology, such as tools for evaluating cognitive abilities and remote monitoring capacity, to trace changes in thinking behavior, thus facilitating timely intervention [64, 65]. RPM supports cognitive decline detection in elderly individuals, as described below and summarized in Fig. (**3**).

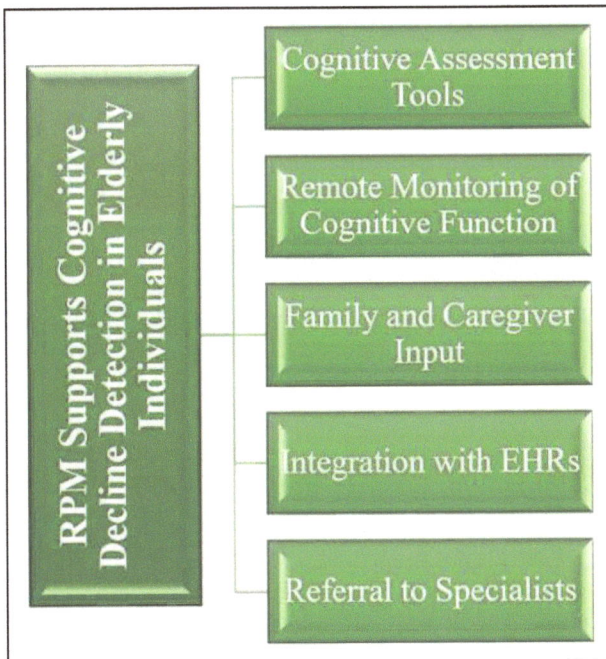

Fig. (3). RPM supports cognitive decline detection in elderly individuals.

Cognitive Assessment Tools

Cognitive assessment tools are incorporated by RPM platforms that are suitable for healthcare providers to analyze several aspects of cognitive functions like memory, attention, language, and executive function. This proactive approach will help in early detection of subtle changes in cognitive functioning as an indication of cognitive decline [66].

Remote Monitoring of Cognitive Function

Continuous cognitive functioning can be remotely monitored by RPM through virtual cognitive assessments, cognitive electronic games, and digital behavior passive monitoring. This suggests that healthcare providers may interpret cognitive deficit markers like more forgetfulness, less involvement in thinking activities or changing ways of communication from the data provided by RPM systems. Remote monitoring thus allows early identification of cognitive disorders and possible intervention to deal with their root causes or risk factors [67, 68].

Family and Caregiver Input

RPM systems' cognitive decline detection may involve family members or caregivers by soliciting their input and observations. Caregivers are another source of information for changes in behavior, memory, or daily functioning that might suggest a decline in cognitive abilities. In addition to these, there are also reporting features for caregivers to report concerns, record observations, or even communicate with healthcare providers so as to facilitate collaboration among caregivers and early detection of cognitive impairment [69, 70].

Referral to Specialists

In situations where cognitive impairment is suspected or detected by RPM, healthcare providers can help ensure prompt referral to specialists like neurologists or geriatricians for further assessment and treatment. Such systems aid in making referrals quicker so that older adults obtain appropriate specialized care and supportive services that are customized to their mental faculties [71].

For remote cognitive assessment by doctors, RPM is concerned with detecting cognitive decline. Collaborating with families and caregivers, continuous monitoring of cognitive function aids in this process of detection. It also collaborates with EHRs and facilitates specialist referrals. In the management of cognitive decline in elderly individuals, RPM plays a role in early detection and intervention, which enhances their overall well-being and quality of life. Thus, as the population that advances in age increases day by day, it will be increasingly vital to look at it from an RPM perspective thus making RPM a must-have part of comprehensive geriatrics care [72, 73].

POST-OPERATIVE CARE

The invaluable support offered to patients by RPM during the postoperative period is a crucial phase in their recovery. RPM uses highly developed technology that helps remotely observe and record vital signs, detect early complications, and reduce the likelihood of re-admission to the hospital [74].

Remote Monitoring of Vital Signs

Modern healthcare leverages remote monitoring of vital signs to follow patients' physiological parameters beyond the conventional clinical environment. Adopted through RPM technology, this technique has various advantages in relation to early detection of health problems, proactive chronic disease management, and better patient results [75].

The monitoring of vital signs from a distance concerns applying wearable outfit that consists of sensors to help track different physiological aspects like heart rate, blood pressure, respiratory rate, oxygen saturation levels, and sometimes even electrocardiogram (ECG) readings when necessary. These devices range from smartwatches to specialized medical-grade monitors and always keep collecting data in real-time while transmitting it wirelessly to healthcare providers' systems for analysis [76].

Real-time data insights into patients' health status are one of the main benefits of vital sign remote monitoring. Healthcare providers can easily detect slight changes or irregularities in their vital signs that may be symptomatic of failing health or a developing condition by Continuously tracking them. This ensures that immediate action is taken, possibly preventing complications or adverse events and leading to better patient results [77, 78].

Remote vital signs monitoring is very useful for patients suffering from long-term conditions such as high blood pressure, heart failure, diabetes, and respiratory problems. These patients need to have their vital signs checked regularly to manage these conditions and avoid worsening symptoms effectively. Through RPM technology, individuals can easily monitor their vitals from home; hence, there is less need for frequent hospital visits, which makes it easier for them to take proactive actions in self-management [79].

Additionally, the idea of personalized medicine can be supported by remote monitoring of vital signs, which gives healthcare providers more personal information about each patient's health. Healthcare providers can customize treatment plans and interventions based on the long-term trends and patterns observed from vital sign data. This approach has resulted in improved healthcare outcomes as well as increased patient satisfaction [80].

This is crucial as it helps in the development of telemedicine and virtual care. With an increase in telehealth services, remote monitoring of vital signs allows patients to participate in virtual consultations with healthcare practitioners, viewing their vital sign data from a distance for guidelines and recommendations. This improves healthcare accessibility, especially to patients living in rural or underserved areas, but also enhances the continuum of care and patient-provider communication [81].

Early Detection of Complications

A crucial element in healthcare management is RPM, which allows early identification of complications. RPM technology involves using wearable devices with sensors to continuously monitor patients' health outside traditional clinical settings. All these physiological indicators, including heart rate, blood pressure, temperature, respiratory rate, and oxygen saturation, are collected in real-time by RPM. By continuously monitoring these indices, the healthcare provider can be alerted to departure from baseline or any unexpected trends that may indicate potential complications [82, 83].

RPM systems are designed to send alerts and notifications when certain thresholds are met to facilitate prompt alerting in the event of alarming changes. Again, data analytics tools that analyze patients' health patterns and trends are part of RPM platforms, thus contributing to early complications detection. Additionally, integrating with EHRs allows for a smooth flow of communication between healthcare providers, which helps in early complications detection through having an all-around view of the patient's progress and previous medical records [84, 85].

Besides, RPM also enables telemedicine visits and remote consultations that allow healthcare providers to review patients' health data and virtually assess them remotely. Timely decision-making and intervention are enabled even when patients are situated remotely or cannot go to healthcare facilities personally *via* teleconsultations. Therefore, RPM technology is essential for early detection of complications because it permits continuous monitoring, can trigger alarms and notices, monitors trends in health information, allows for remote consultations, and makes use of electronic medical records. This proactive monitoring approach enables faster response from healthcare providers, hence better patient outcomes and enhanced patient safety across diverse healthcare settings [86 - 88].

Reduced Hospital Readmissions

Revolutionary post-discharge care and better patient results are the key reasons that make RPM a major strategy for reducing hospital readmissions. The remote monitoring technology of RPM allows healthcare professionals to identify possible complications early enough, thereby reducing the chances of frequent visits to hospitals. RPM uses wearable devices that have sensors for real-time collection of data about vital signs, symptoms, and other health metrics so as to provide a holistic understanding of patients' physiological states [89].

RPM facilitates the close observation of patient recovery progress, enabling health providers to identify potential deterioration or complications before they become critical, thus minimizing hospital admissions. Additionally, RPM systems are meant to raise alarms and send notifications when predetermined thresholds or criteria are met, which may imply healthcare challenges. RPM offers anticipatory monitoring that enables early interventions by health providers, thereby enhancing patient treatment compliance, shortening hospital stays, and preventing readmissions due to medical complications [90].

RPM also allows for remote consultations and telemedicine visits, thereby facilitating virtual assessments by doctors of patients' health information and treatment adjustments as required. These ultimately help ease the burden on healthcare institutions and improve patient care. This happens through a process of hospital readmission reduction, improved patient satisfaction, and general care quality enhancement that takes place across different healthcare settings [91].

DATA ANALYTICS AND ARTIFICIAL INTELLIGENCE

Data analytics and Artificial Intelligence (AI) have greatly transformed healthcare delivery, especially in RPM. This is mainly achieved through early intervention predictive analytics, machine learning algorithms, and personalized treatment plans [92].

Predictive Analytics for Early Intervention

The case of RPM is an example of how predictive analytics can be used for early intervention. It utilizes sophisticated data analysis methods to project likely health states and recognize patients in danger of developing complications before they happen. In RPM, predictive analytics uses patient data such as vital signs, symptoms, medical history, and demographics on a historical and real-time basis to identify patterns and trends that suggest impending health problems [93].

Predictive analytics algorithms can identify patients who may be at risk of experiencing adverse events or deteriorating health conditions by exploring these data points. For instance, minute modifications in vital signs or discrepancies from set ranges can denote the beginning of an infection, deterioration of chronic disease, or drug side effects [94].

Healthcare providers can prevent untoward events and improve patient outcomes by being proactive, beginning intervention at this stage towards treatment, changing the care plan or taking up preventive measures timely. For example, suppose a patient's record of heart failure symptoms shows an upward trend as per predictive analytics algorithms. In that case, doctors can start providing medication reviews, lifestyle changes, or remote monitoring to keep the person from being admitted to the hospital or making their symptoms worse [95].

Again, predictive analytics can assist in prioritizing patient care by determining those who have the greatest chances of having bad outcomes and require immediate attention. By sorting out patients based on their risk profiles, healthcare providers will allocate resources more efficiently, targeting those with the highest need for attention/interventions [92, 96].

Predictive analytics for early intervention can improve proactive and targeted care delivery, enhancing the capabilities of RPM. Predictive analytics assists healthcare providers in intervening at an early stage, improving patient outcomes and the quality of care offered to patients under remote monitoring by using advanced data analysis techniques to forecast potential health issues before they occur [97].

Machine Learning Algorithms

AI is a subset of machine learning algorithms that use this information to improve the usefulness of RPM by examining patients' records and discovering complex patterns, relationships, and correlations. These programs enable machines to draw conclusions based on data without having been explicitly programmed for it, thus enabling them to predict future behaviors, detect trends, and glean insights from huge amounts of data [98]. RPM, machine learning algorithms play a crucial role in several areas which are described below.

Predictive Analytics

Historical and real-time patient data is used in the development of predictive models that predict future health outcomes using machine learning algorithms. These models can determine which patients are at risk of developing complications, forecast readmission rates to hospitals or anticipate changes in someone's wellbeing before they occur. Providers can therefore take an appropriate action by analyzing the trends existing in patients' data thus detecting minor deviations like a precursor for potential health problems thereby contributing towards better results for their customers [99].

Anomaly Detection

Large data sets can be easily tracked to better understand life and nature. The use of these algorithms in RPM, for instance, may help to identify abnormal patterns in vital signs and symptoms as well as other health indicators that require intensive examination. For example, arrhythmias or hypertensive crises may be inferred from anomalies in heartbeat variability or blood pressure readings, thus requiring immediate intervention by health care providers [100].

Personalized Medicine

Machine learning algorithms can be used to create custom treatment plans for patients, taking into account their personal attributes and unique requirements. With the use of these algorithms, it is possible for doctors to treat each patient group in an optimal way through deep analysis of their information such as medical history, genetic data, lifestyle choices, and reactions to different therapies. Personalized treatment plans improve the outcomes of treatments; decrease the side effects of the use of drugs as well as boost patient satisfaction by providing focused care that is tailored to their needs [101].

Clinical Decision Support

Healthcare companies benefit from using machine learning algorithms, which analyze patient information and provide insights or recommendations to support clinical decisions. By providing interpretations for complex datasets, these can help make sense of them even as they are used by healthcare providers. For instance, a diagnostic image might be examined by machine learning algorithms to help radiologists identify anomalies or problematic regions [102].

Machine learning algorithms are generally important for improving remote patient monitoring by allowing predictive analytics, outlier detection, personalized medicine, and clinical decision support. Advanced data analysis, on the other hand, is the driving force behind these algorithms that enables healthcare providers to be proactive, accurate, and patient-centered in their care, which eventually leads to better outcomes and the quality of care for patients under remote monitoring [103].

Personalized Treatment Plans

Individualized treatment proposals based on data analytics and artificial intelligence are changing the face of patient care in RPM. The focus is on patient-specific needs, likes, and distinctiveness, ensuring that each patient has their treatment enhanced for better results. Below is a description of how personalized treatment plans are formulated and executed within an RPM context.

Data-driven Assessment

The creation of a personalized treatment plan is initiated through an adequate evaluation of the patient's medical history, current health condition, genetic data, lifestyle elements, and treatment responses. RPM systems collect and analyze a lot of information about patients, like vital signs, symptoms, medication adherence, and activity levels in order to understand the health profile of a patient [104].

Advanced Analytics

Data analytics algorithms are used for analyzing the recorded patients' data to establish trends, correlations, and patterns that help in personalizing treatment plans. They exploit machine learning methods to discover undisclosed details and predict the best possible remedies according to a patient's specific traits and demands [105, 106].

Risk Stratification

Personalized treatment plans often stratify patients into risk categories according to their physical condition, prognosis, and susceptibility to given health problems. Categorizing patients through their risk profiles helps healthcare providers prioritize interventions and allocate resources more effectively with emphasis on the most deserving ones [106].

Tailored Interventions

Personalized treatment plans recommend tailored interventions, medication regimens, lifestyle modifications and preventive measures based on insights derived from data analytics that are intended to target the individual health needs and goals of the patient. A person with hypertension can get personalized recommendations for dieting, exercising, managing stress, or taking medication so as to enhance blood pressure control and prevent cardiovascular complications [107].

Continuous Monitoring and Adjustment

Whenever the patient's health status, treatment responses, and lifestyle factors change, personalized treatment plans become very dynamic and will continue to be so. RPM systems help healthcare providers monitor patients' data continuously, enabling them to adjust their interventions accordingly and detect any changes in the health status. It is an iterative process in which treatment strategies remain tailored to the patient's changing needs, optimizing outcomes and minimizing adverse events [108].

Patient Empowerment

Personalized treatment plans empower patients to participate actively in their healthcare journey by giving them personalized recommendations, education, and support. RPM systems provide patient-friendly interfaces, mobile applications, and interactive tools so that patients can check their progress toward goals, receive feedback, and communicate with their caregivers. This patient-centered approach enhances engagement among patients, adherence to treatment regimen, and satisfaction with care [109].

When providing remote patient monitoring, personalized care plans make use of data analytics and artificial intelligence to match interventions with the unique requirements, choices, and conditions of every patient. The use of patient data to understand risk levels, suggest appropriate actions, and focus on shared responsibility for the care of these individuals will lead to the customization of treatment options that maximize therapeutic effectiveness and promote better patient outcomes in RPM [110].

REGULATORY FRAMEWORK

The regulatory framework surrounding RPM is essential to ensure the safety, effectiveness, and compliance of these technologies.

FDA Approval Process

The FDA is responsible for controlling medical devices, which include a number of technologies deployed in RPM. The approval or clearance by the FDA may be necessary for manufacturers to market and distribute their products depending on the classification of a given device. Class I devices, for instance, might be exempted from premarket review because they pose very little danger to patients. On the other hand, class II and III devices can only be marketed after they have received clearance from the FDA through the 510(k) premarket notification process or under a more demanding premarket approval (PMA) procedure, respectively. Prior to marketing and use in clinical practice, the Food and Drug Administration assesses whether RPM devices are safe, effective, and perform according to regulatory standards [111].

Compliance with Healthcare Regulations

RPM technologies must consider different healthcare regulations that also cover aspects of patient privacy, data security, reimbursement, and professional licensure in addition to the FDA regulations. Compliance with regulations such as HIPAA ensures the protection of patient's health information and privacy rights. Also, healthcare providers and organizations offering RPM services need to adhere to regulations governing medical practice, telemedicine, and insurance reimbursement [112].

Privacy and Security Considerations

In order to prevent patients' sensitive health information from unauthorized access, disclosure, or misuse, RPM must ensure that privacy and security are maintained as the main concern. Security is also crucial for RPM systems in the sense that any patient data collected has to be safeguarded with appropriate encryption, authentication mechanisms, audit trails, and access controls. Additionally, compliance with HIPAA regulations means that RPM providers have to establish policies and procedures on data protection, confidentiality breach notification, and patient consent. Moreover, following industry standards and best practices like those stipulated by the National Institute of Standards and Technology (NIST) and the International Organization for Standardization (ISO) will help guarantee patients' data availability, confidentiality as well as integrity within the RPM systems [113].

FDA approval, healthcare regulation compliance, and privacy/security concerns form part of the regulatory framework for Remote Patient Monitoring. These regulations must be followed to guarantee the safe, effective, and ethical utilization of RPM technologies in healthcare provision. Regulatory requirements should be met in order to make patients feel confident about RPM, reduce the potential harm associated with it, and enable new practices in clinical medicine to embrace such technology [114].

HEALTHCARE PROVIDER PERSPECTIVE

From the perspective of a healthcare provider, RPM is an innovative way to deliver healthcare services that can help streamline workflows, employ tools for managing patients at a distance, and tackle emerging challenges and opportunities in the healthcare system.

Healthcare providers' workflows can be made more efficient and productive through the integration of RPM systems. The RPM system, by automating the processes of data collection, analysis, and communication, relieves healthcare providers of their burden and enhances proactive patient care management. In addition to this, EHRs are an avenue for clinicians to access and review patient information in familiar systems that streamline documentation, decision-making, and care coordination. Lastly, adjustments can be made to the remote monitoring system following existing patterns for workflow as well as preferences, thereby enabling a smooth transition without interfering with clinical operations [115].

However, healthcare providers also have challenges and chances to encounter in the implementation and optimization of RPM. Some of these challenges are as follows: anxiety over data security, reimbursement constraints, difficulty in adopting technology, and change resistance by healthcare staff and patients. In spite of this, there is a silver lining for overcoming barriers, improving patient outcomes, and enhancing health care delivery. For instance, healthcare providers can use powerful encryption systems, access controls, and HIPAA-compliant practices to handle data privacy and security issues. Furthermore, support for policy changes and payment modifications can motivate the acceptance of RPM, thus leading to its incorporation into clinical practice on a much wider scale. Also, education plus training campaigns can give more power to health professionals in using the RPM tools effectively, as well as involving patients in remote monitoring [116 - 120].

ECONOMIC IMPLICATIONS

The economic implications of RPM are significant, encompassing cost savings for healthcare systems, reductions in hospitalizations, and the promotion of value-based care models.

Cost Savings for Healthcare Systems

Healthcare systems save a lot of costs through RPM because it maximizes resource utilization, minimizes health spending, and reduces the need for costly interventions. Moreover, by keeping track of a patient's health status from afar and recognizing problems early on, RPM reduces avoidable hospitalization rates, emergency department visits, and expensive medical operations. In addition to this, RPM helps manage chronic conditions proactively, reducing disease progression and its accompanying healthcare expenses. Last but not least, virtual consultations, as well as remote follow-ups, become possible across the board for all concerned parties thanks to RPM, which in turn eases the burden on health facilities and their personnel, hence improving operational efficiency while saving money [121, 122].

Reduction in Hospitalizations

RPM's most important economic advantage is the decrease in hospitalization rates, specifically among patients having chronic diseases and intricate medication requirements. RPM reduces the likelihood of flare-ups for individuals with chronic conditions and complications that can be prevented, thus avoiding the necessity to be admitted to a hospital. Furthermore, it assists in early discharge planning as well as post-acute care management that enables patients to heal safely at home while minimizing the chances of having repeated admissions. Consequently, this decrease in hospitalizations leads not only to reduced healthcare expenditures but also to enhanced patient contentment as well as good quality of life [123].

Value-based Care Models

Value-based care models prioritize the delivery of high-quality, cost-effective care that enhances patient outcomes and increases the overall value of healthcare services; it is in this context that RPM aligns with such models. RPM uses preventive care, care coordination, and patient engagement to promote proactive management of chronic conditions, decrease health utilization, and enhance population health outcomes to achieve the goals of value-based care. Moreover, the use of RPM allows healthcare providers to show how important their services are in terms of better patient results, reduced expenses, and more satisfied patients the key criteria for value-based reimbursement models. While healthcare systems move towards value-based terms, RPM is a useful means of attaining improved health outcomes at lesser expenses.

The economic implications of RPM for healthcare systems are substantial and include cost savings, reduced hospitalizations, and the promotion of value-based care models. Healthcare systems can ensure improved efficiency, affordability, and sustainability in care delivery if they use RPM to reduce avoidable admissions while optimizing resource use and enhancing patient outcomes. As RPM continues to evolve and expand, its changing economic impact will considerably influence the future of healthcare delivery and reimbursement [124].

FUTURE TRENDS

The progression of sensor technology marks RPM trends in the future, increased application to other healthcare sectors, and worldwide appropriation. The current developments in sensor technology have made RPM tools more precise, sophisticated, and adaptive, which has resulted in miniaturization, high battery life that can last longer periods, and improved connectivity options. These advancements will improve the precision and reliability of data as well as time analysis, facilitating timely identification of health problems as well as personal interventions. Also, it is expected that RPM will go beyond traditional handling of chronic disorders to cover acute care, postoperative management, mental sickness monitoring systems, maternity-related issues- neonatal health included- as well as preventive wellness programs [125].

Expanding its perspective would allow RPM to cater to a variety of patient needs within many areas of healthcare. Moreover, the widespread acceptance of remote patient monitoring devices is expected to rise steeply due to factors such as mounting healthcare costs, aging populations, and breakthroughs in technology. Nations globally are beginning to see the worth or value of telehealth services for improving medical service delivery, reducing hospitalization rates, and raising patients' satisfaction levels. The COVID-19 pandemic has been a catalyst for the growing utilization and acceptance of RPM technologies, as well as other telehealth and remote monitoring solutions. RPM is expected to play an important role in healthcare systems globally by enhancing patient empowerment, facilitating remote care delivery, and population health management, given the changes in regulatory frameworks and expansion of reimbursement policies [125].

CONCLUSION

In conclusion, RPM is an innovative technology that has considerably shifted the way healthcare services are provided, and it provides a range of opportunities that will help improve patient healthcare, make it more cost-efficient, and enhance population health management. RPM employs advanced sensing technologies to move beyond conventional disease management to address acute cases, postsurgical monitoring, mental health illness, as well preventative wellness programs. The adoption of RPM worldwide is gaining momentum due to rising healthcare costs, the increasing number of older adults globally, and soaring acceptance of telehealth because of the influence of the COVID-19 pandemic on telehealth. The integration of RPM into healthcare systems across the globe ushers in a new epoch of distant care provision, patient empowerment, and value-based healthcare. As regulatory frameworks shift and reimbursement policies widen, RPM will remain central to shaping future healthcare, facilitating improved results, and increasing access to quality healthcare for patients in different populations. RPM is thus more than a paradigm shift or a promising pathway to take toward a more proactive, patient-centric, and sustainable healthcare system.

REFERENCES

[1]   A. Vegesna, M. Tran, M. Angelaccio, and S. Arcona, "Remote Patient Monitoring via Non-Invasive Digital Technologies: A Systematic Review", *Telemed. J. E Health,* vol. 23, no. 1, pp. 3-17, 2017. [http://dx.doi.org/10.1089/tmj.2016.0051] [PMID: 27116181]

[2] M.L. Taylor, E.E. Thomas, C.L. Snoswell, A.C. Smith, and L.J. Caffery, "Does remote patient monitoring reduce acute care use? A systematic review", *BMJ Open*, vol. 11, no. 3, p. e040232, 2021. [http://dx.doi.org/10.1136/bmjopen-2020-040232] [PMID: 33653740]

[3] A. Murdan and J. Ramphul, "LoRa-based Smart Patient Monitoring System," *J. Telecom. Elect. Comp. Eng. (JTEC)*, vol. 15, no. 1, pp. 15–20, 2023.

[4] Correct ref.: Sana F, Isselbacher EM, Singh JP, Heist EK, Pathik B, Armoundas AA. "Wearable devices for ambulatory cardiac monitoring: JACC state-of-the-art review". *Journal of the American College of Cardiology*. 2020 Apr 7;75(13):1582-92

[5] R. L. Bashshur and G. W. Shannon, *History of Telemedicine: Evolution, Context, and Transformation*. New Rochelle, NY: Mary Ann Liebert, Inc., 2009.

[6] N. El-Rashidy, S. El-Sappagh, S.M.R. Islam, H. M El-Bakry, and S. Abdelrazek, "Mobile health in remote patient monitoring for chronic diseases: Principles, trends, and challenges", *Diagnostics (Basel)*, vol. 11, no. 4, p. 607, 2021. [http://dx.doi.org/10.3390/diagnostics11040607] [PMID: 33805471]

[7] M. Abulaiti, Y. Yalikun, K. Murata, A. Sato, M.M. Sami, Y. Sasaki, Y. Fujiwara, K. Minatoya, Y. Shiba, Y. Tanaka, and H. Masumoto, "Establishment of a heart-on-a-chip microdevice based on human iPS cells for the evaluation of human heart tissue function", *Sci. Rep.*, vol. 10, no. 1, p. 19201, 2020. [http://dx.doi.org/10.1038/s41598-020-76062-w] [PMID: 33154509]

[8] Y. Yang, "Remote monitoring of implantable cardioverter-defibrillators from 2006 to 2010: patterns of utilization and the impact of new current procedural terminology codes", 2013. Available from: http://elischolar.library.yale.edu/ysphtdl/1331

[9] Su CR, Hajiyev J, Fu CJ, Kao KC, Chang CH, Chang CT. A novel framework for a remote patient monitoring (RPM) system with abnormality detection. *Health Policy and Technology*. 2019 Jun 1;8(2):157-70. [http://dx.doi.org/10.1016/j.hlpt.2019.05.008]

[10] E.E. Thomas, M.L. Taylor, A. Banbury, C.L. Snoswell, H.M. Haydon, V.M. Gallegos Rejas, A.C. Smith, and L.J. Caffery, "Factors influencing the effectiveness of remote patient monitoring interventions: a realist review", *BMJ Open*, vol. 11, no. 8, p. e051844, 2021. [http://dx.doi.org/10.1136/bmjopen-2021-051844] [PMID: 34433611]

[11] C.J. Hayes, L. Dawson, H. McCoy, M. Hernandez, J. Andersen, M.M. Ali, C.A. Bogulski, and H. Eswaran, "Utilization of Remote Patient Monitoring Within the United States Health Care System: A Scoping Review", *Telemed. J. E Health*, vol. 29, no. 3, pp. 384-394, 2023. [http://dx.doi.org/10.1089/tmj.2022.0111] [PMID: 35819861]

[12] F. Zhang, K.Y. Qu, B. Zhou, Y. Luo, Z. Zhu, D.J. Pan, C. Cui, Y. Zhu, M.L. Chen, and N.P. Huang, "Design and fabrication of an integrated heart-on-a-chip platform for construction of cardiac tissue from human iPSC-derived cardiomyocytes and *in situ* evaluation of physiological function", *Biosensors and Bioelectronics*, vol. 1, no. 179, p. 113080, 2021.

[13] D.M. Hilty, C.M. Armstrong, A. Edwards-Stewart, M.T. Gentry, D.D. Luxton, and E.A. Krupinski, "Sensor, Wearable, and Remote Patient Monitoring Competencies for Clinical Care and Training: Scoping Review", *J. Technol. Behav. Sci.*, vol. 6, no. 2, pp. 252-277, 2021. [http://dx.doi.org/10.1007/s41347-020-00190-3] [PMID: 33501372]

[14] I. Ishaq, D. Carels, G. Teklemariam, J. Hoebeke, F. Abeele, E. Poorter, I. Moerman, and P. Demeester, "IETF Standardization in the Field of the Internet of Things (IoT): A Survey", *Journal of Sensor and Actuator Networks*, vol. 2, no. 2, pp. 235-287, 2013. [http://dx.doi.org/10.3390/jsan2020235]

[15] M. R. Islam, M. R. Islam, and T. A. Mazumder, "Mobile application and its global impact", *Int J Eng Technol*, vol. 10, no. 6, pp. 72-78, 2010.

[16] T.H. Davenport, "From analytics to artificial intelligence", *Journal of Business Analytics,* vol. 1, no. 2, pp. 73-80, 2018.
[http://dx.doi.org/10.1080/2573234X.2018.1543535]

[17] W.R. Smith, A.J. Atala, R.P. Terlecki, E.E. Kelly, and C.A. Matthews, "Implementation Guide for Rapid Integration of an Outpatient Telemedicine Program During the COVID-19 Pandemic", *J. Am. Coll. Surg.,* vol. 231, no. 2, pp. 216-222.e2, 2020.
[http://dx.doi.org/10.1016/j.jamcollsurg.2020.04.030] [PMID: 32360960]

[18] C. Gong, J. Liu, Q. Zhang, H. Chen, and Z. Gong, "The characteristics of cloud computing", *Proceedings of the International Conference on Parallel Processing Workshops,* 2010, pp. 275-279

[19] F.J. Tarazona-Santabalbina, A. Belenguer-Varea, E. Rovira-Daudi, and D. Cuesta-Peredó, "Orthogeriatric care: improving patient outcomes", *Clin. Interv. Aging,* vol. 11, pp. 843-856, 2016.
[http://dx.doi.org/10.2147/CIA.S72436] [PMID: 27445466]

[20] A. Gupta, and G.C. Fonarow, "The Hospital Readmissions Reduction Program—learning from failure of a healthcare policy", *Eur. J. Heart Fail.,* vol. 20, no. 8, pp. 1169-1174, 2018.
[http://dx.doi.org/10.1002/ejhf.1212] [PMID: 29791084]

[21] G.S. Fischer, R.R. Righi, C.A. Costa, G. Galante, and D. Griebler, "R. da R. Righi, C. A. da Costa, G. Galante, and D. Griebler, "Towards evaluating proactive and reactive approaches on reorganizing human resources in IoT-based smart hospitals,"", *Sensors (Basel),* vol. 19, no. 17, p. 3800, 2019.
[http://dx.doi.org/10.3390/s19173800] [PMID: 31480772]

[22] W.H. Shrank, T.L. Rogstad, and N. Parekh, "Waste in the US Health Care System", *JAMA,* vol. 322, no. 15, pp. 1501-1509, 2019.
[http://dx.doi.org/10.1001/jama.2019.13978] [PMID: 31589283]

[23] E.J. Comino, G.P. Davies, Y. Krastev, M. Haas, B. Christl, J. Furler, A. Raymont, and M.F. Harris, "A systematic review of interventions to enhance access to best practice primary health care for chronic disease management, prevention and episodic care", *BMC Health Serv. Res.,* vol. 12, no. 1, p. 415, 2012.
[http://dx.doi.org/10.1186/1472-6963-12-415] [PMID: 23170843]

[24] A.D. van Halteren, M. Munneke, E. Smit, S. Thomas, B.R. Bloem, and S.K.L. Darweesh, "Personalized Care Management for Persons with Parkinson's Disease", *J. Parkinsons Dis.,* vol. 10, no. s1, pp. S11-S20, 2020.
[http://dx.doi.org/10.3233/JPD-202126] [PMID: 32925110]

[25] A.R. Kunduru, "Cloud BPM Application (Appian) Robotic Process Automation Capabilities", *Asian J. Res. Comput. Sci.s,* vol. 16, no. 3, pp. 267-280, 2023.
[http://dx.doi.org/10.9734/ajrcos/2023/v16i3361]

[26] N. Vemuri, N. Thaneeru, and V.M. Tatikonda, "AI-Optimized DevOps for Streamlined Cloud CI/CD",

[27] R.K. Cross, and S. Kane, "Integration of Telemedicine Into Clinical Gastroenterology and Hepatology Practice", *Clin. Gastroenterol. Hepatol.,* vol. 15, no. 2, pp. 175-181, 2017.
[http://dx.doi.org/10.1016/j.cgh.2016.09.011] [PMID: 27989663]

[28] Bokolo Anthony Jnr, "Use of Telemedicine and Virtual Care for Remote Treatment in Response to COVID-19 Pandemic", *J. Med. Syst.,* vol. 44, no. 7, p. 132, 2020.
[http://dx.doi.org/10.1007/s10916-020-01596-5] [PMID: 32542571]

[29] J. F. Imberti, A. Tosetti, D. A. Mei, A. Maisano, and G. Boriani, J. F. Imberti, A. Tosetti, D. A. Mei, A. Maisano, and G. Boriani, "Remote monitoring and telemedicine in heart failure: Implementation and benefits", *Curr Cardiol Rep,* vol. 23, no. 6, pp. 55-55, 2021.
[http://dx.doi.org/10.1007/s11886-021-01487-2]

[30] C. Liddy, I. Moroz, A. Mihan, N. Nawar, and E. Keely, "A Systematic Review of Asynchronous, Provider-to-Provider, Electronic Consultation Services to Improve Access to Specialty Care Available Worldwide", *Telemed. J. E Health,* vol. 25, no. 3, pp. 184-198, 2019.

[http://dx.doi.org/10.1089/tmj.2018.0005] [PMID: 29927711]

[31]   R. Wootton, "Twenty years of telemedicine in chronic disease management – an evidence synthesis", *J. Telemed. Telecare,* vol. 18, no. 4, pp. 211-220, 2012.
[http://dx.doi.org/10.1258/jtt.2012.120219] [PMID: 22674020]

[32]   A. Asiri, S. AlBishi, W. AlMadani, A. ElMetwally, and M. Househ, "The use of telemedicine in surgical care: A systematic review", *Acta Informatica Medica* vol. 26. no. 3, pp. 201-206. 2018.
[http://dx.doi.org/10.5455/aim.2018.26.201-206]

[33]   M.E. Badowski, E.A. Wright, J. Bainbridge, S.M. Michienzi, S.D. Nichols, K.M. Turner, C. Wicke, J. Awad, A. Thompkins, and R.D. Martin, "Implementation and evaluation of comprehensive medication management in telehealth practices", *J. Am. Coll. Clin. Pharm.,* vol. 3, no. 2, pp. 520-531, 2020.
[http://dx.doi.org/10.1002/jac5.1210]

[34]   C. M. Contreras, G. A. Metzger, J. D. Beane, P. H. Dedhia, A. Ejaz, and T. M. Pawlik, "Telemedicine: Patient-provider clinical engagement during the COVID-19 pandemic and beyond", *J Gastrointest Surg,* vol. 24, no. 7, pp. 1692-1697, 2020.
[http://dx.doi.org/10.1007/s11605-020-04623-5]

[35]   L. Shawwa, "The Use of Telemedicine in Medical Education and Patient Care", *Cureus,* vol. 15, no. 4, p. e37766, 2023.
[http://dx.doi.org/10.7759/cureus.37766] [PMID: 37213963]

[36]   N. Zwar, M. Harris, R. Griffiths, M. Roland, S. Dennis, G. Powell Davies, and T. Harris, "A systematic review of chronic disease management", *Aust Prim Health Care Res Inst,* 2006. . Available from: http://aphcri.anu.edu.au/projects/network/systematic-review-chronic-disease-management

[37]   U. Alam, O. Asghar, S. Azmi, and R. A. Malik, U. Alam, O. Asghar, S. Azmi, and R. A. Malik, "General aspects of diabetes mellitus", *Handb Clin Neurol,* vol. 126, pp. 211-222, 2014.
[http://dx.doi.org/10.1016/B978-0-444-53480-4.00015-1]

[38]   L. Dayer, S. Heldenbrand, P. Anderson, P.O. Gubbins, and B.C. Martin, "Smartphone medication adherence apps: Potential benefits to patients and providers", *J. Am. Pharm. Assoc. (Wash. D.C.),* vol. 53, no. 2, pp. 172-181, 2013.
[http://dx.doi.org/10.1331/JAPhA.2013.12202] [PMID: 23571625]

[39]   V. Sharma, M. Feldman, and R. Sharma, "Telehealth Technologies in Diabetes Self-management and Education", *J. Diabetes Sci. Technol.,* vol. 18, no. 1, pp. 148-158, 2024.
[http://dx.doi.org/10.1177/19322968221093078] [PMID: 35485769]

[40]   E.B. Kirkland, E. Johnson, C. Bays, J. Marsden, R. Verdin, D. Ford, K. King, and K.R. Sterba, "Diabetes Remote Monitoring Program Implementation: A Mixed Methods Analysis of Delivery Strategies, Barriers and Facilitators", *Telemedicine Reports,* vol. 4, no. 1, pp. 30-43, 2023.
[http://dx.doi.org/10.1089/tmr.2022.0038] [PMID: 36950477]

[41]   T. Shaik, X Tao, N Higgins, L Li, R Gururajan, X Zhou, and U.R. Acharya, "Remote patient monitoring using artificial intelligence: Current state, applications, and challenges", *Wiley Interdisciplinary Reviews: Data Mining and Knowledge Discovery,* vol. 13, no. 2, p. e1485, 2023.

[42]   R. Eenheid, "Studiecoördinatiecentrum, Hypertensie en Cardiovasculaire Essential hypertension", 2003. Available from: https://www.thelancet.com/

[43]   F.H. Messerli, B. Williams, and E. Ritz, "Essential hypertension", 2007. Available from: https://www.thelancet.com
[http://dx.doi.org/10.1016/S0140-6736(07)61299-9]

[44]   M.M. Ibrahim, and A. Damasceno, "Hypertension in developing countries", In: *The Lancet* vol. 380. Elsevier B.V., 2012, no. 9841, pp. 611-619.
[http://dx.doi.org/10.1016/S0140-6736(12)60861-7]

[45]   N.M. Kaplan, R.G. Victor, and N.M. Kaplan, *Kaplan's clinical hypertension.* Wolters Kluwer Health/Lippincott Williams & Wilkins, 2010.

[46] E.I. Anyaegbu, and V.R. Dharnidharka, "Hypertension in the Teenager", *Pediatr. Clin. North Am.,* vol. 61, no. 1, pp. 131-151, 2014.
[http://dx.doi.org/10.1016/j.pcl.2013.09.011] [PMID: 24267462]

[47] H. Fröhlich, "Theory of the superconducting state. I. The ground state at the absolute zero of temperature", *Adv Phys,* vol. 3, no. 4, pp. 325-362, 1954.

[48] N.M. Kaplan, and L.H. Opie, "Series Controversies in Cardiology 2 Controversies in hypertension", 2006. Available from: www.thelancet.com

[49] J.I.E. Hoffman, S. Kaplan, and R.R. Liberthson, "Prevalence of congenital heart disease", *Am. Heart J.,* vol. 147, no. 3, pp. 425-439, 2004.
[http://dx.doi.org/10.1016/j.ahj.2003.05.003] [PMID: 14999190]

[50] D. J. P. Barker, *Fetal origins of coronary heart disease,* 1995.
[http://dx.doi.org/10.1136/bmj.311.6998.171]

[51] O. Paul, "A Longitudinal Study of Coronary Heart Disease", 1963. Available from: http://ahajournals.org
[http://dx.doi.org/10.1161/01.CIR.28.1.20]

[52] van Wheel C, van Grunsven P. Resistance to prescribing and to antibiotics. The Lancet. 1999;354(9184):1052., *PIIS0140673698102799,* 1999.

[53] E. Marijon, M. Mirabel, D.S. Celermajer, and X. Jouven, "Rheumatic heart disease", In: *The Lancet.* Elsevier B.V., 2012, pp. 953-964.
[http://dx.doi.org/10.1016/S0140-6736(11)61171-9]

[54] A. Bookman, and D. Kimbrel, "Families and elder care in the twenty-first century", 2011. Available from: www.futureofchildren.org
[http://dx.doi.org/10.1353/foc.2011.0018]

[55] F. G. Miskelly, "Assistive technology in elderly care", *Age Ageing,* vol. 30, no. 6, pp. 455-458, 2001.
[http://dx.doi.org/10.1093/ageing/30.6.455]

[56] X. Wang, J. Ellul, and G. Azzopardi, "Elderly Fall Detection Systems: A Literature Survey", *Front. Robot. AI,* vol. 7, p. 71, 2020.
[http://dx.doi.org/10.3389/frobt.2020.00071] [PMID: 33501238]

[57] L.P. Serrano, K.C. Maita, F.R. Avila, R.A. Torres-Guzman, J.P. Garcia, A.S. Eldaly, C.R. Haider, C.L. Felton, M.R. Paulson, M.J. Maniaci, and A.J. Forte, "Benefits and challenges of remote patient monitoring as perceived by health care practitioners: a systematic review", *The Permanente Journal,* vol. 27, no. 4, p. 100, 2023.

[58] T. Xu, Y. Zhou, and J. Zhu, "New advances and challenges of fall detection systems: A survey", *Appl. Sci. (Basel),* vol. 8, no. 3, p. 418, 2018.
[http://dx.doi.org/10.3390/app8030418]

[59] X. Yu, "Approaches and principles of fall detection for elderly and patient", *Proc 10th IEEE Int Conf e-Health Netw Appl Serv (HealthCom),* 2008pp. 42-47
[http://dx.doi.org/10.1109/HEALTH.2008.4600107]

[60] W. Y. Lam and P. Fresco, "Medication Adherence Measures: An Overview", In: *BioMed Research International* Hindawi Publishing Corporation, 2015.
[http://dx.doi.org/10.1155/2015/217047]

[61] B. Noah, M.S. Keller, S. Mosadeghi, L. Stein, S. Johl, S. Delshad, V.C. Tashjian, D. Lew, J.T. Kwan, A. Jusufagic, and B.M. Spiegel, "Impact of remote patient monitoring on clinical outcomes: an updated meta-analysis of randomized controlled trials", *NPJ digital medicine,* vol. 1, no. 1, p. 20172, 2018.

[62] H.Y.K. Ko, N.K. Tripathi, C. Mozumder, S. Muengtaweepongsa, and I. Pal, "Real-Time Remote Patient Monitoring and Alarming System for Noncommunicable Lifestyle Diseases", *Int. J. Telemed.*

Appl., vol. 2023, pp. 1-13, 2023.
[http://dx.doi.org/10.1155/2023/9965226] [PMID: 38020047]

[63]   A. Parihar, J.B. Prajapati, B.G. Prajapati, B. Trambadiya, A. Thakkar, and P. Engineer, "Role of IOT in healthcare: Applications, security & privacy concerns", *Intelligent Pharmacy,* vol. 2, no. 5, pp. 707-714, 2024.
[http://dx.doi.org/10.1016/j.ipha.2024.01.003]

[64]   B. Jimmy, and J. Jose, *Patient Medication Adherence: Measures in Daily Practice,* 2011.
[http://dx.doi.org/10.5001/omj.2011.38]

[65]   A. Revathi, R. Kaladevi, K. Ramana, R.H. Jhaveri, M. Rudra Kumar, and M. Sankara Prasanna Kumar, "Early Detection of Cognitive Decline Using Machine Learning Algorithm and Cognitive Ability Test", *Secur. Commun. Netw.,* vol. 2022, pp. 1-13, 2022.
[http://dx.doi.org/10.1155/2022/4190023]

[66]   R. Rosli, M.P. Tan, W.K. Gray, P. Subramanian, and A.V. Chin, "Cognitive assessment tools in Asia: a systematic review", *Int. Psychogeriatr.,* vol. 28, no. 2, pp. 189-210, 2016.
[http://dx.doi.org/10.1017/S1041610215001635] [PMID: 26450414]

[67]   S.A. Polevaya, E.V. Eremin, N.A. Bulanov, A.V. Bakhchina, A.V. Kovalchuk, and S.B. Parin, ""Event-related telemetry of heart rate for personalized remote monitoring of cognitive functions and stress under conditions of everyday activity," Sovremennye tehnologii v", *Sovrem. Tekhnologii Med.,* vol. 11, no. 1, pp. 109-114, 2019.
[http://dx.doi.org/10.17691/stm2019.11.1.13]

[68]   M. Lee, R.K. Mishra, A. Momin, N. El-Refaei, A.B. Bagheri, M.K. York, M.E. Kunik, M. Derhammer, B. Fatehi, J. Lim, R. Cole, G. Barchard, A. Vaziri, and B. Najafi, "Smart-Home Concept for Remote Monitoring of Instrumental Activities of Daily Living (IADL) in Older Adults with Cognitive Impairment: A Proof of Concept and Feasibility Study", *Sensors (Basel),* vol. 22, no. 18, p. 6745, 2022.
[http://dx.doi.org/10.3390/s22186745] [PMID: 36146095]

[69]   P.S. Foong, C.A. Lim, J. Wong, C.S. Lim, S.T. Perrault, and G.C.H. Koh, "You Cannot Offer Such a Suggestion': Designing for Family Caregiver Input in Home Care Systems", *Conference on Human Factors in Computing Systems - Proceedings,* 2020
[http://dx.doi.org/10.1145/3313831.3376607]

[70]   V.L. Tiase, W. Hull, M.M. McFarland, K.A. Sward, G. Del Fiol, C. Staes, C. Weir, and M.R. Cummins, "Patient-generated health data and electronic health record integration: a scoping review", *JAMIA Open,* vol. 3, no. 4, pp. 619-627, 2021.
[http://dx.doi.org/10.1093/jamiaopen/ooaa052] [PMID: 33758798]

[71]   M.P. Patel, P. Schettini, C.P. O'Leary, H.B. Bosworth, J.B. Anderson, and K.P. Shah, "Closing the Referral Loop: an Analysis of Primary Care Referrals to Specialists in a Large Health System", *J. Gen. Intern. Med.,* vol. 33, no. 5, pp. 715-721, 2018.
[http://dx.doi.org/10.1007/s11606-018-4392-z] [PMID: 29532299]

[72]   A. Coulter, A. Noone, and M. Goldacre, "General practitioners' referrals to specialist outpatient clinics. I. Why general practitioners refer patients to specialist outpatient clinics," *BMJ*, vol. 299, no. 6694, pp. 304–306, Jul. 1989.

[73]   M.T. Donohoe, R.L. Kravitz, D.B. Wheeler, R. Chandra, A. Chen, and N. Humphries, "Reasons for outpatient referrals from generalists to specialists", *J. Gen. Intern. Med.,* vol. 14, no. 5, pp. 281-286, 1999.
[http://dx.doi.org/10.1046/j.1525-1497.1999.00324.x] [PMID: 10337037]

[74]   Jones SB, Schumann R, Jones DB. Post-anesthesia care unit: management of anesthetic and surgical complications. Morbid Obesity. 2010 Jan 1:155.
http://ndl.ethernet.edu.et/bitstream/123456789/24712/1/7.pdf#page=173

[75]   F.T.Z. Khanam, A. Al-Naji, and J. Chahl, "Remote monitoring of vital signs in diverse non-clinical

and clinical scenarios using computer vision systems: A review", *Appl. Sci. (Basel),* vol. 9, no. 20, p. 4474, 2019.
[http://dx.doi.org/10.3390/app9204474]

[76] C. Li, J. Cummings, J. Lam, E. Graves, and W. Wu, "Radar remote monitoring of vital signs", *IEEE Microw. Mag.,* vol. 10, no. 1, pp. 47-56, 2009.
[http://dx.doi.org/10.1109/MMM.2008.930675]

[77] N. Kalid, A. A. Zaidan, B. B. Zaidan, O. H. Salman, M. Hashim, and H. Muzammil, "Based real time remote health monitoring systems: A review on patients prioritization and related 'big data' using body sensors information and communication technology," *J. Med. Sys.,* vol. 42, no. 2, pp. 1–30, 2018.

[78] N. Selvaraj, "Long-term remote monitoring of vital signs using a wireless patch sensor," In: *IEEE Healthcare Innovation Conference (HIC)*, Seattle, WA, USA, 2014, pp. 83-86.
[http://dx.doi.org/10.1109/HIC.2014.7038880]

[79] I. Mastoris, E.M. DeFilippis, T. Martyn, A.A. Morris, H.G. Van Spall, and A.J. Sauer, "Remote Patient Monitoring for Patients with Heart Failure: Sex- and Race-based Disparities and Opportunities", In: *Cardiac Failure Review*. vol. 9. Radcliffe Medical Media, 2023.
[http://dx.doi.org/10.15420/cfr.2022.22]

[80] C. Li, and J. Wang, "S. Wang, and Y. Zhang, "A review of IoT applications in healthcare,"", *Neurocomputing,* vol. 565, 2024.
[http://dx.doi.org/10.1016/j.neucom.2023.127017]

[81] A. Haleem, M. Javaid, R. P. Singh, and R. Suman, "Telemedicine for healthcare: Capabilities, features, barriers, and applications", *Sensors International,* vol. 2, KeAi Communications Co., 2021.
[http://dx.doi.org/10.1016/j.sintl.2021.100117]

[82] S.W. Moon, J.J. Kim, D.G. Cho, and J.K. Park, "Early detection of complications: anastomotic leakage", *J. Thorac. Dis.,* vol. 11, no. S5, suppl. Suppl. 5, pp. S805-S811, 2019.
[http://dx.doi.org/10.21037/jtd.2018.11.55] [PMID: 31080662]

[83] D.J. Sugarbaker, M.T. Jaklitsch, R. Bueno, W. Richards, J. Lukanich, S.J. Mentzer, Y. Colson, P. Linden, M. Chang, L. Capalbo, E. Oldread, S. Neragi-Miandoab, S.J. Swanson, and L.S. Zellos, "Prevention, early detection, and management of complications after 328 consecutive extrapleural pneumonectomies", *J. Thorac. Cardiovasc. Surg.,* vol. 128, no. 1, pp. 138-146, 2004.
[http://dx.doi.org/10.1016/j.jtcvs.2004.02.021] [PMID: 15224033]

[84] F. Healey, D.S. Sanders, T. Lamont, J. Scarpello, and T. Agbabiaka, "Early detection of complications after gastrostomy: summary of a safety report from the National Patient Safety Agency", *BMJ,* vol. 340, no. may04 2, p. c2160, 2010.
[http://dx.doi.org/10.1136/bmj.c2160] [PMID: 20442227]

[85] H.M.K. Ghomrawi, M.K. O'Brien, M. Carter, R. Macaluso, R. Khazanchi, M. Fanton, C. DeBoer, S.C. Linton, S. Zeineddin, J.B. Pitt, M. Bouchard, A. Figueroa, S. Kwon, J.L. Holl, A. Jayaraman, and F. Abdullah, "Applying machine learning to consumer wearable data for the early detection of complications after pediatric appendectomy", *NPJ Digit. Med.,* vol. 6, no. 1, p. 148, 2023.
[http://dx.doi.org/10.1038/s41746-023-00890-z] [PMID: 37587211]

[86] S. M. Marshall, and A. Flyvbjerg, *Clinical review Prevention and early detection of vascular complications of diabetes,* 2006.

[87] E. Latifah, K. Siregar, and D. Delmaifanis, "The Role of Digital Health in the Early Detection and Management of Obstetric Complications in the Community: A Systematic Review", *Open Access Maced J Med Sci,* vol. 11, no. F, pp. 143-155, 2023.
[http://dx.doi.org/10.3889/oamjms.2023.11391]

[88] M. Ellebæk, and N. Qvist, "Early detection and the prevention of serious complications of anastomotic leakage in rectal cancer surgery", *Tech. Coloproctol.,* vol. 18, no. 1, pp. 1-2, 2014.
[http://dx.doi.org/10.1007/s10151-013-1025-8] [PMID: 23633242]

[89]   R.B. Zuckerman, S.H. Sheingold, E.J. Orav, J. Ruhter, and A.M. Epstein, "Readmissions, Observation, and the Hospital Readmissions Reduction Program", *N. Engl. J. Med.,* vol. 374, no. 16, pp. 1543-1551, 2016.
[http://dx.doi.org/10.1056/NEJMsa1513024] [PMID: 26910198]

[90]   D. Zhang, I. Gurvich, J. A. Van Mieghem, E. Park, R. Young, and M. Williams, "Hospital Readmissions Reduction Program: An economic and operational analysis," *Manag. Sci.,* vol. 62, no. 11, pp. 3351–3371, Nov. 2016.

[91]   C.K. McIlvennan, Z.J. Eapen, and L.A. Allen, "Hospital readmissions reduction program", *Circulation,* vol. 131, no. 20, pp. 1796-1803, 2015.
[http://dx.doi.org/10.1161/CIRCULATIONAHA.114.010270] [PMID: 25986448]

[92]   M.G. Kibria, K. Nguyen, G.P. Villardi, O. Zhao, K. Ishizu, and F. Kojima, "Big Data Analytics, Machine Learning, and Artificial Intelligence in Next-Generation Wireless Networks", *IEEE Access,* vol. 6, pp. 32328-32338, 2018.
[http://dx.doi.org/10.1109/ACCESS.2018.2837692]

[93]   N. Mehta, A. Pandit, and S. Shukla, "Transforming healthcare with big data analytics and artificial intelligence: A systematic mapping study", *J. Biomed. Inform.,* vol. 100, p. 103311, 2019.
[http://dx.doi.org/10.1016/j.jbi.2019.103311] [PMID: 31629922]

[94]   S. Bose, S.K. Dey, and S. Bhattacharjee, "Big data, data analytics, and artificial intelligence in accounting: An overview", In: *Handbook of Big Data Research Methods.* Edward Elgar Publishing Ltd., 2023, pp. 32-51.
[http://dx.doi.org/10.4337/9781800888555.00007]

[95]   A.M. Rahmani, E. Azhir, S. Ali, M. Mohammadi, O.H. Ahmed, M. Yassin Ghafour, S. Hasan Ahmed, and M. Hosseinzadeh, "Artificial intelligence approaches and mechanisms for big data analytics: a systematic study", *PeerJ Comput. Sci.,* vol. 7, p. e488, 2021.
[http://dx.doi.org/10.7717/peerj-cs.488] [PMID: 33954253]

[96]   S.B. Golas, M. Nikolova-Simons, R. Palacholla, J. op den Buijs, G. Garberg, A. Orenstein, and J. Kvedar, "Predictive analytics and tailored interventions improve clinical outcomes in older adults: a randomized controlled trial", *NPJ Digit. Med.,* vol. 4, no. 1, p. 97, 2021.
[http://dx.doi.org/10.1038/s41746-021-00463-y] [PMID: 34112921]

[97]   "World Health Organization", In: *Monitoring the building blocks of health systems a handbook of indicators and their measurement strategies.* World Health Organization, 2010.

[98]   B. Mahesh, "Machine Learning Algorithms-A Review", *Int. J. Sci. Res.,* vol. 9, 2018.
[http://dx.doi.org/10.21275/ART20203995]

[99]   V. Kumar, and M. L, "Predictive Analytics: A Review of Trends and Techniques", *Int. J. Comput. Appl.,* vol. 182, no. 1, pp. 31-37, 2018.
[http://dx.doi.org/10.5120/ijca2018917434]

[100] V. Chandola, A. Banerjee, and V. Kumar, "Anomaly detection: A survey," *ACM Computing Surveys,* vol. 41, no. 3, Art. no. 15, pp. 1–58, 2009.

[101] L.H. Goetz, and N.J. Schork, "Personalized medicine: motivation, challenges, and progress", *Fertil. Steril.,* vol. 109, no. 6, pp. 952-963, 2018.
[http://dx.doi.org/10.1016/j.fertnstert.2018.05.006] [PMID: 29935653]

[102] B.W. Mamlin, J.M. Overhage, W. Tierney, P. Dexter, and C.J. McDonald, "Clinical Decision Support Within the Regenstrief Medical Record System", In: *Clinical Decision Support Systems* Springer New York, 2007, pp. 190-214.
[http://dx.doi.org/10.1007/978-0-387-38319-4_9]

[103] R.T. Sutton, D. Pincock, D.C. Baumgart, D.C. Sadowski, R.N. Fedorak, and K.I. Kroeker, "An overview of clinical decision support systems: benefits, risks, and strategies for success", *NPJ Digit. Med.,* vol. 3, no. 1, p. 17, 2020.

[http://dx.doi.org/10.1038/s41746-020-0221-y] [PMID: 32047862]

[104] Z. Wen, S. Wang, D. M. Yang, Y. Xie, M. Chen, J. Bishop, and G. Xiao, "Deep learning in digital pathology for personalized treatment plans of cancer patients," *Sem. Diag. Patho.*, vol. 40, no. 2, pp. 109–119, Mar. 2023.
[http://dx.doi.org/10.1053/j.semdp.2023.02.003]

[105] Drancourt N, Roger-Leroi V, Martignon S, Jablonski-Momeni A, Pitts N, Doméjean S. Carious lesion activity assessment in clinical practice: A systematic review. *Clinical Oral Investigations.* 2019 Apr 10;23(4):1513-24.
[http://dx.doi.org/10.1007/s00784-019-02839-7]

[106] I. Sánchez-Garzón, J. Fdez-Olivares, E. Onaindía, G. Milla, J. Jordán, and P. Castejón, "A multi-agent planning approach for the generation of personalized treatment plans of comorbid patients", In: *Lecture Notes in Computer Science (including subseries Lecture Notes in Artificial Intelligence and Lecture Notes in Bioinformatics)* Springer Verlag, 2013, pp. 23-27.
[http://dx.doi.org/10.1007/978-3-642-38326-7_4]

[107] S.N. Mohsin, A. Gapizov, C. Ekhator, N.U. Ain, S. Ahmad, M. Khan, C. Barker, M. Hussain, J. Malineni, A. Ramadhan, and R. Halappa Nagaraj, "The Role of Artificial Intelligence in Prediction, Risk Stratification, and Personalized Treatment Planning for Congenital Heart Diseases", *Cureus,* vol. 15, no. 8, p. e44374, 2023.
[http://dx.doi.org/10.7759/cureus.44374] [PMID: 37664359]

[108] M. L. Pedersen, "Diabetes care in the dispersed population of Greenland. A new model based on continued monitoring, analysis and adjustment of initiatives taken", In: *International Journal of Circumpolar Health* vol. 78. Taylor and Francis Ltd., 2019.
[http://dx.doi.org/10.1080/22423982.2019.1709257]

[109] J.E. Prey, J. Woollen, L. Wilcox, A.D. Sackeim, G. Hripcsak, S. Bakken, S. Restaino, S. Feiner, and D.K. Vawdrey, "Patient engagement in the inpatient setting: a systematic review", *J. Am. Med. Inform. Assoc.,* vol. 21, no. 4, pp. 742-750, 2014.
[http://dx.doi.org/10.1136/amiajnl-2013-002141] [PMID: 24272163]

[110] E. Hickmann, P. Richter, and H. Schlieter, "All together now – patient engagement, patient empowerment, and associated terms in personal healthcare", *BMC Health Serv. Res.,* vol. 22, no. 1, p. 1116, 2022.
[http://dx.doi.org/10.1186/s12913-022-08501-5] [PMID: 36056354]

[111] M. S. Lipsky and L. K. Sharp, "From idea to market: the drug approval process," J. Ame. Board. Fam. Prac., vol. 14, no. 5, pp. 362–367, 2001. http://www.jabfm.org/

[112] J. Kwon, and M.E. Johnson, "Security practices and regulatory compliance in the healthcare industry", *J. Am. Med. Inform. Assoc.,* vol. 20, no. 1, pp. 44-51, 2013.
[http://dx.doi.org/10.1136/amiajnl-2012-000906] [PMID: 22955497]

[113] P. McCole, E. Ramsey, and J. Williams, "Trust considerations on attitudes towards online purchasing: The moderating effect of privacy and security concerns", *J. Bus. Res.,* vol. 63, no. 9-10, pp. 1018-1024, 2010.
[http://dx.doi.org/10.1016/j.jbusres.2009.02.025]

[114] P.C. Kumar, M. Chetty, T.L. Clegg, and J. Vitak, "Privacy and security considerations for digital technology use in elementary schools", In: *Conference on Human Factors in Computing Systems - Proceedings* Association for Computing Machinery, 2019.
[http://dx.doi.org/10.1145/3290605.3300537]

[115] M. Choummanivong, S. Karimi, J. Durham, V. Sychareun, V. Flenady, D. Horey, and F. Boyle, "Stillbirth in Lao PDR: a healthcare provider perspective", *Glob. Health Action,* vol. 13, no. sup2, p. 1786975, 2020.
[http://dx.doi.org/10.1080/16549716.2020.1786975] [PMID: 32741353]

[116] N. Jinga, C. Mongwenyana, A. Moolla, G. Malete, and D. Onoya, "Reasons for late presentation for

antenatal care, healthcare providers' perspective", *BMC Health Serv. Res.,* vol. 19, no. 1, p. 1016, 2019.
[http://dx.doi.org/10.1186/s12913-019-4855-x] [PMID: 31888616]

[117]   W. Agyemang-Duah, C.M. Mensah, P. Peprah, F. Arthur, and E.M. Abalo, "Facilitators of and barriers to the use of healthcare services from a user and provider perspective in Ejisu-Juaben municipality, Ghana", *J. Public Health (Berl.),* vol. 27, no. 2, pp. 133-142, 2019.
[http://dx.doi.org/10.1007/s10389-018-0946-0]

[118]   K. Innes, J. Morphet, A.P. O'Brien, and I. Munro, "Caring for the mental illness patient in emergency departments – an exploration of the issues from a healthcare provider perspective", *J. Clin. Nurs.,* vol. 23, no. 13-14, pp. 2003-2011, 2014.
[http://dx.doi.org/10.1111/jocn.12437] [PMID: 24313388]

[119]   S. Srivastava, and R.K. Singh, "Exploring integrated supply chain performance in healthcare: a service provider perspective", *Benchmarking (Bradf.),* vol. 28, no. 1, pp. 106-130, 2021.
[http://dx.doi.org/10.1108/BIJ-03-2020-0125]

[120]   D Marynowski-Traczyk, and M. Broadbent, "What are the experiences of emergency department nurses in caring for clients with a mental illness in the emergency department?", *Australasian Emergency Nursing Journal,* vol. 14, no. 3, pp. 172-9, 2011.

[121]   E. Glaeser, and J. Gyourko, "The economic implications of housing supply", In: *Journal of Economic Perspectives.* American Economic Association, 2018, pp. 3-29.
[http://dx.doi.org/10.1257/jep.32.1.3]

[122]   O. Heffetz, and R.H. Frank, "Chapter 3 - Preferences for Status: Evidence and Economic Implications", *Handbook of Social Economics,* vol. 1, pp. 69-91, 2011.

[123]   S. Wiggins, and S. Proctor, *How Special Are Rural Areas? The Economic Implications of Location for Rural Development.* Overseas Development Institute, 2001.
[http://dx.doi.org/10.1111/1467-7679.00142]

[124]   A.P. Dhawan, W.J. Heetderks, M. Pavel, S. Acharya, M. Akay, A. Mairal, B. Wheeler, C.C. Dacso, T. Sunder, N. Lovell, M. Gerber, M. Shah, S.G. Senthilvel, M.D. Wang, and B. Bhargava, "Current and Future Challenges in Point-of-Care Technologies: A Paradigm-Shift in Affordable Global Healthcare With Personalized and Preventive Medicine", *IEEE J. Transl. Eng. Health Med.,* vol. 3, pp. 1-10, 2015.
[http://dx.doi.org/10.1109/JTEHM.2015.2400919] [PMID: 27170902]

[125]   L.P. Malasinghe, N. Ramzan, and K. Dahal, "Remote patient monitoring: a comprehensive study", *J. Ambient Intell. Humaniz. Comput.,* vol. 10, no. 1, pp. 57-76, 2019.
[http://dx.doi.org/10.1007/s12652-017-0598-x]

CHAPTER 5

AI's Inroad into Medication Enhancement

Sunita[1], **Shaweta Sharma**[2], **Shekhar Singh**[3], **S. Govindarajan**[4] and **Akhil Sharma**[5,*]

[1] *Metro College of Health Sciences and Research, Greater Noida, Uttar Pradesh, India*

[2] *School of Medical and Allied Sciences, Galgotias University Plot No. 2, Yamuna Expy, Opposite Buddha International Circuit, Sector 17A, Greater Noida, Uttar Pradesh, India*

[3] *Faculty of Pharmacy, Babu Banarasi Das Northern India Institute of Technology, Lucknow, Uttar Pradesh, India*

[4] *Department of Civil Engineering, Aditya University, Surampalem, India*

[5] *R.J. College of Pharmacy, Raipur, Gharbara, Tappal, Khair, Uttar Pradesh, India*

Abstract: AI and pharmaceutical improvement crossroads are an incredible opportunity in healthcare that can transform drug discovery, development, and delivery. AI-based approaches such as predictive modeling, pattern recognition, and mining of biomedical literature are some of the methodologies that can be accelerated for the identification of promising drug candidates. AI empowers drug design and synthesis by analyzing unstructured data and representing complex biological systems–such as protein folding. Automated laboratory processes (*i.e.*, drug testing or synthesis) lead to faster and more efficient cycles of research. Virtual screening, de novo drug design, and repurposing existing drugs are some of the ways AI applications can help in medication to result in more precise and effective therapies. Predictive analysis facilitates the evaluation of treatment responses whereas real-time monitoring systems guarantee the safety of drugs *via* early detection of adverse drug reactions. Targeted drug delivery systems enhance drug delivery and effectiveness, leading to better patient outcomes. Such advancements not only accelerate the exploration of drug discovery but also lead to better diagnostic accuracy, patient safety, and resource distribution to give rise to an economical health care model. However, the application of AI for drug development has its obstacles, including concerns about data privacy, ethics, and transparency in AI algorithms. To unlock the full potential promise of AI in healthcare, these roadblocks must be overcome. The next steps are further streamlining of AI algorithms to improve precision, greater incorporation of AI in clinical decision support, and the development of regulatory frameworks to ensure the safe and ethical use of AI across various facets of patient care. In this paper, we briefly outline how AI has transformed aspects of medication enhancement from the perspective of benefits to patient-oriented care; and express how its current challenges will nevertheless facilitate advances and opportunities in the future of healthcare.

* **Corresponding author Akhil Sharma:** R.J. College of Pharmacy, Raipur, Gharbara, Tappal, Khair, Uttar Pradesh, India; E-mail: xs2akhil@gmail.com

Akhil Sharma, Neeraj Kumar Fuloria, Pankaj Kumar Singh & Shaweta Sharma (Eds.)
All rights reserved-© 2025 Bentham Science Publishers

Keywords: Artificial intelligence, Discovery, De novo drug design, Healthcare, High-throughput screening, Machine learning, Medication, Nanotechnology, Pharmacovigilance, Personalized medicine, Predictive analytics, Patients, Precision, Robotics, Repurposing, Targeted.

INTRODUCTION

Artificial Intelligence (AI) in the health care industry means utilizing state-of-the-art computer programs and methods to examine challenging medical information, perform activities usually performed by humans, and assist in clinical judgment. With technologies such as machine learning, natural language processing, computer vision, and robotics, among others, they can deduce information from data, decipher patterns, and provide insights at rates much faster than humans [1].

Various fields in healthcare apply AI, such as interpreting medical images, drug discovery, personalizing treatment recommendations, predictive analytics, virtual health assistants, and automating administrative duties. To help doctors detect diseases, anticipate patients' prognoses, and design curative approaches that suit individuals with different backgrounds, AI systems process huge amounts of data from patients' Electronic Health Records (EHRs), medical imaging scans, genetic profiles, wearable devices, and other sources [2].

AI has the potential to completely change healthcare administration by increasing diagnostic accuracy, leading to more effective treatment modalities, improved operational efficiencies, and ultimately, better patient care outcomes. However, this comes with issues such as data privacy, regulatory compliance, algorithm transparency, bias mitigation, and ethical aspects, among other difficult questions that must be addressed continually to guarantee the responsible and fair implementation of AI within any health system [3].

There is an improvement in medication whereby drugs can be made to function better, safer, and easier to get. Enhanced medications also have the potential to improve treatment outcomes by enabling better targeting of diseases. Through AI-facilitated innovative drug discovery techniques, drugs can be tailored toward disease pathways, thus increasing their efficiency and possibly enabling reduced reliance on higher doses or a combination of different medicines [4].

Attempts to enhance drugs aim at reducing the negative impact of pharmaceutical therapies. Enhanced medications are designed to decrease the frequency and intensity of side effects by improving the drug formulations or focusing on particular biological pathways, thus making them safer and more bearable for patients. Improvements in medication enhancement strategy lead to the growth of personalized medicine where treatment is aligned with individual factors like genomics, biomarkers, and behavior patterns. Thus, it enables accurate dosage determination as well as the choice of therapeutic interventions aimed at maximizing patient benefits while minimizing adverse outcomes [5, 6].

In the management of chronic diseases and prevention of their progression, improved medicines play a vital role. This kind of medication improvement may be able to slow down or stop the development of diseases by making drugs that are focused on reducing damage to the body. Medicines have typically been designed with due consideration to addressing specific disorders that are not currently covered within the medical sphere or those disorders for which there are limited therapeutic options. Innovations in technology and research have made it possible to develop better medications that can treat patients who were previously untreatable or undertreated due to certain conditions, thus filling up a void in healthcare provision [7, 8].

Enhancing drugs for optimization can make them less expensive and thereby reduce the need for frequent dosage or some adjunctive therapies and hospitalization. Enhanced medications improve treatment efficiency in health care, resulting in a balanced allocation of resources among healthcare systems. Medication enhancement is vital to advancing healthcare by improving treatment efficacy, safety, and accessibility aimed at unmet medical needs with a view to encouraging personalized, patient-centered care. This goal can be achieved only if there is greater investment in research and innovation towards medication enhancement, which will enable people's life spans to rise globally [9, 10].

Healthcare is being transformed by artificial intelligence across all levels, and this change is ultimately causing a revolution in the manner we diagnose, treat, and manage diseases. AI-supported diagnostics algorithms have significantly improved the way medical images are understood, ranging from X-rays to MRI scans. This has led to much more accurate and faster recognition of abnormalities that had not been seen before. As such, there is earlier diagnosis as well as intervention in conditions like cancer or neurological disorders. Also, AI has caused drug discovery and development processes to be completely different, hence considerably shortening the time frame involved in launching new drugs into the market [11].

AI can analyze large sets of data, determine which drugs may be useful, foresee how they will perform, and suggest molecular structures that could be optimized for better results. The system also enables medication customization by analyzing patients' genetic profiles, laboratory test results, or diagnoses. This innovative approach helps achieve better treatment outcomes with fewer side effects compared to conventional healthcare delivery strategies [12].

More importantly, healthcare providers gain a lot of knowledge from AI-powered clinical decision support systems that help them in treatment planning and risk assessment. Also, patients can take care of their chronic conditions at home because of AI-based remote monitoring and telemedicine solutions that enhance access to health care and reduce costs. Integration of AI into health offers the potential of improving diagnostic precision, speeding up drug discovery, facilitating personalized medicine, enhancing clinical judgment-making, and improving patient experiences, thus heralding a transformative era in healthcare service delivery [13].

AI TECHNOLOGIES DRIVING MEDICATION ENHANCEMENT

AI technologies are driving significant advancements in medication enhancement, revolutionizing various aspects of drug discovery, development, and delivery which are discussed below in detail.

Predictive Modeling

Translating data into future events is the core idea behind predictive modeling. By integrating historical information and current variables, predictive modeling uses data mining, machine learning algorithms, and statistical procedures to estimate forthcoming results in different domains such as healthcare, finance, marketing, and weather forecasting. Therefore, it helps decision-making processes by giving an insight into what will happen in the future concerning trend patterns and events [14, 15].

In healthcare, predictive modeling holds immense potential to improve patient outcomes, enhance clinical decision-making, and optimize healthcare delivery. By analyzing vast amounts of patient data, including Electronic Health Records (EHRs), medical imaging, genetic profiles, and demographic information, predictive models can assist healthcare providers in several areas:

Risk Stratification and Disease Prediction

Predictive models are employed to evaluate individual patients' susceptibility to developing certain diseases or medical conditions. They can, therefore, classify patients according to their risk level by analyzing information about patients and identifying the risks involved. A case in point is when predictive models gauge the chances of one getting a cardiovascular disease considering factors such as age, gender, blood pressure, cholesterol levels, and way of life; this will enable healthcare providers to institute intercessions that correspond with minimizing cardiovascular risks [16].

Treatment Response Prediction

Predictive modeling determines how patients will respond to particular treatments or interventions. Predictive models, on the other hand, use a combination of patient attributes, biomarkers, genetic data, and medical histories to predict whether or not treatments will succeed or fail. As such, predictive models allow healthcare providers to individualize treatment plans for patients based on their probability of success. For instance, predictive models may be employed to identify cancer patients who are most likely to respond positively to a specific chemotherapy regimen so as to minimize unintended side effects and optimize therapeutic outcomes [17, 18].

Hospital Readmission Prediction

Forecasting the probability of hospital readmission after being discharged is done using predictive models. Predictive models can identify patients at high risk of readmission through the analysis of demographics, clinical characteristics, comorbidity, and social determinants of health so that healthcare providers may implement targeted interventions like care coordination, patient education, and follow-up care to reduce readmission rates and improve patient outcomes [19, 20].

Resource Allocation and Capacity Planning

Healthcare institutions utilize predictive modeling to optimize resource allocation and capacity planning. Predictive models can forecast patient volumes, emergency room visits, and hospital admissions based on historical patient data, seasonal trends, and demographic patterns. This allows healthcare organizations to mobilize their resources more effectively, predict staffing requirements, and improve the efficiency of healthcare delivery workflows [21, 22].

Pattern Recognition

The significance of pattern recognition algorithms in medicine development cannot be overstated. These algorithms enable the identification and interpretation of complex patterns in biological data, chemical structures, and drug responses. With the help of high-level computational methods, these algorithms reveal important information that can guide drug discovery, development, and optimization efforts [23].

Drug Target Identification

In medical enhancement, the use of pattern recognition is significant in identifying potential drug objectives. This approach involves delving into huge biological datasets, which scrutinizes gene expression profiles, protein interactions, and disease pathways for repeat patterns indicative of therapeutic targets that look promising. Pattern recognition algorithms can locate proteins, receptors, or genetic pathways that influence disease progression by identifying patterns in molecular signatures known to be associated with specific diseases. These targets, when discovered, stand as research points for efforts required in finding drugs; this guides scientists toward creating precise and effective therapies aimed at modulating disease mechanisms [24 - 26].

Bioinformatics Analysis

Bioinformatics is an area where pattern recognition algorithms are inescapable; they help to untangle complexities found in genetic sequences, protein structures, and other biological data. By examining DNA sequences, RNA expression profiles, and protein-protein interactions, these techniques for pattern recognition can reveal undiscovered patterns that offer insight into disease mechanisms and potential drug targets. Some of the pattern recognition algorithms, for example, can identify sequence motifs or structural patterns in genetic data indicative of genes or pathways that are associated with disease. Such findings guide the creation of innovative medicines targeting precise genetic mistakes or diseases' signs and symptoms, thus paving the way for personalized medications [27, 28].

Image Analysis

Pattern recognition algorithms in pharmaceutical research are used to examine medical images, such as microscopy images or structural data, to understand molecular structures or cellular patterns that will help in drug development. Characterizing drug compounds, understanding their impacts on life systems, and eavesdropping on mechanisms of action, among others, are some of the ways these algorithms help researchers by detecting patterns in images. For instance, pattern recognition algorithms can identify morphological features or spatial arrangements in cellular images that correlate with drug efficacy or toxicity. By correlating image patterns with biological responses, researchers gain valuable insights into the interactions between drugs and cells, thus facilitating the optimization of drug candidates and the prediction of their pharmacological properties [29, 30].

Pattern recognition algorithms are essential for drug improvement; they help find potential drug targets, analyze complex biological data, and interpret imaging data that pertains to drug development. The innovation in drug discovery, personalized medicine, and therapeutic optimization is driven by these algorithms, which discover hidden patterns and elucidate underlying mechanisms, thus leading to a better understanding of healthcare, resulting in improved patient outcomes [31].

Mining Biomedical Literature

The extraction of valuable insights and knowledge from vast repositories of scientific articles, journals, and databases in the field of biomedicine is a very systematic way of mining biomedical literature. This process employs computerized methods, including NLP algorithms, to evaluate and understand text-based information. First, relevant datasets are accessed from PubMed, MEDLINE, and PubMed Central as sources that cover various scientific literature on genetics, pharmacology, clinical research, *etc* [32, 33].

The next step is to remove and normalize the data using preprocessing techniques, followed by information extraction methods geared towards finding important biomedical entities like proteins, genes, diseases, and drugs from the literature. The processed text is then analyzed using text-mining algorithms to determine patterns, relationships, and trends in the literature. These findings help in medical research, leading to a better understanding of gene mutation-disease associations, drug targets for the new generation pharmaceuticals, and even disease mechanisms [34].

Visualization techniques play a significant role in interpreting and exploring results, thereby enabling researchers to explore the data more deeply. This makes mining biomedical literature an important resource for biomedical research and healthcare that can transform massive scientific publications into actionable knowledge [35].

Extracting Insights from Unstructured Data

Extracting insights from unstructured data is about analyzing and drawing out meaningful information from data that does not have a predefined data model or organization. In terms of improving medication, unstructured data includes clinical notes, patient records, medical literature, social media posts, and research articles. Below are the processes where insights can be extracted to enhance medication-related.

Sentiment Analysis

Sentiment analysis is a system that has been used to analyze unstructured text data taken from sources such as patient reviews and social media posts to determine feelings, thoughts, and emotions about drugs. Through sentiment analysis, healthcare providers can discern the preferences of patients, get to know their concerns and understand issues pertaining to medication adherence and satisfaction. This information can be applied to improve patient engagement strategies as well as optimize medication management systems [36, 37].

Image Analysis and Computer Vision

Medical evaluation data, such as X-ray, Magnetic Resonance Imaging (MRI), and histopathology slides, contain vital information on how the ailment is progressing, the response to treatment, and drug effectiveness. Computer vision algorithms are used to extract quantitative features, detect abnormalities, and classify treatment patterns. Information can be derived from unstructured images to guide therapy, track patients' progress, and evaluate drug performance [38].

Data Integration and Fusion

Structured data from EHRs, clinical databases, and genomic repositories is commonly integrated with unstructured data to enhance understanding. This can involve merging different types of information, such as text-based data, numbers, and images, to enable a thorough examination of linkages, correlations, and patterns across medication use, patient demographics, or therapeutic results. Data integration methods support the assimilation of divergent sources to generate a complete picture of medical processes [39].

Predictive Modeling and Pattern Recognition

Unstructured data is applied to machine learning algorithms used in developing predictive models, thus enabling the identification of patterns and assisting medication improvement activities. Predictive analytics involves training models on historical data, which can enable the prediction of adverse events, forecast drug responses, and customize treatment based on individual patient characteristics. The detection of recurrent patterns or exceptions in unorganized data using pattern recognition techniques helps to identify insights into medicine use and trends [40].

Image Analysis for Drug Discovery

Deep learning methods have changed image analysis in drug discovery, bringing about efficient ways of generating meaningful information from complex biomedical images. In drug discovery, image analysis is important in several stages, such as compound screening, target Identification, and efficacy assessment. Deep learning is applied to image analysis for drug discovery, as described below [41, 42].

Compound Screening and Target Identification

Deep learning models, especially Convolutional Neural Networks (CNNs), are used to analyze images of chemical compounds and forecast their biological activities. Through training on enormous amounts of compound images and their confronting biological activities, CNNs are able to learn how to find recurring imagery as well as structural features related to particular medications or organic effects. This allows for the screening of compounds in a high-throughput manner so as to identify potential drug candidates with desired pharmacological properties [43].

Cellular Imaging and High-Content Screening (HCS)

The potential candidates for drug testing are identified, and cellular morphology and function changes are assessed by carrying out high-content screening, which involves the automated analysis of cellular images. Deep learning models can be used to analyze HCS image data for phenotypes of cells, quantify morphometric alterations in cells, and recognize certain cells of interest. With the aid of annotated datasets of cellular images, CNNs can correctly categorize cells, find subcellular structures, and foresee what impacts probable drugs will have on cell pathways, thereby resulting in the discovery of new therapeutic entities [44].

Disease Modeling and Biomarker Identification

The histopathology images are analyzable by deep learning models to identify the associated histological features with disease states; CNNs trained on histopathology datasets can classify tissue samples, detect pathological changes, and predict disease outcomes. Apart from that, deep learning techniques will also be useful in assessing molecular imaging data such as Positron Emission Tomography (PET) or Magnetic Resonance Imaging (MRI) for the identification of disease progression biomarkers and treatment response evaluations. This would enable us to identify possible targets for drugs and assess the therapeutic efficacy in preclinical and clinical studies [44].

Drug Repurposing and Combination Therapy

Current deep learning models are able to inspect and deduce fresh indications for existing medications or even identify the drugs' mixture that could be applied together. By examining large biomedical image databases, CNNs can detect phenotypic similarities of various diseases as well as foresee the interaction of drug impacts on cellular pathways. The other task that can be done by artificial intelligence is personalized treatment strategy through analyzing organoids derived from patients or xenografts. In this way, precision medicine initiatives are made possible by deep learning techniques [45].

Protein Folding Prediction

In bioinformatics and structural biology, the problem of predicting protein folding has far-reaching effects on our knowledge about drug discovery, how proteins work, and why diseases develop. Protein folding is a process where a linearly arranged sequence of amino acids attains its three-dimensional native structure that is essential for biological function. However, it remains difficult to predict the native three-dimensional (3D) structure for a protein-based solely on its amino acid sequence due to the intricate mechanisms like van der Waals forces, hydrogen bonds, electrostatic attraction, or hydrophobicity that affect this event [46].

A principal advantage of deep learning-based protein folding prediction is its capacity to catch non-linear links and complicated relationships between amino acids in the protein sequence. With deep learning models, hierarchical representations of protein sequences are learned, and it can automatically reveal those essential features and patterns that cause protein folding. Deep learning models can be trained on large datasets consisting of experimentally determined structures for proteins from where they generalize well, thereby achieving high precision in predicting unknown structures for new proteins [47].

Among the architectures that have been proposed for predicting protein folding are Recurrent Neural Networks (RNNs), Long Short-Term Memory Networks (LSTMs), and attention-based models. These models can take the primary sequence of amino acids as input and predict various aspects of protein structure, such as secondary structure elements (alpha helices, beta sheets), tertiary structure, or quaternary structure interactions [48].

The power of machine learning algorithms for the purpose of predicting protein folding patterns is capable of reshaping drug invention and development by enabling rapid and accurate prediction of protein structures as well as interactions. Thus, by accurately determining protein structure, investigators can understand more about how proteins work and, therefore, identify molecules that could be targeted with drugs to treat a particular disease or condition. Moreover, deep learning models can assist in the fabrication of artificial proteins with specific characteristics, thus making it easier to develop novel biotech and pharmaceutical tools [49].

Automated Laboratory Processes

Robotic technology is increasingly being used to automate laboratory processes, leading to transformations in conducting experiments, collecting data, and analyzing. Laboratory automation systems employ robots to carry out monotonous tasks with high accuracy and repeatability, thus allowing researchers more time and resources for difficult and thought-provoking issues [50]. Robotics is transforming laboratory processes, as described below.

Sample Handling and Preparation

The employment of robotics systems in sample handling and preparation tasks has resulted in automating functions like pipetting, dilution, mixing, and aliquoting. Automated liquid handling robots that can accurately dispense the exact volume of liquids into multiwell plates can minimize human errors and discrepancies. This makes it possible to conduct experiments repeatedly with similar results and quickly screen compounds for high-throughput drug discovery, genomics research, or biomarker analysis [51].

Laboratory Instrumentation

Robotics technology has been used to integrate lab instruments to automate data collection and analysis workflows. Automated analytical instruments like Liquid Chromatography-Mass Spectrometry (LC-MS) systems and High-performance Liquid Chromatography (HPLC) systems have robotic samplers and autosamplers, thereby enabling successive injection of samples into an auto-analyzer for continuous processing without any manual intervention. This enhances the efficiency of analytical workflows and speeds up the rate at which new scientific discoveries are made [52].

Cell Culture and Assay Automation

Robotic platforms are applied to automate the working of cells in biomedical research and drug formulation. Automated cell culture systems can perform tasks such as seeding, media exchange, and incubation; this enables the continuous growth of cells and sustenance of cell lines with limited human involvement. The robotics-aided assay platforms can carry out intricate biochemical and cell-based assays to fast-track the screening of new drugs for toxicity target identification procedures [53].

High-Throughput Screening (HTS)

High-throughput screening facilities need robotics systems for the rapid identification of large compound libraries with biological targets of interest. Automated screening platforms that use robotics technology on a massively parallel basis dispensing compounds, performing assays, and analyzing data are among the tasks carried out by these platforms. Thus, thousands to millions of compounds can be screened within a short time frame. The latter speeds up novel drug candidate discovery and leads to optimization toward therapeutic development [54].

Data Management and Analysis

By integrating robotics systems with advanced software for managing and analyzing data, experimental workflows have been automated, and data interpretation has been made easier. To ensure that the integrity of data is preserved, lab experiments can be monitored by automated Laboratory Information Management Systems (LIMS) in real-time. Robotics-integrated data analysis platforms enable fast processing and analysis of big datasets resulting from automated experimentations advancing scientific discoveries and decision-making [55, 56].

The use of robotic technologies in the laboratory has increased the efficiency of some work done by repetition, thereby leading to higher levels of research activities and improved data-based quality control systems. Scientific innovation and developments, such as drug discovery and biotechnology advancements, among others, are predicted to be key to further developing robot technology [56].

Drug Synthesis and Testing

The discovery and development of drugs involves drug synthesis and testing processes, which help determine the safety, pharmacokinetic properties, and efficacy of potential drugs. Robotics occupies an important place in the automation and facilitation of drug synthesis and testing. This eases or simplifies the identification of new therapeutic agents and their further optimization. Robotics is transforming drug synthesis and testing as described below.

Automated Synthesis Platforms

Robotic systems automate the synthesis of chemical compounds to enable the generation of highly diversified and fast libraries for screening purposes. The automated synthesis platforms can carry out several chemical reactions, such as peptide synthesis, organic synthesis, and combinatorial chemistry, with high reproducibility and accuracy. By automating the synthetic workflows, robotics speeds up the search for new drug candidates and simplifies the refinement of lead compounds for further medicinal chemistry development [57].

In Vitro Assay Automation

The use of robotics in carrying out *in vitro* assays to assess the biological activity and toxicity of drugs is important. Companies have come up with machines that perform automated assays capable of handling cell culture, reagent dispensing, plate washing, and data acquisition activities, thereby making the fast conductance of various biochemical and cellular assays possible. Over a century ago, it was demonstrated that automating these operations increased reproducibility, which is important in preclinical research screening for new therapeutic drugs to reach the market sooner and at lower costs [58].

Medicinal Chemistry Optimization

The optimization of drug candidates through SAR studies and lead optimization campaigns is facilitated by robotics-assisted synthesis and testing platforms. By generating analogs and derivatives of lead compounds with alterations in their chemical structure, automated synthesis systems can modify the developed molecules. In contrast, the potency, selectivity, and pharmacokinetic properties of the new compounds are tested by automated screening platforms. This iterative process allows medicinal chemists to explore chemical space systematically to identify better drug-like candidates [59].

Data Management and Analysis

Data management and analysis software that is integrated with robotics simplifies the process of data collection, storage, and analysis during drug synthesis and testing. Automated laboratory information management systems (LIMS) can track sample information, experimental parameters, and results in real-time to ensure data integrity and traceability. Analysis platforms for data that are integrated with robotics facilitate quick processing and analysis of big data sets, thus enabling faster decision-making processes and revealing knowledge in the field of pharmaceutical research [60, 61].

APPLICATIONS OF AI IN MEDICATION ENHANCEMENT

Applications of AI in medication enhancement are shown in Fig. (1) and discussed below.

Virtual Screening

Virtual screening is an extensively implemented computational technique in identifying potential drug candidates from a vast library of chemical compounds using computer algorithms and molecular modelling methods without the need to test them experimentally. It functions by employing computer algorithms and molecular modelling techniques to forecast the possibility of a compound connecting with a certain target, such as a protein receptor or enzyme [62].

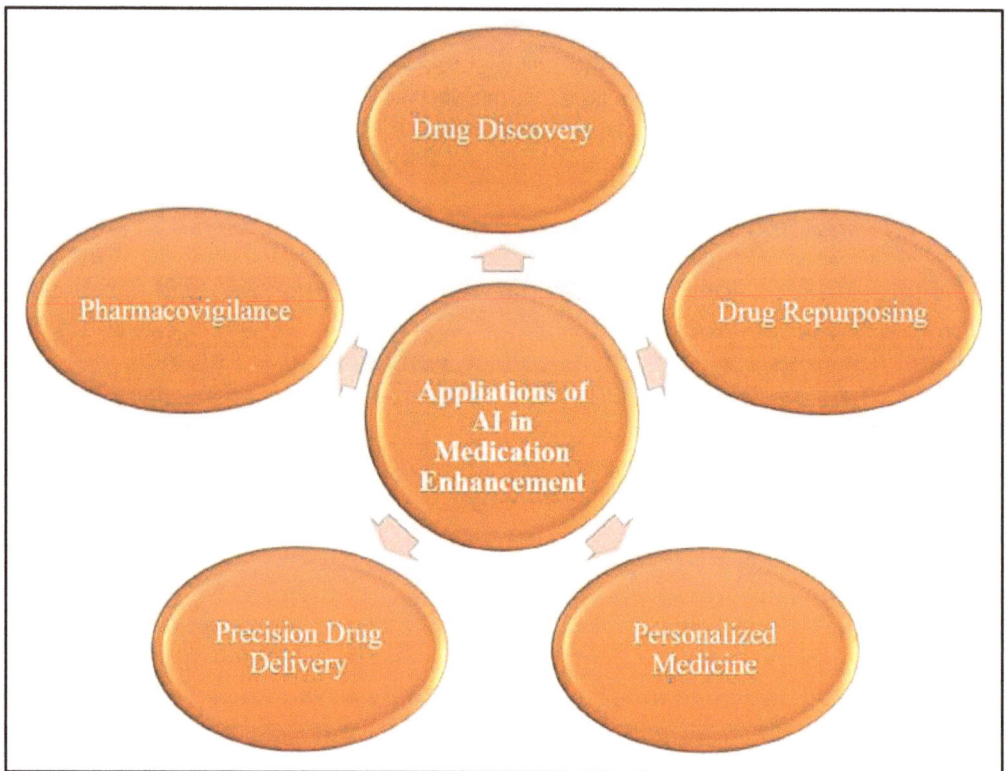

Fig. (1). Applications of AI in medication enhancement.

This method consists of database screening, which involves screening large compound databases for molecules based on their predicted binding affinity and pharmacological properties. Furthermore, ligand-based screening depends on the similarity between candidate compounds and known ligands. In contrast, structure-based screening uses computational models of the three-dimensional structure of the target protein to predict binding affinity [63].

Virtual screening can be used in different drug discovery stages, such as lead identification, hit-to-lead optimization, and even drug repurposing. In spite of its speed and cost-effectiveness benefits, virtual screening has challenges associated with model accuracy and the need for experimental validation of predicted hits. Nevertheless, it remains an important tool that contributes to the rapid identification of novel therapeutics and leads to optimization for subsequent development [64].

De novo Drug Design

Drug design and synthesis can be done using computer programs that help design new chemicals that will have the desired effects. In contrast to traditional procedures necessitating screening of libraries, de novo drug design, as the name suggests, involves the generation of novel molecules from scratch that are meant to act on specific targets or pathways in biology. This is achieved through the use of computational algorithms and molecular modeling techniques aimed at coming up with molecules with optimum affinity for binding, specificity, and pharmacokinetic properties [65].

In de novo drug design, researchers specify the chemical features and structural properties that need to be present in a target molecule, including its dimensions, outline, and functional groups. Then, computational algorithms generate potential molecules that meet these conditions by putting together molecular pieces or examining chemical space for new frameworks and building blocks. Predictive models and scoring functions are used to estimate their binding probability to the target and the chance that they may become drug candidates for these proposed molecules [66].

In drug discovery, *de novo* drug design plays a role at different levels, from lead identification to lead optimization and beyond. It enables researchers to navigate through huge areas of chemical space in order to develop new agents with unique mechanisms of action as well as therapeutic potential. With the help of computational models and algorithms, this method speeds up the process of finding new drugs and saves time and resources used during traditional drug discovery techniques [67].

De novo drug design still has its share of problems, such as the necessity for valid computer models, complex predictions on drugs' likelihood, and testing for the realness of promised pharmaceuticals. However, it is important to remember that this method remains a valuable tool in the arsenal of drug discovery experts, with prospects for finding innovative therapeutics and fulfilling unmet medical needs in several disease areas [68].

Identification of New Uses for Existing Drugs

Drug repurposing, also called drug repositioning or reprofiling, is the process of finding new applications for existing drugs that go beyond their original intended use. This method takes advantage of the vast amounts of safety and pharmacokinetic data available on approved drugs to speed up the drug discovery and development cycle. Instead of having to start all over again, scientists look into current molecules in search of alternatives to be used in treating different diseases or conditions [69, 70].

The process of discovering new applications for existing drugs generally relies on a combination of experimental and computational approaches. Through bioinformatics and network analysis, computational methods study big data sets featuring gene expression profiles, drug-target interactions, and disease pathways. With the help of these databases, scientists can find out which emerging diseases may be treated by certain drugs that modify biologically related processes or targets [71, 72].

Drug repurposing heavily relies on experimental validation, where drug candidates identified are subjected to preclinical and clinical studies aimed at evaluating their effectiveness, safety, and pharmacokinetics in the new indication. This can entail *in vitro* tests, animal models, and clinical trials to assess a drug's therapeutic potential and understand its mechanism of action in relation to the new disease [73, 74].

Drug repurposing can be advantageous compared to conventional drug discovery techniques since it lowers the cost of development, shortens the time required for development, and reduces risks associated with failure. By using previously developed drugs for new purposes, scientists can avoid toiling with certain predicaments that may accompany the designing of novel chemical entities, including toxicity tests and optimization of pharmacokinetic characteristics. Moreover, recycled medicines could also take advantage of regulatory approvals and commercial manufacturing processes already in place, shortening their go-to-market period [75, 76].

Drug repurposing is applicable in different therapeutic fields, such as infectious diseases, cancer, neurological disorders, and orphan diseases. For instance, thalidomide has been repurposed to treat multiple myeloma, sildenafil has been used to manage pulmonary hypertension, and minoxidil has been used to promote hair growth. With progress in computational and experimental methods, drug reutilization persists as an encouraging approach to identifying new therapies and addressing unmet medical needs [77, 78].

Predictive Analytics for Treatment Response

Predictive analytics for treatment response utilize sophisticated data analysis methods to forecast specific medical treatments or interventions that patients react to. This is done by exploiting huge datasets that consist of patient demography, past medical history, and genetic information, among others, to enhance predictive analytics models in the identification of patterns and links that are helpful in forecasting treatment results more accurately. The details enable healthcare providers to personalize treatment plans, optimize therapeutic interventions, and improve patient outcomes [79].

Oncology is one area in which predictive analytics for treatment response is widely used. Predictive models in oncology predict the probability of response to chemotherapy, immunotherapy, or targeted therapy based on tumor characteristics and patient factors. By studying genomic information, tumor mutations, and biomarker profiles, patients can be divided into subgroups with differing reactions to treatment using predictive models that help clinicians choose the best therapy for a given individual [80].

Oncology, among other fields, uses predictive analytics. For example, in cardiology, using predictive models that can predict the risk of adverse cardiovascular events and help in the management of patients with heart diseases to identify those who are most likely to benefit from interventions like statin therapy or cardiac catheterization. In psychiatry, predictive analytics can be used to inform patients about anticipated responses to antidepressants or antipsychotics based on genetic markers, symptom severity, and treatment history so that clinicians can tailor treatment plans for individual patients [81].

For the development and implementation of treatment response prediction analytics models, clinicians must collaborate with data scientists and healthcare informaticists. In this process, issues such as data quality, confidentiality, and security are very important because their validity depends on good-quality data. To ensure that they have clinical purpose and relevance for different populations of patients, these predictive models should be constantly checked and adjusted as necessary [82].

Targeted Drug Delivery Systems

The utilization of precision drug delivery for a targeted drug delivery system is summarized in Table **1**.

Table 1. Utilization of precision drug delivery for targeted drug delivery system.

Precision Drug Delivery Systems	Description
Nanoparticles	These are designed to encapsulate drugs in nanosize and then deliver them to specific locations within the body, such as tumors or diseased tissues. This minimizes systemic exposure [83].

Precision Drug Delivery Systems	Description
Liposomes	Drug-containing aqueous cores or lipid bilayers are examples of lipid-based blisters, which can be modified on their surfaces to target specific cells or tissues for drug delivery [84].
Polymer-based Drug Delivery Systems	Polymeric materials can release drugs at a controlled rate at their desired site of action by responding to pH changes, temperature fluctuations, or enzyme activities [85].
Antibody-Drug Conjugates (ADCs)	Monoclonal antibodies are attached to cytotoxic drugs so as to achieve targeted delivery into cells that reveal identified surface antigens, thus minimizing off-target effects and improving therapeutic efficacy [86].
Microneedle Arrays	Drug delivery can be accurately and painlessly done by using an array of minuscule needles assembled on a patch or a device that pierces the skin to get into the bloodstream or subdermal tissues [87].
Implantable Drug Delivery Devices	Biodegradable or non-biodegradable implants can be directly put into organs or tissues to give out medicines for a long period, thus making it possible to have focused therapy with minimal body exposure [88].
Inhalation Drug Delivery Systems	Among the devices that deliver drugs to the lungs directly *via* inhalation, they allow for local therapy of respiratory conditions or systemic drug delivery with the rapid onset of action [89].
Magnetic Drug Targeting	Magnetic nanoparticles and drug carriers are incorporated with medicines that can be moved under the control of outer magnetic Fields, which allow for accurate establishment and increased medicinal transport efficacy [90].

Further improvement of these precision drug delivery systems can be done by integrating AI algorithms that optimize parameters of drug delivery, predict patients' responses, and personalize treatment strategies. AI is capable of analyzing complex datasets like patient demographics, genetic information, and clinical outcomes in order to individualize drug delivery systems for patients, improve therapeutic efficacy, and minimize side effects. Combining AI with targeted drug delivery systems has the potential to advance precision medicine, thereby improving disease conditions in different patients [91].

Early Detection of Adverse Drug Reactions

AI and machine learning technologies foster revolutionary change in pharmacovigilance through early Adverse Drug Reactions (ADR) detection, which significantly improves detection, prediction, and prevention. In this regard, AI's role is diverse and comes with several benefits that help to improve patient safety and healthcare results [92, 93].

AI's most significant contribution to pharmacovigilance is its ability to process large and unending data sources faster. Using advanced algorithms and computing power, AI systems can instantly analyze electronic health records, patient reports, medical literature, and other related data sources. This enables healthcare providers to continuously monitor drug safety and detect emerging potential ADRs almost immediately [93].

Additionally, AI is also beneficial for the timely detection of ADRs through complex analysis of huge data sets to find connections between different adverse events. For example, if there are slight changes in patients' details or if certain treatments seem to be causing symptoms they have not exhibited before, an AI system can raise a red flag on possible ADRs that could worsen into more severe conditions. This early response mechanism allows healthcare providers to act promptly, alter their interventions appropriately, and avoid harm posed by unwanted results on patients [94].

In addition, AI can determine ADRs before they happen, enabling proactive preventive measures to be taken. By studying historical records and identifying risk factors linked to individual drugs or types of patients, AI models can predict the probability of side effects, which is useful information for determining drug prescriptions and monitoring protocols. This forecasting ability makes it possible for healthcare providers to act in advance to prevent ADRs and improve the safety of patients [95].

Machine Learning algorithms in pharmacovigilance are vital as they keep on learning and improve their capacity to anticipate and identify ADRs precisely as time passes. On the other hand, using annotated information on known ill-effects events for training purposes, ML models can learn complex patterns and associations that let them detect potential ADRs with high accuracy. This ongoing process of learning makes AI systems more sensitive and specific, thus making them effective tools for the early detection and monitoring of ADRs [96].

There are several benefits to using AI in pharmacovigilance, such as facilitating real-time monitoring of drug safety, enabling rapid identification of potential ADRs, and helping detect emerging trends and patterns related to ADRs. AI is revolutionizing pharmacovigilance through automation, analysis of large datasets, and utilization of sophisticated computational techniques that enhance patient safety and provide better healthcare outcomes [97].

Real-time Monitoring of Drug Safety

In fact, the significance of AI in pharmacovigilance for real-time monitoring of drug safety is immense and complex, with several functionalities that promote early identification, evaluation, and control of adverse events connected to pharmaceutical products. By using AI technologies such as machine learning and

NLP, pharmacovigilance experts can draw relevant information from multiple data sources and take immediate action on potential safety issues [98].

Automated adverse event detection is among the main features that AI promotes in pharmacovigilance. By using NLP, AI can automatically extract key information from unstructured data sources like electronic health records, social media, and medical literature. In this way, it is possible to quickly identify textual data containing adverse events, thereby helping pharmacovigilance professionals instantly track drug safety through different channels [99].

Determining signs is an important function of AI in the context of signal detection. In fact, machine-learning algorithms can identify subtle relationships between drug exposure and reported adverse drug events, enabling the early discovery of safety signals that may not be identified through manual analysis alone. This ability enables pharmacovigilance professionals to proactively investigate and respond to emerging safety concerns before they escalate [100].

Moreover, AI also helps in data triage by sifting and organizing huge amounts of information according to the urgency of various cases. Automating case prioritization through AI allows pharmacovigilance experts to concentrate their time and effort on handling urgent reports that need immediate action taken. This facilitates improved flow in the pharmacovigilance process, ensuring timely resolution of important safety concerns [101].

Another important function that AI can perform in pharmacovigilance is predictive analytics. Machine learning models can analyze factors such as patient demographics, medical history, and drug properties to determine the likelihood of adverse events. To improve patient outcomes and alleviate potential safety concerns, pharmacovigilance professionals may implement proactive risk management strategies by identifying patients with more susceptibility to unwanted effects [102].

Furthermore, AI helps pharmacovigilance professionals continuously monitor drug safety and respond quickly to any emerging signals. AI also helps pharmacovigilance teams by giving them insights into safety trends and patterns in real-time, enabling proactive patient safety measures and improved healthcare results.

Pharmacovigilance through AI is integral to real-time drug safety surveillance through automation, analysis of big data, and timely insights that enhance patient care outcomes. By using AI technologies, pharmacovigilance professionals can identify and manage possible safety concerns linked to pharmaceutical products, thus improving public health and patients' well-being as a whole [103].

BENEFITS OF AI IN MEDICATION ENHANCEMENT

The benefits of AI in medication enhancement are significant and multifaceted. They impact various stages of the healthcare process, which is summarized in Fig. (2).

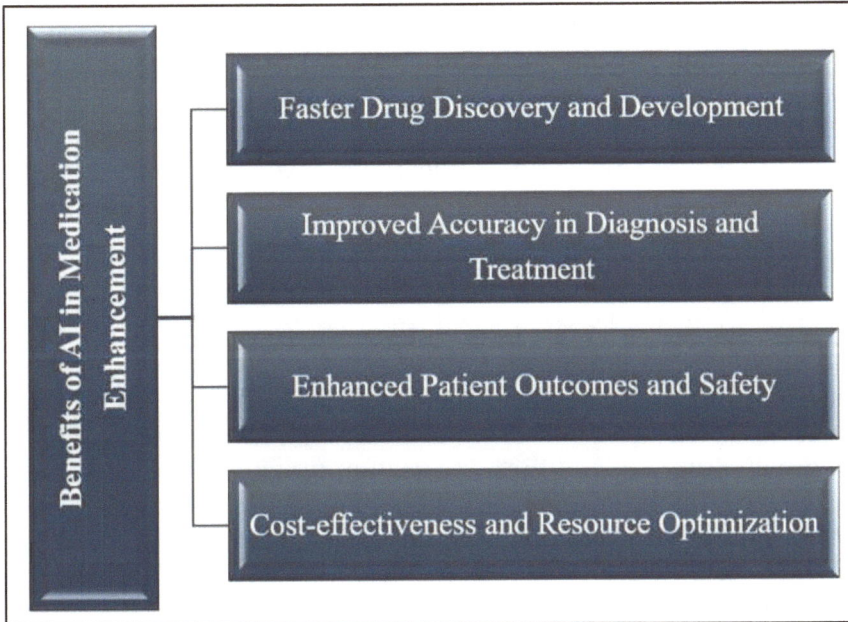

Fig. (2). Benefits of AI in medication enhancement.

Faster Drug Discovery and Development

By scrutinizing enormous quantities of biological information, AI facilitates drug development by identifying possible drug targets, forecasting compound interactions, and enhancing molecular structures. Machine learning algorithms are another way for scientists to discover novel therapeutic agents more quickly by using existing drug databases and scientific literature. This consequently reduces the time it takes for a drug to be developed and increases the chances of new medications becoming available [104].

Improved Accuracy in Diagnosis and Treatment

For example, AI diagnostic tools may analyze patient records, genetic data, and medical imaging. Machine learning algorithms can identify patterns in patient information that human doctors might not notice, leading to earlier diagnosis of diseases and more customized treatment plans. Furthermore, decision support systems propelled by AI can suggest accurate drugs and dosage routines for individual patients after considering aspects like age or prior medication history [105].

Enhanced Patient Outcomes and Safety

AI can improve patient outcomes and safety by enhancing medication selection and dosing. AI-based personalized treatment plans can help minimize the chances of suffering from adverse drug reactions (ADRs) or drug interactions that can impact therapy outcomes and lead to reduced admissions in hospitals. Monitoring systems with AI capability also enable health professionals to identify early signs of response to treatment or complications, thus taking necessary actions within good time, such as adjusting medications for better medication regimens [106].

Cost-effectiveness and Resource Optimization

Consequently, AI technologies are contributing to cost savings and resource optimization within the healthcare system. This is due to AI's streamlining of drug discovery processes and improving diagnostic accuracy to minimize the time and resources used in research and development, hence lowering the cost of developing new drugs. In addition, medication usage can be optimized by AI-driven decision support systems, which can also lead to a reduction in unnecessary prescriptions and healthcare waste, resulting in better resource allocation and more economical care provision by medical facilities [107].

The benefits of incorporating AI in drug development include faster processing of new drugs, more precise diagnosis and patient-centered therapy, better outcomes and safety for patients, and economic efficiency with optimal resource use. Medical facilities can completely change the way they manage medication by employing artificial intelligence technologies, which will help enhance quality, efficiency, and access to medical care [108].

FUTURE DIRECTIONS AND OPPORTUNITIES

Collaboration among stakeholders such as healthcare providers, technology developers, policymakers, and patient advocacy groups is therefore crucial in navigating these challenges and ethical considerations. In doing this it will involve addressing factors like data privacy and security, AI algorithms' biases, regulatory compliance, and equity in access to AI-driven healthcare, thereby maximizing the benefits of AI while reducing risks related to medication enhancement through technology and responsible use of AI for health care delivery [109].

AI can change the way in which drugs are discovered and developed so that medications will be more efficient and personalized. For instance, new AI-based drug design techniques like virtual screening, de novo drug design, and predictive modeling could facilitate the discovery of novel drugs and optimize properties for specific targets or patient populations. Furthermore, when it comes to diseases affecting a wide range of patients, AI-assisted approaches to drug repurposing as well as combination therapy will give room to new uses of existing medicines, thus enhancing outcomes in treatment [110, 111].

With the increased integration of AI in the healthcare sector, societal and ethical implications must be addressed to ensure responsible use of technology. This encompasses concerns such as data privacy and security, AI algorithmic bias, decision-making transparency and accountability, and equal access to AI-based healthcare services. Hence, stakeholder collaboration is needed to build an ethics framework that can lead to regulation guidelines and governance mechanisms for the responsible adoption of AI in drug improvement and the provision of medical services [112].

With the integration of AI into medication enhancement, there are promising opportunities to improve clinical practice, advance drug discovery, transform healthcare delivery, and address societal and ethical implications. The future of AI in medication enhancement is poised to revolutionize health care and improve patient outcomes globally by leveraging potential AI-driven technologies and promoting stakeholder collaboration [113].

CONCLUSION

In conclusion, the incorporation of artificial intelligence into medicine improvement is a game changer in the field. AI can handle vast amounts of data, create insights, and improve clinical judgment, thereby making it a possible revolutionizing tool in drug creation, diagnosis of diseases, treatments, and healthcare provision. AI-driven advances in drug design can fast-track researchers' identification of new medications, customized treatment protocols, and better patient results. Besides, AI incorporation into everyday clinical practice allows medical practitioners to make more precise diagnoses, adapt therapeutic strategies according to a particular patient, and, therefore, improve the quality of care. AI-based technologies can overcome long-standing issues in drug safety, including side effects and medication errors, through real-time monitoring of drug safety, early identification of adverse events, and proactive risk management solutions. Healthcare organizations can make the best use of drugs and reduce healthcare costs as well as improve operational efficiency by using artificial intelligence (AI) algorithms and predictive analytics in medicine. Furthermore,

AI-based telemedicine portals, digital assistants, and remote monitoring devices will foster patient involvement, increase healthcare accessibility, and bolster seamless transitions between different healthcare delivery settings. AI is making significant strides in drug enhancement; ethical issues, regulatory hurdles, and societal consequences must, however, be taken into account for responsible and fair use of technology to be achieved. This encompasses protecting patient privacy and data security, reducing bias in AI algorithms, increasing transparency and accountability for decision-making procedures, and ensuring that AI-driven healthcare services are made available to all. The use of AI in medication optimization is a new horizon that promises substantial advancements in health care. It has the possibility of making significant improvements in patient outcomes, bettering drug safety, and transforming health care delivery itself. Embracing the opportunities offered by AI technologies and tackling their associated challenges also enables stakeholders to exploit their capability to revolutionize medication management, which can subsequently improve the quality of healthcare globally.

ACKNOWLEDGEMENTS

Authors are highly thankful to their Universities/Colleges for providing library facilities for the literature survey.

REFERENCES

[1]   O. Ali, W. Abdelbaki, A. Shrestha, E. Elbasi, M.A.A. Alryalat, and Y.K. Dwivedi, "A systematic literature review of artificial intelligence in the healthcare sector: Benefits, challenges, methodologies, and functionalities", *Journal of Innovation & Knowledge,* vol. 8, no. 1, p. 100333, 2023.
[http://dx.doi.org/10.1016/j.jik.2023.100333]

[2]   A. Bohr, and K. Memarzadeh, "The rise of artificial intelligence in healthcare applications", In: *Artificial Intelligence in Healthcare.* Elsevier, 2020, pp. 25-60.
[http://dx.doi.org/10.1016/B978-0-12-818438-7.00002-2]

[3]   Davenport T, Kalakota R. The potential for artificial intelligence in healthcare. Future healthcare journal. 2019 Jun 1;6(2):94-8.
[http://dx.doi.org/10.7861/futurehosp.6-2-94]

[4]   L.K. Vora, A.D. Gholap, K. Jetha, R.R.S. Thakur, H.K. Solanki, and V.P. Chavda, "Artificial Intelligence in Pharmaceutical Technology and Drug Delivery Design", *Pharmaceutics,* vol. 15, no. 7, p. 1916, 2023.
[http://dx.doi.org/10.3390/pharmaceutics15071916] [PMID: 37514102]

[5]   K.S. Vidhya, A. Sultana, N.K. M, and H. Rangareddy, "Artificial Intelligence's Impact on Drug Discovery and Development From Bench to Bedside", *Cureus,* vol. 15, no. 10, p. e47486, 2023.
[http://dx.doi.org/10.7759/cureus.47486] [PMID: 37881323]

[6]   A. Haleem, M. Javaid, R. Pratap Singh, and R. Suman, "Medical 4.0 technologies for healthcare: Features, capabilities, and applications", *Internet of Things and Cyber-Physical Systems,* vol. 2, pp. 12-30, 2022.
[http://dx.doi.org/10.1016/j.iotcps.2022.04.001]

[7]   K. Alosaimi, H. Alwafi, Y. Alhindi, A. Falemban, A. Alshanberi, N. Ayoub, and S. Alsanosi,

"Medication Adherence among Patients with Chronic Diseases in Saudi Arabia", *Int. J. Environ. Res. Public Health,* vol. 19, no. 16, p. 10053, 2022.
[http://dx.doi.org/10.3390/ijerph191610053] [PMID: 36011690]

[8] E. Unni, "Medicine Use in Chronic Diseases", *Pharmacy (Basel),* vol. 11, no. 3, p. 100, 2023.
[http://dx.doi.org/10.3390/pharmacy11030100] [PMID: 37368426]

[9] F. Jiang, Y. Jiang, H. Zhi, Y. Dong, H. Li, S. Ma, Y. Wang, Q. Dong, H. Shen, and Y. Wang, "Artificial intelligence in healthcare: past, present and future", *Stroke Vasc. Neurol.,* vol. 2, no. 4, pp. 230-243, 2017.
[http://dx.doi.org/10.1136/svn-2017-000101] [PMID: 29507784]

[10] F. Jiang, Y. Jiang, H. Zhi, Y. Dong, H. Li, S. Ma, Y. Wang, Q. Dong, H. Shen, and Y. Wang, "Artificial intelligence in healthcare: past, present and future", *Stroke Vasc. Neurol.,* vol. 2, no. 4, pp. 230-243, 2017.
[http://dx.doi.org/10.1136/svn-2017-000101] [PMID: 29507784]

[11] M. Y. Shaheen, "Applications of Artificial Intelligence (AI) in healthcare: A review", *ScienceOpen Preprints,* 2021.
[http://dx.doi.org/10.14293/S2199-1006.1.SOR-.PPVRY8K.v1]

[12] A. Panesar, "Machine Learning and AI for Healthcare", *Apress Media,* vol. LLC, 2019.
[http://dx.doi.org/10.1007/978-1-4842-3799-1]

[13] "IoT and AI in healthcare: A systematic literature review", *Issues Inf Syst,* vol. 19, no. 1, pp. 33-41, 2018.
[http://dx.doi.org/10.48009/3_iis_2018_33-41]

[14] C. Wang, T. He, H. Zhou, Z. Zhang, and C. Lee, "Artificial intelligence enhanced sensors - enabling technologies to next-generation healthcare and biomedical platform", *Bioelectron. Med.,* vol. 9, no. 1, p. 17, 2023.
[http://dx.doi.org/10.1186/s42234-023-00118-1] [PMID: 37528436]

[15] C. Sarkar, B. Das, V.S. Rawat, J.B. Wahlang, A. Nongpiur, I. Tiewsoh, N.M. Lyngdoh, D. Das, M. Bidarolli, and H.T. Sony, "Artificial Intelligence and Machine Learning Technology Driven Modern Drug Discovery and Development", *Int. J. Mol. Sci.,* vol. 24, no. 3, p. 2026, 2023.
[http://dx.doi.org/10.3390/ijms24032026] [PMID: 36768346]

[16] S. Patil, and H. Shankar, "International Journal of Multidisciplinary Sciences and Arts Transforming Healthcare", *Harnessing the Power of AI in the Modern Era,* vol. 2, no. 1, 2023.
[http://dx.doi.org/10.47709/ijmdsa.vxix.xxxx]

[17] A.A. Kashif, B. Bakhtawar, A. Akhtar, S. Akhtar, N. Aziz, and M.S. Javeid, "Treatment Response Prediction in Hepatitis C Patients using Machine Learning Techniques", *International Journal of Technology, Innovation and Management (IJTIM),* vol. 1, no. 2, pp. 79-89, 2021. [IJTIM].
[http://dx.doi.org/10.54489/ijtim.v1i2.24]

[18] H. Bartelink, A. Begg, J. C. Martin, M. van Dijk, L. van 't Veer, P. van der Vaart, and M. Verheij, "Towards prediction and modulation of treatment response", *Radiother Oncol,* vol. 50, no. 1, pp. 1-11, 1999.
[http://dx.doi.org/10.1016/S0167-8140(99)00009-2]

[19] O. Hasan, D.O. Meltzer, S.A. Shaykevich, C.M. Bell, P.J. Kaboli, A.D. Auerbach, T.B. Wetterneck, V.M. Arora, J. Zhang, and J.L. Schnipper, "Hospital readmission in general medicine patients: a prediction model", *J. Gen. Intern. Med.,* vol. 25, no. 3, pp. 211-219, 2010.
[http://dx.doi.org/10.1007/s11606-009-1196-1] [PMID: 20013068]

[20] E. Mahmoudi, N. Kamdar, N. Kim, G. Gonzales, K. Singh, and A.K. Waljee, "Use of electronic medical records in development and validation of risk prediction models of hospital readmission: systematic review", *BMJ,* vol. 369, p. m958, 2020.
[http://dx.doi.org/10.1136/bmj.m958] [PMID: 32269037]

[21]   D. Gyulai, B. Kádár, and L. Monostori, "Capacity planning and resource allocation in assembly systems consisting of dedicated and reconfigurable lines", In: *Procedia CIRP*. Elsevier B.V., 2014, pp. 185-191.
[http://dx.doi.org/10.1016/j.procir.2014.10.028]

[22]   B.M. Steenkamer, H.W. Drewes, R. Heijink, C.A. Baan, and J.N. Struijs, "Defining Population Health Management: A Scoping Review of the Literature", *Popul. Health Manag.*, vol. 20, no. 1, pp. 74-85, 2017.
[http://dx.doi.org/10.1089/pop.2015.0149] [PMID: 27124406]

[23]   A. R. Webb, and K. D. Copsey, *Statistical Pattern Recognition,* 3rd ed. Hoboken, NJ, USA: Wiley, 2011. Available from: www.wiley.com/go/statistical_pattern_recognition

[24]   D. Ochoa, A. Hercules, M. Carmona, D. Suveges, A. Gonzalez-Uriarte, C. Malangone, A. Miranda, L. Fumis, D. Carvalho-Silva, M. Spitzer, J. Baker, J. Ferrer, A. Raies, O. Razuvayevskaya, A. Faulconbridge, E. Petsalaki, P. Mutowo, S. Machlitt-Northen, G. Peat, E. McAuley, C.K. Ong, E. Mountjoy, M. Ghoussaini, A. Pierleoni, E. Papa, M. Pignatelli, G. Koscielny, M. Karim, J. Schwartzentruber, D.G. Hulcoop, I. Dunham, and E.M. McDonagh, "Open Targets Platform: supporting systematic drug–target identification and prioritisation", *Nucleic Acids Res.*, vol. 49, no. D1, pp. D1302-D1310, 2021.
[http://dx.doi.org/10.1093/nar/gkaa1027] [PMID: 33196847]

[25]   V.V. Kravchenko, G.F. Kaufmann, J.C. Mathison, D.A. Scott, A.Z. Katz, D.C. Grauer, M. Lehmann, M.M. Meijler, K.D. Janda, and R.J. Ulevitch, "Modulation of gene expression via disruption of NF-kappaB signaling by a bacterial small molecule", *Science,* vol. 321, no. 5886, pp. 259-263, 2008.
[http://dx.doi.org/10.1126/science.1156499] [PMID: 18566250]

[26]   J.N.Y. Chan, C. Nislow, and A. Emili, "Recent advances and method development for drug target identification", *Trends Pharmacol. Sci.,* vol. 31, no. 2, pp. 82-88, 2010.
[http://dx.doi.org/10.1016/j.tips.2009.11.002] [PMID: 20004028]

[27]   M. Goujon, H. McWilliam, W. Li, F. Valentin, S. Squizzato, J. Paern, and R. Lopez, "A new bioinformatics analysis tools framework at EMBL-EBI", *Nucleic Acids Res,* vol. 38, pp. W695-W699, 2010.
[http://dx.doi.org/10.1093/nar/gkq313]

[28]   P.C.Y. Woo, Y. Huang, S.K.P. Lau, and K.Y. Yuen, "Coronavirus genomics and bioinformatics analysis", *Viruses,* vol. 2, no. 8, pp. 1804-1820, 2010.
[http://dx.doi.org/10.3390/v2081803] [PMID: 21994708]

[29]   M. Petrou, and C. Petrou, *Image Processing: The Fundamentals,* 2nd ed. Chichester, UK: Wiley, 2010.
[http://dx.doi.org/10.1002/9781119994398]

[30]   C.-H. Teh, and R. T. Chin, "On image analysis by the methods of moments", In: *IEEE Trans Pattern Anal Mach Intell* vol. 10. , 1988, no. 4, pp. 496-513.
[http://dx.doi.org/10.1109/34.3913]

[31]   J.M. Prats-Montalbán, A. de Juan, and A. Ferrer, "Multivariate image analysis: A review with applications", *Chemom. Intell. Lab. Syst.,* vol. 107, no. 1, pp. 1-23, 2011.
[http://dx.doi.org/10.1016/j.chemolab.2011.03.002]

[32]   Available from: http://eprints.cdlr.strath.ac.uk/2611/ G. G. Chowdhury, "Natural language processing," 2003.
[http://dx.doi.org/10.1002/aris.1440370103]

[33]   S. Zhao, C. Su, Z. Lu, and F. Wang, "Recent advances in biomedical literature mining", *Brief. Bioinform.,* vol. 22, no. 3, p. bbaa057, 2021.
[http://dx.doi.org/10.1093/bib/bbaa057] [PMID: 32422651]

[34]   B. de Bruijn and J. Martin, "Getting to the (c)ore of knowledge: Mining biomedical literature," *Inter.*

J. Med. Inform., vol. 67, no. 1–3, pp. 7–18, Dec. 2002.

[35] H. Shatkay and R. Feldman, "Mining the biomedical literature in the genomic era: An overview," *J. Comp. Bio.*, vol. 10, no. 6, 2003.

[36] B. Shukla, S. K. Khatri, and P. K. Kapur, *Eds. In: Proceedings of the 4th International Conference on Reliability, Infocom Technologies and Optimization (ICRITO 2015),* Trends and Future Directions, Amity University, Noida, India, 2015. ISBN: 978-93-84935-45-0.

[37] https://upg-bulletin-se.ro/wp-content/uploads/2020/05/4.Bucur-3-2019.pdf Bucur C. Using machine learning techniques to gain insights from enterprise unstructured data. Economic Insights-Trends and Challenges. 2019;8(3):33-43.

[38] T. F. Cootes and C. J. Taylor, "Statistical models of appearance for medical image analysis and computer vision," In: *Proc. SPIE 4322, Medical Imaging: Image Processing,* San Diego, CA, USA, 3 Jul. 2001.
[http://dx.doi.org/10.1117/12.431093]

[39] C. Bachmann, B. Abdulhai, M.J. Roorda, and B. Moshiri, "Multisensor data integration and fusion in traffic operations and management", *Transp. Res. Rec.,* vol. 2308, no. 1, pp. 27-36, 2012.
[http://dx.doi.org/10.3141/2308-04]

[40] E. Tu, N. Kasabov, and J. Yang, "Mapping temporal variables into the NeuCube for improved pattern recognition, predictive modelling and understanding of stream data", *arXiv,* 2016. Available from: https://arxiv.org/abs/1603.05594

[41] Y. LeCun, Y. Bengio, and G. Hinton, "Deep learning", *Nature,* vol. 521, no. 7553, pp. 436-444, 2015.
[http://dx.doi.org/10.1038/nature14539] [PMID: 26017442]

[42] C. Scheeder, F. Heigwer, and M. Boutros, "Machine learning and image-based profiling in drug discovery", *Curr. Opin. Syst. Biol.,* vol. 10, pp. 43-52, 2018.
[http://dx.doi.org/10.1016/j.coisb.2018.05.004] [PMID: 30159406]

[43] M. A. Farha, E. D. Brown, and E. Brown, "Strategies for target identification of antimicrobial natural products," 2016.
[http://dx.doi.org/10.1039/C5NP00127G]

[44] F. Zanella, J.B. Lorens, and W. Link, "High content screening: seeing is believing", *Trends Biotechnol.,* vol. 28, no. 5, pp. 237-245, 2010.
[http://dx.doi.org/10.1016/j.tibtech.2010.02.005] [PMID: 20346526]

[45] A.S. Correia, F. Gärtner, and N. Vale, "Drug combination and repurposing for cancer therapy: the example of breast cancer", *Heliyon,* vol. 7, no. 1, p. e05948, 2021.
[http://dx.doi.org/10.1016/j.heliyon.2021.e05948] [PMID: 33490692]

[46] S. Takada, "Gō-ing for the prediction of protein folding mechanisms", *Proc Natl Acad Sci USA,* vol. 96, 1999no. 21, pp. 11698-11700.
[http://dx.doi.org/10.1073/pnas.96.21.11698]

[47] I. Dubchak, S. Muchnik, S. R. Holbrook, and S.-H. Kim, "Prediction of protein folding class using global description of amino acid sequence", *Proc Natl Acad Sci USA,* vol. 92, 1995no. 19, pp. 8700-8704.
[http://dx.doi.org/10.1073/pnas.92.19.8700]

[48] D. Baker, "Protein folding, structure prediction and design", *Biochem. Soc. Trans.,* vol. 42, no. 2, pp. 225-229, 2014.
[http://dx.doi.org/10.1042/BST20130055] [PMID: 24646222]

[49] J. N. Onuchic and P. G. Wolynes, "Theory of protein folding," *Curr. Opn. Struc. Bio*, vol. 14, no. 1. pp. 70–75, 2004.
[http://dx.doi.org/10.1016/j.sbi.2004.01.009]

[50] F. Biermann, J. Mathews, B. Nießing, N. König, and R.H. Schmitt, "Automating laboratory processes

by connecting biotech and robotic devices—an overview of the current challenges, existing solutions, and ongoing developments", *Processes (Basel),* vol. 9, no. 6, p. 966, 2021.
[http://dx.doi.org/10.3390/pr9060966]

[51]   H. Fleischer, R.R. Drews, J. Janson, B.R. Chinna Patlolla, X. Chu, M. Klos, and K. Thurow, "Application of a Dual-arm robot in complex sample preparation and measurement processes", *SLAS Technol.,* vol. 21, no. 5, pp. 671-681, 2016.
[http://dx.doi.org/10.1177/2211068216637352] [PMID: 27000132]

[52]   J.A. Tweed, Z. Gu, H. Xu, G. Zhang, P. Nouri, M. Li, and R. Steenwyk, "Automated sample preparation for regulated bioanalysis: an integrated multiple assay extraction platform using robotic liquid handling", *Bioanalysis,* vol. 2, no. 6, pp. 1023-1040, 2010.
[http://dx.doi.org/10.4155/bio.10.55] [PMID: 21083206]

[53]   M. E. Kempner, A. Felder, B. L. Smith, C. J. Johnson, and D. T. Williams, "Kempner-Felder-2002: A review of cell culture automation", 2002.

[54]   Michael S, Auld D, Klumpp C, Jadhav A, Zheng W, Thorne N, Austin CP, Inglese J, Simeonov A. A robotic platform for quantitative high-throughput screening. Assay and drug development technologies. 2008 Oct 1;6(5):637-57.
[http://dx.doi.org/10.1089/adt.2008.150]

[55]   H. Balta, J. Bedkowski, S. Govindaraj, K. Majek, P. Musialik, D. Serrano, K. Alexis, R. Siegwart, and G. De Cubber, "Integrated data management for a fleet of search-and-rescue robots", *J. Field Robot.,* vol. 34, no. 3, pp. 539-582, 2017.
[http://dx.doi.org/10.1002/rob.21651]

[56]   M. Andronie, G. Lăzăroiu, O.L. Karabolevski, R. Ştefănescu, I. Hurloiu, A. Dijmărescu, and I. Dijmărescu, "Remote big data management tools, sensing and computing technologies, and visual perception and environment mapping algorithms in the internet of robotic things", *Electronics (Basel),* vol. 12, no. 1, p. 22, 2022.
[http://dx.doi.org/10.3390/electronics12010022]

[57]   M. Andronie, G. Lăzăroiu, M. Iatagan, I. Hurloiu, R. Ştefănescu, A. Dijmărescu, and I. Dijmărescu, "Big data management algorithms, deep learning-based object detection technologies, and geospatial simulation and sensor fusion tools in the internet of robotic Things", *ISPRS Int. J. Geoinf.,* vol. 12, no. 2, p. 35, 2023.
[http://dx.doi.org/10.3390/ijgi12020035]

[58]   P. Nelson, C. Linegar, and P. Newman, "Building, curating, and querying large-scale data repositories for field robotics applications", In: *Proc 10th Int Conf Field and Service Robotics (FSR)* Toronto, Canada, 2015, pp. 517-531.
[http://dx.doi.org/10.1007/978-3-319-27702-8_34]

[59]   A.B. Henson, P.S. Gromski, and L. Cronin, "Designing algorithms to aid discovery by chemical robots", *ACS Cent. Sci.,* vol. 4, no. 7, pp. 793-804, 2018.
[http://dx.doi.org/10.1021/acscentsci.8b00176] [PMID: 30062108]

[60]   Vijaykumar, and Saravanakumar, "Future robotics database management system along with cloud TPS", *Int. J. Cloud Comput.: Serv. Archit.,* vol. 1, no. 3, pp. 103-113, 2011.
[http://dx.doi.org/10.5121/ijccsa.2011.1308]

[61]   J.P. Hughes, S. Rees, S.B. Kalindjian, and K.L. Philpott, "Principles of early drug discovery", *Br. J. Pharmacol.,* vol. 162, no. 6, pp. 1239-1249, 2011.
[http://dx.doi.org/10.1111/j.1476-5381.2010.01127.x] [PMID: 21091654]

[62]   Lin X, Li X, Lin X. A review on applications of computational methods in drug screening and design. Molecules. 2020 Mar 18;25(6):1375.

[63]   P. D. Lyne, "Box 1. Benchmark datasets for virtual screening", *Drug Discovery Today,* 2002. Available from: www.drugdiscoverytoday.com

[64]   Singh NK, Maiti NJ, Mishra M, Raj S, Rakshit G, Ghosh R, Roy S. Virtual Screening and Lead Discovery. Computational Methods for Rational Drug Design. 2025 Jan 20:97-121.
[http://dx.doi.org/10.1002/9781394249190.ch5]

[65]   V.D. Mouchlis, A. Afantitis, A. Serra, M. Fratello, A.G. Papadiamantis, V. Aidinis, I. Lynch, D. Greco, and G. Melagraki, "Advances in de novo drug design: From conventional to machine learning methods", *Int. J. Mol. Sci.,* vol. 22, no. 4, p. 1676, 2021.
[http://dx.doi.org/10.3390/ijms22041676] [PMID: 33562347]

[66]   T. Blaschke, A. A. Garcia, M. R. B. P. Gasteiger, L. R. S. Rachman, and M. H. F. Z. Montague, "REINVENT 2.0—an AI tool for de novo drug design", *J Chem Inf Model,* vol. 60, 2020no. 8, pp. 3780-3786. Available from: https://github.com/MolecularAI/Reinvent

[67]   M. Popova, O. Isayev, and A. Tropsha, "Deep reinforcement learning for de novo drug design", *Sci Adv,* vol. 4, 2018no. 7, p. eaap7885.
[http://dx.doi.org/10.1126/sciadv.aap7885]

[68]   A. Gupta, A.T. Müller, B.J.H. Huisman, J.A. Fuchs, P. Schneider, and G. Schneider, "Generative recurrent networks for De Novo drug design", *Mol. Inform.,* vol. 37, no. 1-2, p. 1700111, 2018.
[http://dx.doi.org/10.1002/minf.201700111] [PMID: 29095571]

[69]   S. Pushpakom, F. Iorio, P.A. Eyers, K.J. Escott, S. Hopper, A. Wells, A. Doig, T. Guilliams, J. Latimer, C. McNamee, A. Norris, P. Sanseau, D. Cavalla, and M. Pirmohamed, "Drug repurposing: progress, challenges and recommendations", *Nat. Rev. Drug Discov.,* vol. 18, no. 1, pp. 41-58, 2019.
[http://dx.doi.org/10.1038/nrd.2018.168] [PMID: 30310233]

[70]   V. Parvathaneni, N.S. Kulkarni, A. Muth, and V. Gupta, "Drug repurposing: a promising tool to accelerate the drug discovery process", *Drug Discov. Today,* vol. 24, no. 10, pp. 2076-2085, 2019.
[http://dx.doi.org/10.1016/j.drudis.2019.06.014] [PMID: 31238113]

[71]   Z. Gao, H. Li, H. Zhang, X. Liu, L. Kang, X. Luo, W. Zhu, K. Chen, X. Wang, and H. Jiang, "PDTD: a web-accessible protein database for drug target identification", *BMC Bioinformatics,* vol. 9, no. 1, p. 104, 2008.
[http://dx.doi.org/10.1186/1471-2105-9-104] [PMID: 18282303]

[72]   R. Borges, "We need a global system to help identify new uses for existing drugs", *BMJ,* vol. 348, no. feb27 1, p. g1806, 2014.
[http://dx.doi.org/10.1136/bmj.g1806] [PMID: 24578516]

[73]   D. E. Pankevich, B. M. Altevogt, J. Dunlop, F. H. Gage, and S. E. Hyman, "Improving and accelerating drug development for nervous system disorders", *Neuron,* vol. 84, no. 3, pp. 546-553, 2014.
[http://dx.doi.org/10.1016/j.neuron.2014.10.007]

[74]   S. Kraljevic, P. J. Stambrook, and K. Pavelic, "Accelerating drug discovery," *EMBO Reports,* vol. 5, no. 9, pp. 837–842, Sep. 2004.

[75]   R.C. Wang, and Z. Wang, "Precision Medicine: Disease Subtyping and Tailored Treatment", *Cancers (Basel),* vol. 15, no. 15, p. 3837, 2023.
[http://dx.doi.org/10.3390/cancers15153837] [PMID: 37568653]

[76]   S.G. Nicholls, B.J. Wilson, D. Castle, H. Etchegary, and J.C. Carroll, "Personalized medicine and genome-based treatments: Why personalized medicine ≠ individualized treatments", *Clin. Ethics,* vol. 9, no. 4, pp. 135-144, 2014.
[http://dx.doi.org/10.1177/1477750914558556]

[77]   C. Fiocchi, "Tailoring treatment to the individual patient - will inflammatory bowel disease medicine be personalized?", *Dig. Dis.,* vol. 33, suppl. Suppl. 1, pp. 82-89, 2015.
[http://dx.doi.org/10.1159/000437086] [PMID: 26368553]

[78]   S.J. Ruberg, and L. Shen, "Personalized medicine: Four perspectives of tailored medicine", *Stat. Biopharm. Res.,* vol. 7, no. 3, pp. 214-229, 2015.

[http://dx.doi.org/10.1080/19466315.2015.1059354]

[79]   M. S. Ibrahim, and S. Saber, "Machine learning and predictive analytics: Advancing disease prevention in healthcare", *J Contemp Healthc Anal,* vol. 7, no. 1, pp. 53-71, 2023. Available from: https://publications.dlpress.org/index.php/jcha/article/view/16

[80]   J. Gudin, S. Mavroudi, A. Korfiati, K. Theofilatos, D. Dietze, and P. Hurwitz, "Reducing opioid prescriptions by identifying responders on topical analgesic treatment using an individualized medicine and predictive analytics approach", *J. Pain Res.,* vol. 13, pp. 1255-1266, 2020. [http://dx.doi.org/10.2147/JPR.S246503] [PMID: 32547186]

[81]   N.J. Wesdorp, T. Hellingman, E.P. Jansma, J.H.T.M. van Waesberghe, R. Boellaard, C.J.A. Punt, J. Huiskens, and G. Kazemier, "Advanced analytics and artificial intelligence in gastrointestinal cancer: a systematic review of radiomics predicting response to treatment", *Eur. J. Nucl. Med. Mol. Imaging,* vol. 48, no. 6, pp. 1785-1794, 2021. [http://dx.doi.org/10.1007/s00259-020-05142-w] [PMID: 33326049]

[82]   S.B. Golas, M. Nikolova-Simons, R. Palacholla, J. op den Buijs, G. Garberg, A. Orenstein, and J. Kvedar, "Predictive analytics and tailored interventions improve clinical outcomes in older adults: a randomized controlled trial", *NPJ Digit. Med.,* vol. 4, no. 1, p. 97, 2021. [http://dx.doi.org/10.1038/s41746-021-00463-y] [PMID: 34112921]

[83]   D. Beydoun, R. Amal, G. Low, and S. Mcevoy, "Role of nanoparticles in photocatalysis," 1999.

[84]   G. Bozzuto, and A. Molinari, "Liposomes as nanomedical devices", *Int. J. Nanomedicine,* vol. 10, pp. 975-999, 2015. [http://dx.doi.org/10.2147/IJN.S68861] [PMID: 25678787]

[85]   X. Guo, L. Wang, X. Wei, and S. Zhou, "Polymer-based drug delivery systems for cancer treatment", *J. Polym. Sci. A Polym. Chem.,* vol. 54, no. 22, pp. 3525-3550, 2016. [http://dx.doi.org/10.1002/pola.28252]

[86]   L. Ducry, Eds., Antibody-Drug Conjugates. New York, NY, USA: Humana Press, 2013.

[87]   R.F. Donnelly, T.R.R. Singh, M.J. Garland, K. Migalska, R. Majithiya, C.M. McCrudden, P.L. Kole, T.M.T. Mahmood, H.O. McCarthy, and A.D. Woolfson, "Hydrogel-forming microneedle arrays for enhanced transdermal drug delivery", *Adv. Funct. Mater.,* vol. 22, no. 23, pp. 4879-4890, 2012. [http://dx.doi.org/10.1002/adfm.201200864] [PMID: 23606824]

[88]   S.A. Stewart, J. Domínguez-Robles, R.F. Donnelly, and E. Larrañeta, "Implantable polymeric drug delivery devices: Classification, manufacture, materials, and clinical applications", *Polymers (Basel),* vol. 10, no. 12, p. 1379, 2018. [http://dx.doi.org/10.3390/polym10121379] [PMID: 30961303]

[89]   Q. T. Zhou, S. S. Y. Leung, P. Tang, T. Parumasivam, Z. H. Loh, and H. K. Chan, "Inhaled formulations and pulmonary drug delivery systems for respiratory infections", *Adv Drug Deliv Rev,* vol. 85, pp. 83-99, 2015. [http://dx.doi.org/10.1016/j.addr.2014.10.022]

[90]   A.S. Lübbe, C. Alexiou, and C. Bergemann, "Clinical applications of magnetic drug targeting", *J. Surg. Res.,* vol. 95, no. 2, pp. 200-206, 2001. [http://dx.doi.org/10.1006/jsre.2000.6030] [PMID: 11162046]

[91]   D.R. Serrano, F.C. Luciano, B.J. Anaya, B. Ongoren, A. Kara, G. Molina, B.I. Ramirez, S.A. Sánchez-Guirales, J.A. Simon, G. Tomietto, and C. Rapti, "Artificial intelligence (AI) applications in drug discovery and drug delivery: Revolutionizing personalized medicine", *Pharmaceutics,* vol. 16, no. 10, p. 1328, 2024.

[92]   R. Liu and P. Zhang, "Towards early detection of adverse drug reactions: combining pre-clinical drug structures and post-market safety reports," *BMC Med. Inform. Dec. Mak,* vol. 19, no. 279, 2019. [http://dx.doi.org/10.1186/s12911-019-0999-1]

[93]   Ahire YS, Patil JH, Chordiya HN, Deore RA, Bairagi VA. Advanced applications of artificial

intelligence in pharmacovigilance: Current trends and future perspectives. *J Pharm Res.* 2024 Jan;23(1):23-33.

[94]   M. Hashiguchi, S. Imai, K. Uehara, J. Maruyama, M. Shimizu, and M. Mochizuki, "Factors affecting the timing of signal detection of adverse drug reactions", *PLoS One,* vol. 10, no. 12, p. e0144263, 2015.
[http://dx.doi.org/10.1371/journal.pone.0144263] [PMID: 26641634]

[95]   H.M.R. Alrwayli, B.G.S. Alanazi, M.M.S. Alanazi, A.D. Alanazi, A.I.A. Alenezi, M.J.N. Alruwili, M.A.E. Alanazi, A.T.A. Alanazi, F.H.F. Alanazi, M.M.R. Alruwaili, and S.M.F. Alenazi, "Laboratory tests for the early detection of adverse drug reaction", *Saudi J. Med. Pharm. Sci.,* vol. 9, no. 12, pp. 835-838, 2023.
[http://dx.doi.org/10.36348/sjmps.2023.v09i12.009]

[96]   S. Yang, and S. Kar, "Application of artificial intelligence and machine learning in early detection of Adverse Drug Reactions (ADRs) and drug-induced toxicity", *Artificial Intelligence Chemistry,* vol. 1, no. 2, p. 100011, 2023.
[http://dx.doi.org/10.1016/j.aichem.2023.100011]

[97]   S. Singh, R. Kumar, S. Payra, and S.K. Singh, "Artificial intelligence and machine learning in pharmacological research: bridging the gap between data and drug discovery", *Cureus,* vol. 15, no. 8, p. e44359, 2023.
[http://dx.doi.org/10.7759/cureus.44359] [PMID: 37779744]

[98]   T. A. Lieu, M. L. Ray, R. D. Olson, J. A. Hinman, and J. M. Goldenberg, "Real-time vaccine safety surveillance for the early detection of adverse events", *Med Care,* vol. 45, no. 10, pp. 918-924, 2007.
[http://dx.doi.org/10.1097/MLR.0b013e3180616c0a]

[99]   T. A. Lieu, M. L. Ray, R. D. Olson, J. A. Hinman, J. M. Goldenberg, and A. A. Barron, "Real-time vaccine safety surveillance for the early detection of adverse events", *Med Care,* vol. 45, no. 10, pp. 918-924, 2007.
[http://dx.doi.org/10.1097/MLR.0b013e3180616c0a]

[100] S. Kalogiannidis, D. Kalfas, O. Papaevangelou, G. Giannarakis, and F. Chatzitheodoridis, "The role of artificial intelligence technology in predictive risk assessment for business continuity: A case study of greece", *Risks,* vol. 12, no. 2, p. 19, 2024.
[http://dx.doi.org/10.3390/risks12020019]

[101] C.C. Freifeld, J.S. Brownstein, C.M. Menone, W. Bao, R. Filice, T. Kass-Hout, and N. Dasgupta, "Digital drug safety surveillance: monitoring pharmaceutical products in twitter", *Drug Saf.,* vol. 37, no. 5, pp. 343-350, 2014.
[http://dx.doi.org/10.1007/s40264-014-0155-x] [PMID: 24777653]

[102] L.K. Vora, A.D. Gholap, K. Jetha, R.R.S. Thakur, H.K. Solanki, and V.P. Chavda, "Artificial intelligence in pharmaceutical technology and drug delivery design", *Pharmaceutics,* vol. 15, no. 7, p. 1916, 2023.
[http://dx.doi.org/10.3390/pharmaceutics15071916] [PMID: 37514102]

[103] H. Edrees, W. Song, A. Syrowatka, A. Simona, M.G. Amato, and D.W. Bates, "Intelligent telehealth in pharmacovigilance: A future perspective", *Drug Saf.,* vol. 45, no. 5, pp. 449-458, 2022.
[http://dx.doi.org/10.1007/s40264-022-01172-5] [PMID: 35579810]

[104] K. Williams, E. Bilsland, A. Sparkes, W. Aubrey, M. Young, L.N. Soldatova, K. De Grave, J. Ramon, M. de Clare, W. Sirawaraporn, S.G. Oliver, and R.D. King, "Cheaper faster drug development validated by the repositioning of drugs against neglected tropical diseases", *J. R. Soc. Interface,* vol. 12, no. 104, p. 20141289, 2015.
[http://dx.doi.org/10.1098/rsif.2014.1289] [PMID: 25652463]

[105] D.A. Keesler, and V.H. Flood, "Current issues in diagnosis and treatment of von Willebrand disease", *Res. Pract. Thromb. Haemost.,* vol. 2, no. 1, pp. 34-41, 2018.
[http://dx.doi.org/10.1002/rth2.12064] [PMID: 30046704]

[106] A.M. Burgener, "Enhancing communication to improve patient safety and to increase patient satisfaction", *Health Care Manag. (Frederick)*, vol. 36, no. 3, pp. 238-243, 2017.
[http://dx.doi.org/10.1097/HCM.0000000000000165] [PMID: 28657914]

[107] M.J. Siedner, M.B. Bwana, M.Y.S. Moosa, M. Paul, S. Pillay, S. McCluskey, I. Aturinda, K. Ard, W. Muyindike, P. Moodley, J. Brijkumar, T. Rautenberg, G. George, B. Johnson, R.T. Gandhi, H. Sunpath, and V.C. Marconi, "The REVAMP trial to evaluate HIV resistance testing in sub-Saharan Africa: a case study in clinical trial design in resource limited settings to optimize effectiveness and cost effectiveness estimates", *HIV Clin. Trials*, vol. 18, no. 4, pp. 149-155, 2017.
[http://dx.doi.org/10.1080/15284336.2017.1349028] [PMID: 28720039]

[108] H.G. Eichler, S.X. Kong, W.C. Gerth, P. Mavros, and B. Jönsson, "Use of cost-effectiveness analysis in health-care resource allocation decision-making: how are cost-effectiveness thresholds expected to emerge?", *Value Health*, vol. 7, no. 5, pp. 518-528, 2004.
[http://dx.doi.org/10.1111/j.1524-4733.2004.75003.x] [PMID: 15367247]

[109] A. Verma, P. Bhattacharya, N. Madhani, C. Trivedi, B. Bhushan, S. Tanwar, G. Sharma, P.N. Bokoro, and R. Sharma, "Blockchain for industry 5.0: Vision, opportunities, key enablers, and future directions", *IEEE Access*, vol. 10, pp. 69160-69199, 2022.
[http://dx.doi.org/10.1109/ACCESS.2022.3186892]

[110] P. Budhwar, S. Chowdhury, G. Wood, H. Aguinis, G.J. Bamber, J.R. Beltran, P. Boselie, F. Lee Cooke, S. Decker, A. DeNisi, P.K. Dey, D. Guest, A.J. Knoblich, A. Malik, J. Paauwe, S. Papagiannidis, C. Patel, V. Pereira, S. Ren, S. Rogelberg, M.N.K. Saunders, R.L. Tung, and A. Varma, "Human resource management in the age of generative artificial intelligence: Perspectives and research directions on ChatGPT", *Hum. Resour. Manage. J.*, vol. 33, no. 3, pp. 606-659, 2023.
[http://dx.doi.org/10.1111/1748-8583.12524]

[111] B. Bhushan, A. Kumar, A.K. Agarwal, A. Kumar, P. Bhattacharya, and A. Kumar, "Towards a secure and sustainable internet of medical things (IoMT): Requirements, design challenges, security techniques, and future trends", *Sustainability (Basel)*, vol. 15, no. 7, p. 6177, 2023.
[http://dx.doi.org/10.3390/su15076177]

[112] S. Phuyal, D. Bista, and R. Bista, "Challenges, opportunities and future directions of smart manufacturing: A state of art review", *Sustainable Futures*, vol. 2, p. 100023, 2020.
[http://dx.doi.org/10.1016/j.sftr.2020.100023]

[113] I. Gibson, D. Rosen, and B. Stucker, *Additive manufacturing technologies: 3D printing, rapid prototyping, and direct digital manufacturing.* 2nd ed. Springer: New York, 2015.
[http://dx.doi.org/10.1007/978-1-4939-2113-3]

CHAPTER 6

IoT's Role in Revolutionizing Pillbox Technology

Shekhar Singh[1], Akhil Sharma[2], Sunita[3], Sumit Chowdary Mukund[4] and **Shaweta Sharma[5,*]**

[1] *Faculty of Pharmacy, Babu Banarasi Das Northern India Institute of Technology, Lucknow, Uttar Pradesh, India*

[2] *R.J. College of Pharmacy, Raipur, Gharbara, Tappal, Khair, Uttar Pradesh, India*

[3] *Metro College of Health Sciences and Research, Greater Noida, Uttar Pradesh, India*

[4] *Department of Civil Engineering, Aditya University, Surampalem, India*

[5] *School of Medical and Allied Sciences, Galgotias University Plot No. 2, Yamuna Expy, Opposite Buddha International Circuit, Sector 17A, Greater Noida, Uttar Pradesh, India*

Abstract: The incorporation of Internet of Things (IoT) technology into pillboxes means that there has been a great advancement in the field of drug management. Pill organizers have long been the main way to organize medicines. However, they mostly do not tackle adherence issues leading to poor treatment outcomes. Nevertheless, IoT-enabled smart pillboxes have completely transformed medication management by capitalizing on connectedness and data analytics to boost adherence and patient engagement. The chapter discusses the changes that have taken place in pill box technology from simple holders to IoT-based systems and the benefits and implications of these developments. Some of these include IoT integration, which provides wireless connections, sensors for real-time monitoring, and cloud-based data analysis, among others. There are various features such as personalized medication reminders, remote monitoring, and feedback that aid people in taking their prescribed medications as per the advice given by their doctors, thus lowering medication errors through enhanced adherence. Additionally, the use of Internet of Things technology in pillboxes provides patients with real-time feedback on their adherence behavior, and hence, they become more active participants in the management of their healthcare. The future of IoT-enabled pillbox technology with AI also anticipates personalization of medicine administration and expansion into other areas of healthcare. This chapter ends by calling for more research, collaboration, and policy support needed for enhancing the widespread adoption of IoT-based healthcare solutions and optimizing medication consumption to promote better patient care outcomes.

* **Corresponding author Shaweta Sharma:** School of Medical and Allied Sciences, Galgotias University Plot No. 2, Yamuna Expy, Opposite Buddha International Circuit, Sector 17A, Greater Noida, Uttar Pradesh, India; E-mail: shawetasharma@galgotiasuniversity.edu.in

Keywords: Artificial intelligence, Clinical, Chronic, Compliance, Disease, Digital health, Healthcare, Internet of things, Post-operation, Privacy, Patient, Personalized medicine, Recovery, Remote patient monitoring, Security, Wearable devices.

INTRODUCTION

Medication management has become more complicated in today's healthcare. Patients have a difficult time adhering to them, which leads to negative health outcomes and increased expenditures on healthcare. Luckily, technology advancements have been made, especially in the Internet of Things that could help promote medication management further. This chapter discusses how IoT has revolutionized medication management through its integration into pillbox technology [1, 2].

IoT is a network of interconnected devices embedded with sensors, software, and other technologies that enable them to exchange data and communicate over the Internet. In various industries, including healthcare, IoT has gained immense popularity as it enables remote monitoring, data collection, and analysis for improved patient care and operational efficiency [3 - 5].

IoT has greatly transformed pillbox technology from a mere container for the arrangement of drugs to an intelligent product. In particular, smartness is achieved by adding sensors, making it connectible, and installing mobile applications that work with it to monitor and control compliance with medication. Thus, theseapplications have features such as automated reminders, tracking dosing and synchronizing information with healthcare providers [6].

The most important thing about IoT-connected pillbox technology is that it increases the levels of adherence to medication. Smart pillboxes offer notifications and reminders to help patients follow the prescription times that have been personalized for them. Additionally, real-time monitoring features allow doctors to intervene early in case of non-adherence; this has the effect of improving treatment outcomes generally [7, 8].

IoT-enabled pillboxes allow monitoring of the medication adherence of patients from afar, enabling healthcare providers to determine whether they are adhering to prescribed medication. This kind of remote support system allows for immediate changes in therapy, thus helping to reduce chances for complications and hospital stays. Furthermore, patients are more confident knowing their healthcare team's continuous involvement with their lives, thus leading to a higher degree of participation and pleasure [9, 10].

The integration of IoT in pillbox technology has various challenges and issues that must be addressed despite its potential as a transformative tool. These include concerns over the safety of data, compatibility with existing medical systems, and the elderly or technically unsophisticated who seek to reach it. Collaboration involving healthcare providers, developers of technology, regulatory bodies, and patients is needed to address these challenges [11].

However, the incorporation of IoT in pillbox technology has a number of problems and factors that should be considered. It should be noted that these may include issues about data protection and security, compatibility with other health systems, and availability to older people or those who are not technically advanced. Dealing with those difficulties necessitates the engagement of a wide range of participants such as healthcare professionals, computer scientists, government authorities in charge of regulations, and patients themselves [11, 12].

The inclusion of IoT in pill box technology is a deviation from the usual method of handling medicine; thus, it provides contemporary ways through which medication adherence can be improved, remote monitoring can be done, and data can support a decision-making process. By connecting people with real-time information and using analytics, smart pillboxes can change patient care, resulting in improved treatment results. Nevertheless, for this potential to be realized, several obstacles that touch on confidentiality issues and others pertaining to interoperation must be addressed. Through cooperation among interested parties in this area, everyone may fully exploit these advantages tied to an IoT-incorporated pillbox technology, hence transforming healthcare delivery across the globe [13, 14].

PILLBOX TECHNOLOGY EVOLUTION

Historical Perspective on Medication Adherence and the Need for Innovative Solutions

Medication adherence in the health care system remains a challenge as patients follow prescription treatment patterns. Medication non-compliance results in worsened health outcomes, escalated medical service expenses, and an erosion in quality of life. Even with progress made in medical practice, aiming at optimal compliance is still impossible. This historical review looks at medication adherence and presents the factors that impact it alongside the identification of creative measures required to tackle this matter decisively [15 - 18].

In ancient times, people used to administer medications in the form of herbal mixtures, lotions, and mysterious liquids; therefore, this concept has existed since then. Although these remedies were not based on scientific research and were subject to different interpretations, they were necessary to be obeyed. Practices such as Hippocrates' admonition to "not harm" underscored the importance of patient compliance with treatment protocols [19, 20].

The advent of modern pharmacotherapy in the 19th and 20th centuries marked a significant milestone in healthcare. The discovery of antibiotics, vaccines, and other life-saving medications revolutionized the treatment of infectious diseases and chronic conditions. However, with the proliferation of pharmaceuticals came the challenge of ensuring patient adherence to complex medication regimens [21].

A notable achievement in healthcare was the arrival of modern pharmacotherapy in the 19th and 20th centuries. With these discoveries, antibiotics, vaccines, and other life-saving drugs were found to be useful in treating infectious diseases as well as chronic illnesses. Despite this breakthrough, problems of complex medication regimens that patient adherence may not be easy solutions have been brought about by a growing number of pharmaceuticals being manufactured [22].

Substandard care results from poor adherence to the medication that is associated with it, causing high hospital admissions and death rates. This gives rise to the progression of diseases, increasing drug resistance, and complications that weigh heavily on healthcare organizations and society in its entirety. The economic implications of non-adherence to medications are significant, with estimations indicating billions of dollars worth of avoidable health expenses yearly. Hospitalizations, emergency visits, and preventable complications highlight the pressing need for addressing adherence barriers through novel interventions [23, 24].

Improvements in technology, particularly the IoT, give hope for better medication adherence. Smart pillboxes, wearable devices, and mobile health applications provide innovative means to enhance medication management through real-time monitoring and improved communication between patients and their healthcare providers. Personalized approaches are employed for medication adherence in order to meet the needs of individual patients. This technique also uses artificial intelligence algorithms, predictive analytics, and behavioral science principles to develop focused interventions aimed at addressing individual adherence barriers and optimizing treatment outcomes [25, 26].

Medication adherence has always been a significant problem in healthcare, with implications reaching far into patient outcomes and the cost of healthcare. It, however, remains a complex and multifaceted endeavor to achieve optimal adherence despite decades of research and intervention efforts. Nonetheless, advances in technology and personalized medicine provide novel strategies to address barriers to adherence as well as improve therapeutic outcomes. Healthcare stakeholders can lead the way towards a tomorrow where medication adherence is improved by embracing creative solutions and adopting collaborative approaches that ensure patients derive maximum benefits from pharmacotherapy [27].

Challenges of Medication Adherence in Chronic Disease Management

The considerable effects of medication adherence on patients' health outcomes, as well as healthcare systems, make managing chronic diseases a difficult task. This is attributed to the sheer complexity of treatment regimens, which often necessitate patients having to handle more than one drug, with each requiring its own dosing, administration, and side effect schedules. Adding to this, polypharmacy occurs when individuals are given various drugs for different chronic illnesses or complications, resulting in a greater pill burden and an escalating rate of non-adherence [28].

Furthermore, patients' perception of prescription efficiency and the presence of adverse effects can impair adherence since patients may stop taking medicines or change their drugs due to side effects experienced or doubt concerning the efficacy of their medication. Also, access and cost are serious obstacles since sometimes patients may face financial difficulties in purchasing medicine and also experience complications when trying to get it, probably from distant, underserved localities or poverty-stricken environments. Moreover, low health literacy is a major impediment as many patients have challenges understanding how to take medications that are prescribed to them, managing the medications they use, and what it means to adhere [29, 30].

In addition, social support and mental conditions such as depression and anxiety will also play the most important role in encouraging a patient, thus self-motivation and belief in oneself by submitting to medical care. These challenges are exacerbated by stigmatization that is linked with specific chronic diseases and cultural beliefs on medications, thereby contributing to medication nonadherence among affected populations. Effective communication between providers and patients is key in addressing these issues. However, it frequently fails due to insufficient education of patients, lack of clear instructions, or inadequate support from medical practitioners, all of which impede adherence initiatives [31].

To combat these challenges and enhance drug adherence in chronic disease management, it is necessary to consider a comprehensive approach that includes patient education, simplified treatment regimens, and such support services as medication reminders and adherence monitoring, addressing the problems of cost and access, promoting shared decision-making, overcoming the barriers that exist between patients and health care providers. Proactive targeting of these challenges through customized interventions enables healthcare providers to make patients better self-managers of their chronic conditions with improved health outcomes [29, 32].

Comparison of Traditional Pillboxes and Smart Pillboxes

The comparison highlights the differences between traditional pillboxes and smart pillboxes [33], emphasizing the advanced features and capabilities offered by smart pillboxes in improving medication adherence and management, which are summarized in Table **1**.

Table 1. Comparison of traditional pillboxes and smart pillboxes.

Aspect	Traditional Pillboxes	Smart Pillboxes
Design	Simple plastic containers with compartments for each day of the week or multiple times per day.	Typically sleek and compact design with compartments for each dose, often with additional features such as digital displays and alarms [34].
Functionality	Basic storage for organizing medications.	Advanced features such as automated reminders, dose tracking, and real-time monitoring [35].
Reminder System	None	Built-in alarms, LED lights, or smartphone notifications to remind users to take their medication [36].
Adherence Tracking	Not applicable	Ability to track medication adherence through digital records and data synchronization with healthcare providers [37].
Connectivity	No connectivity features.	Integrated with smartphone apps or connected to Wi-Fi for data synchronization and remote monitoring [38].
Data Analysis	No data analysis capabilities.	Data-driven insights into medication adherence patterns, trends, and outcomes [39].
Accessibility	Easy to use, but may not accommodate complex medication regimens.	Can accommodate complex medication regimens and provide customized reminders and notifications [40].
Cost	Typically, it is low-cost or even free.	Higher initial investment due to advanced features, but potential long-term cost savings through improved adherence and health outcomes [41].
Privacy and Security	Limited privacy and security features.	May include encryption and authentication measures to protect patient data [42].
User Interface	Simple and straightforward.	User-friendly interface with options for customization and personalization [43].
Maintenance	Minimal maintenance is required.	May require periodic software updates or battery replacements [44].

(Table 1) cont.....

Aspect	Traditional Pillboxes	Smart Pillboxes
Integration with Healthcare Systems	Not integrated with healthcare systems.	Potential integration with electronic health records (EHRs) and healthcare provider platforms for seamless communication and data sharing [45].

ADVANTAGES OF SMART PILLBOXES IN IMPROVING MEDICATION ADHERENCE

Smart pillboxes offer numerous advantages in improving medication adherence compared to traditional pillboxes [46]. The advantages of smart pillboxes are summarized in Fig. (**1**).

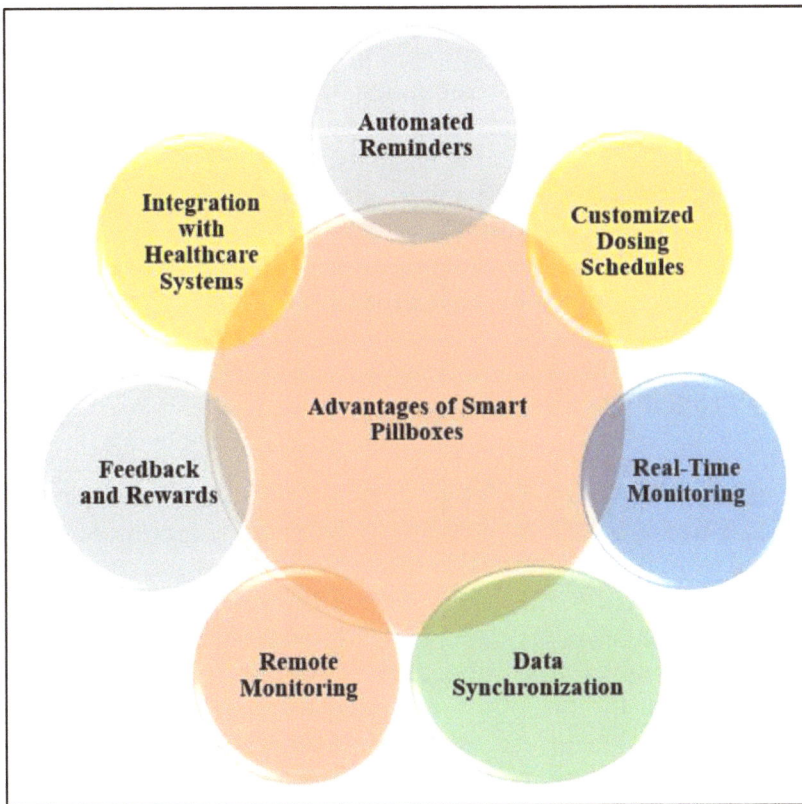

Fig. (1). Advantages of smart pillboxes in improving medication adherence.

Automated Reminders

This technology coins medication adherence through automated reminders, one of the most common features of smart pillboxes. They are built in such a way that they produce sounds of different natures and content, such as alarms, vibrations,

LED lights, and mobile notifications. These reminders guide people through their medication regimen fluently using different flows, such as the symphony of vibrating alerts, LED light flashes, and even gentle sound notifications from phones or other smart devices. They play an important role in informing users when to take their medications and provide structure and order among the complexities of life on a daily basis [47].

These reminders adapt to accommodate individual preferences and routines, making it easy for them to fit within different ways of life so that taking medicine becomes something routine rather than a chore. They go beyond being just functional, acting as beacons of reassurance and encouragement, which bring inner peace to people dealing with long-term illnesses or complex treatment schedules [48, 49].

Again, the ability of smart pillbox reminders to work together with other people goes beyond individuals and lets remote monitoring provide caregivers and healthcare providers with invaluable insights. These reminders foster a shared responsibility for improving drug adherence through timely interventions and support. As such, automatic reminders are leading in the field of medication adherence solutions as they use technology to make people powerful and healthy and change the way of thinking about proactive self-care in today's world [50, 51].

Customized Dosing Schedules

The tailored treatment regimens of smart pillboxes in individualized dosing schedules reflect a personalized approach to medication management. Users may adjust their dose timings with unprecedented accuracy *via* intuitive interfaces and advanced programming capacities, thus guaranteeing the highest levels of compliance and therapeutic efficiency. Other than simple time-based reminders, this customization enables users to configure the following: frequency of dosage, intervals, and even combinations of medicines as per their prescribed regimens. If you take one tablet in the morning or a more complex regime that has several drugs that have to be taken at varying times during the day, smart pillboxes give users complete control over their medicinal intake, too [52, 53].

Customized dosing schedules are valuable in that they can take into account the complications of everyday living and ailments. These plans relate to everyday routines and personal inclinations, making them blend well with life's fabric, hence minimizing interruptions and enhancing adherence. For example, synchronizing medication doses with meal times, work schedules, or any other daily activities will allow users to adjust their dosing schedules accordingly, thus promoting self-rule and empowerment as far as their health is concerned [54].

Customized dosing schedules are versatile, extending beyond convenience to optimize the outcome of treatment. One way through which smart pillboxes facilitate adherence to prescribed protocols is the tailoring of medication regimens to individual needs. Apart from ensuring that therapeutic agents reach patients in a timely manner, this ensures that too little or too much medicine is used, reducing risks associated with under or over-dosing during treatment processes [55].

When integrated with remote monitoring capabilities, personalized dosing schedules enable healthcare providers and caregivers to monitor medication adherence in real time, offering crucial data on patient compliance and response to treatment. Such a collaborative way of administering medicine allows medical teams to intervene early whenever there are deviations from the recommended instructions that are meant for the best results, thus improving the condition of patients [56].

At its core, smart pillboxes that offer personalized dosing schedules represent a new way of taking medicines for patients involving technology to individualize treatment regimens, increase users' involvement level, and improve therapeutic results. These timetables enable the independence of drug administration by individuals, heralding an age of accurate medication where therapy guidelines are customized according to each patient's specific requirements and situations [57, 58].

Real-Time Monitoring

Smart pillboxes with integrated real-time monitoring capabilities are expected to signal a revolution in how we handle medication, giving users and carers unique viewpoints and aids. Additionally, the devices offer constant drug ingestion tracking by simply merging into digital platforms and employing connectivity features that facilitate instant response and interference. In addition, real-time monitoring goes beyond the conventional adherence approaches by making use of sensors, data analytics, and wireless communications, thereby ushering in a new era of proactive healthcare management [59].

The major concept behind real-time monitoring is the capture and analysis of data on medication adherence when it occurs. Such capabilities provide holistic comprehension of user behavior and adherence patterns, such as determining an instance where a dose has been taken or identifying compliance trends over time. The minute details empower people to have educated choices about their health and medicine management but also allow for timely interventions in cases of deviation from prescribed regimens [60].

Medication management, with the help of real-time monitoring, has been made a collaborative process that caters to remote monitoring and intervention. Caregivers can receive missing dose notifications or deviation from medication-taking patterns through private online networks and mobile apps. Timely intervention is facilitated by this system as reminders or support is given to patients regarding their treatment plans in order to improve the adherence and health outcomes concerned [61].

Data from real-time monitoring can be used to give information about personalized interventions and predictive analytics. Based on adherence patterns and medication-taking behavior, health professionals can identify non-adherence risk factors and provide appropriate interventions. This active process will not only boost drug adherence but also minimize the incidence of adverse effects as well as hospitalization, hence enhancing care quality and patient outcomes [62].

Data Synchronization

Smart pillboxes with data synchronization features are revolutionizing medication management by allowing for continuous interaction among users, caregivers, and healthcare providers. These devices enable drug adherence data to be transmitted correctly and safely from one platform or device to another within seconds using their advanced capabilities of synchrony. The use of data synchronization as a means of medication management process through cloud computing, wireless connectivity, and interoperability will enhance communication among the staff members, streamline medicine prescriptions, facilitate orders for medical procedures, and therefore improve patients' health results [63 - 65].

Data synchronization basically means that medication adherence data can be aligned on different digital platforms and devices. Be it a smartphone application, an online portal, or an electronic health record system, all parties involved in this approach are able to get the most recent information regarding drug intake, compliance patterns, and treatment outcomes by synchronizing everything. Therefore, there is a smooth flow of data that favors teamwork, leading to collaboration among patients, families, and health practitioners so that they can make informed decisions about medicine administration and patients' well-being [66].

Data synchronization allows personalized interventions and support mechanisms that rely on real-time adherence data. Healthcare providers can identify incidences for intervention through adherence patterns and medication-taking behaviors and align the strategies with specific needs. Timely reminders, counseling, or adjusting treatment plans are examples of how synchronized actions seek to optimize adherence as well as health outcomes through proactive involvement with the patients [67, 68].

Communication and information sharing among healthcare teams are enhanced by synchronization, thereby enabling seamless care coordination and collaboration. Interoperable systems and secure data exchange protocols facilitate healthcare providers' access to medication adherence data across different care settings, thus ensuring continuity of care and avoiding gaps in treatment. This multidisciplinary approach to medication management promotes patient safety by minimizing medication errors and refining the general quality of care provided [69, 70].

The synchronization of data in smart pillboxes is a primary component of contemporary healthcare, and it leads to easy sharing and cooperation among medical practitioners. The alignment of digital channels and appliances brings on board all the stakeholders involved, such as patients, caregivers, and general healthcare providers, who want to see that there are improvements in adherence levels toward medication by patients. As medical services continue to change, the synchronization of information will increasingly become important in streamlining drug use procedures and changing the way patients receive care [71].

Remote Monitoring

Medication management is being revolutionized by smart pillboxes that have remote monitoring capabilities, which allow caregivers and healthcare providers to keep track of medication adherence from afar. Such devices facilitate real-time remote monitoring through the uninterrupted transmission of adherence data using wireless connections, providing important information about patient behavior and treatment outcomes. This is especially useful for patients who need continuous assistance, such as those with complex medication regimens or chronic diseases [72].

The use of remote monitoring helps track medication adherence by allowing caregivers and healthcare providers to follow up on when patients are taking their prescribed drug doses and identify any deviations from the routine. Through the use of digital platforms and secure communication channels, it is possible to access adherence data from anywhere, which ensures that timely interventions and support can be provided. Remote monitoring is a means by which healthcare teams can take action in anticipation of patient behavior toward optimizing adherence through reminders, counseling, or adjustment of treatment plans [73].

Remote monitoring is vital in promoting communication and cooperation between healthcare stakeholders. This way, a common approach to medication management can be evolved. Sharing of adherence data among caregivers, specialists, and other members of the healthcare team can be seamless through interoperable systems and secure exchange protocols. It also promotes continuity of care through interdisciplinary collaboration, ensuring informed decision-making that leads to better patient outcomes.

Additionally, remote monitoring is another key area that helps in patient empowerment and engagement. It makes the patients feel responsible for their health by fostering a sense of accountability for taking medication as prescribed. Because they are aware that someone else is watching, many people would be more compliant with their treatment schedules and take an active part in their healthcare. This collaboration between doctors and patients is crucial to achieving long-term compliance and better treatment results [71].

Feedback and Rewards

The smart pillboxes have an ingenious way of incentivizing and reinforcing adherence to medication. Real-time data is shown on the level of adherence by these systems as they give ideas into the behavior of taking drugs. Feedback and reward systems influenced by behavioral psychology principles like gamification and positive reinforcement encourage users' compliance with their medicine intake schedules, thereby enhancing health outcomes [74].

Smart pillboxes use feedback mechanisms that help users know if they take their drugs as prescribed. If it is by visual cues, individualized messages, or reports of adherence, the users get timely responses about their medication consumption patterns. This feedback is useful as a way of self-monitoring and self-management, empowering them to monitor their progress and make well-informed decisions regarding their health [75].

Additionally, feedback systems can reward programs by being coupled with them to give further incentives for adherence. When users are offered rewards that they can touch – like points badges or virtual prizes, they get motivated to keep on adhering to their medication schedules. These rewards make one feel good about oneself as a result of the act of faithfully following the drug-taking plan, which is represented by an improved flow of events in behavior over time [76].

Customization of feedback and reward systems to meet individual needs is possible. This is done by setting attainable adherence goals or customizing rewards that are based on user preferences, thus making these systems adjust to the unique motivations and requirements of each user. In turn, this customization improves motivation and efficacy, giving rise to sustainable change in behavior and better medication conformity [77].

Apart from being motivating factors, feedback and rewards can also bring about a sense of community and social support. Users can connect with their peers who are facing similar challenges, such as sharing adherence achievements or participating in challenges or competitions. Therefore, this reinforcing camaraderie further strengthens the user's long-term commitment to taking medication [78].

Basically, the feedback and rewards systems provided by smart pill boxes are a powerful tool in promoting medication adherence and improving health outcomes. With real-time feedback, tangible incentives, and personalized support, these systems allow individuals to take charge of their health and remain consistent with their medication regimens. In an ever-evolving healthcare landscape, feedback and reward systems will increasingly become critical for optimizing medication management and cultivating a culture of proactive self-care [79].

Integration with Healthcare Systems

The pivotal feature of smart pillboxes is the integration with healthcare systems that facilitates seamless communication and collaboration between patients, caregivers, and healthcare providers in order to make it possible for them to have their needs met easily. They improve medication management by linking up with EHR, pharmacy systems, and telehealth platforms, thereby enabling comprehensive healthcare delivery [80].

Smart pillboxes connected to healthcare systems can retrieve and change the patients' medication records in real time. The smooth transfer of data provides healthcare providers with correct and recently updated patient information on drug regimens, leading to informed choices and personalized management. Unlike verifying medicine prescriptions, detecting probable medicines interferences, or monitoring treatment compliance, integration with healthcare systems helps in making drugs safe as well as ensuring that patients are treated effectively [81].

Interfacing with EHR systems makes medication-related information easier to document and manage. Administrative load is reduced by smart pillboxes that automatically record adherence data and sync it into patients' electronic records, thereby ensuring continuity of care across multiple healthcare environments. This interoperability promotes teamwork among healthcare providers, enabling seamless coordination of care as well as improving healthcare delivery quality and efficiency [82].

In addition, being linked with pharmacy systems allows automated refill requests to be made and prescription synchronization to take place, which is key to medication management and adherence. Smart pillboxes can even send notifications to users or healthcare providers as soon as medicine refills are required, simplifying the whole process of refilling medicines and hence minimizing the dangers associated with treatment discontinuation. Also, automating medication management tasks *via* integration with pharmacy systems improves convenience for patients while enhancing compliance with prescribed regimens [83].

To support remote monitoring and virtual care provision, smart pillboxes can interface with telehealth platforms, as well as EHR and pharmacy integration. Healthcare providers can use secure communication channels to monitor patients' medication adherence from a distance while also facilitating timely interventions such as virtual medication reviews. This technology helps improve access to care for individuals who have limited mobility or are unable to access traditional healthcare services, and it also encourages patient participation in their treatment plans.

Advantages of smart pillboxes in enhancing drug adherence include automated reminders, personalized dosing programs, real-time monitoring, data syncing, remote monitoring, feedback loops, and integration with healthcare systems. Such advanced features assist users in better handling their medications, thereby improving treatment adherence while at the same time enhancing their health outcomes [84].

IoT-enabled features in pillbox technology represent a significant advancement in medication management, leveraging connectivity and smart capabilities to enhance adherence and improve health outcomes, as summarized in Fig. (2).

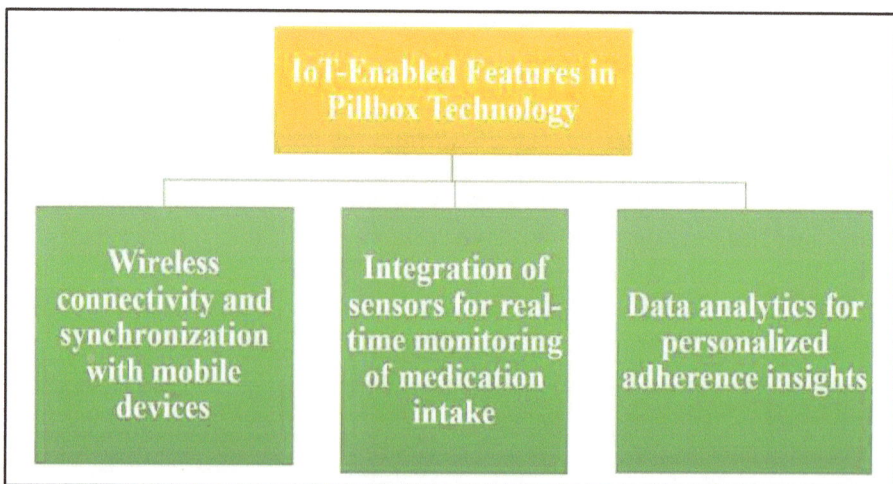

Fig. (2). IoT-enabled features in pillbox technology.

ROLE OF CLOUD COMPUTING IN FACILITATING REMOTE MONITORING AND DATA MANAGEMENT

Cloud computing is very important for remote monitoring and data management in different sectors, such as health. Cloud computing, in the smart pillbox technology, facilitates a continuous flow of medication adherence records, access to adherence information from remote locations, and efficient management of data. Cloud computing facilitates remote monitoring and data management in pillbox technology, which is discussed below.

Data Storage and Accessibility

Smart pillboxes are used to collect adherence data in medication storage, and cloud computing is the scalable and secure platform for this purpose. Such information concerning compliance is sent to the virtual servers, which protect it and make it available in all locations with Internet access. Remote accessibility to compliance details allows users of these devices, caretakers, or medics timely observations or responses [85, 86].

Concurrent Synchronization

Cloud computing allows for the instant synchronization of medication adherence data between cloud-based servers and smart pillboxes, thereby ensuring immediate updating of adherence data, which in turn assists in real-time monitoring of drug taking by end users as well as health personnel who can then get prompt notifications or alerts about missed doses or deviations from the prescribed regimen [87].

Scalability and Flexibility

Scalability and flexibility are features of cloud computing that allow for the management of vast amounts of medication adherence data that is produced by smart pillboxes. As a result, cloud-based servers can handle more data and users, allowing uninterrupted access to information on adherence with no need for additional hardware or infrastructure investments [88].

Data Security and Privacy

To protect medication adherence data stored in the cloud, cloud computing providers put in place strong security measures that include encryption and access controls, as well as compliance with the Health Insurance Portability and Accountability Act (HIPAA) for healthcare data. Using secure cloud infrastructure, smart pillbox manufacturers can guarantee the privacy, authenticity, and availability of medication adherence data [89].

Analytics and Insights

Cloud computing is not limited to enabling advanced analytics and data processing capabilities that can be used to derive actionable insights from medication adherence data. In addition, by using cloud-based analytic tools coupled with machine-learning algorithms, smart pillbox manufacturers are capable of examining adherence patterns, identifying these trends, and providing personalized insights for both users and healthcare professionals. This enhances the ability to make targeted interventions as well as support strategies for enhancing adherence to medication, leading to better health outcomes [90, 91].

Cloud computing is crucial when it comes to supporting smart pillboxes remotely. With secure, scalable, and accessible storage solutions, cloud computing offers real-time synchronization, data analysis, and remote monitoring capabilities that can increase medication adherence and improve health outcomes for patients [92].

ADVANTAGES OF IOT-ENABLED PILLBOXES

The advantages of IoT-enabled pillboxes encompass a range of benefits that significantly improve medication management and health outcomes and depicted in Fig. (**3**).

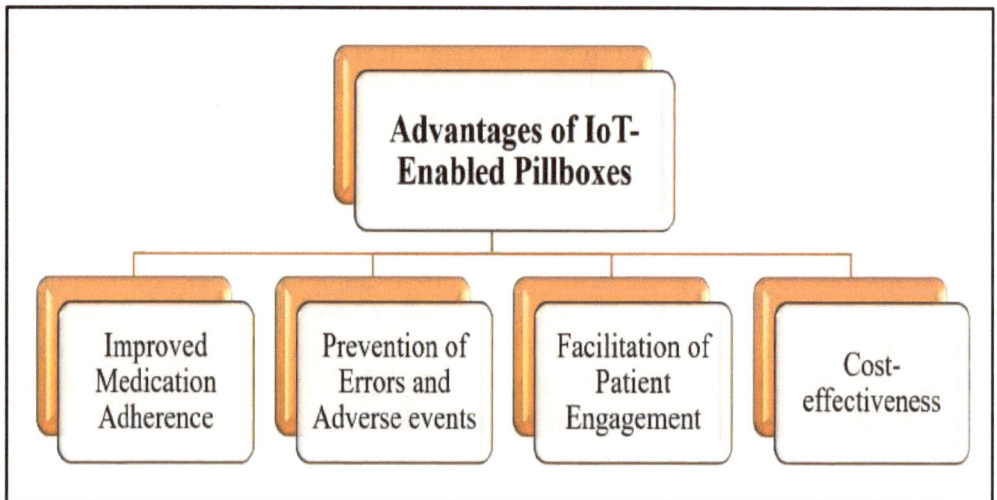

Fig. (3). Advantages of IoT-enabled pillboxes.

Improved Medication Adherence

Healthcare management has been improved through the use of IoT pillboxes, which have improved medication adherence. In enhancing adherence to doses and, ultimately, treatment outcomes, these pillboxes combine personalized reminders with real-time monitoring as well as data analytics. Missed doses are evaded by constant reminders that are offered *via* mobile gadgets that are connected to the internet, thus ensuring regular adherence to the recommended drug schedules in a timely manner [93].

Monitoring in real-time, as enabled by sensors within the pillbox, detects drug intake or missing doses and gives instant feedback to users as well as caregivers. This also helps in handling adherence challenges early enough. Additionally, IoT pillboxes provide individualized insights and encouragement on medication schedules, thereby allowing patients to take control of their treatment regimen and care for themselves [94].

All these contribute toward ensuring that adherence is sustained on a long-term basis by fostering accountability and engagement in medication management. Pillboxes connected to the IoT assist in this regard through remote access to adherence data, which allows users, caregivers, and healthcare providers to work together in order to provide comprehensive support and intervention strategies. In addition, IoT-enabled pillboxes can improve treatment efficacy, thereby enabling patients to take control of their health and well-being [95].

Prevention of Medication Errors and Adverse Events

The advantage of IoT pillboxes is that they can prevent the occurrence of medication errors and adverse events that result from improper use of drugs. The safety aspects of these IoT-enabled pill boxes are highly valued in the management of medicine as they have been designed with features such as real-time alerts and drug verification systems to reduce harmful errors and reactions. As a matter of fact, IoT pillboxes offer timely notifications and reminders, reducing the chances of missed doses or incorrect dosing and ensuring adherence to prescribed medication regimens. These include sensors and barcode scanning capabilities that an IoT-enabled pill box can use to verify the intake of medications to avoid mistakes like taking the wrong dosage or medicine in general [96].

In case of possible drug interactions or contraindications, IoT pillboxes will signal users and caregivers to contact health providers or pharmacists for further instructions. Again, the IoT pillboxes foster communication between patients and healthcare givers, hence enabling remote monitoring and interventions if non-adherence occurs or when medication concerns arise. The use of IoT-enabled pillboxes to prevent medication errors and adverse events boosts safety and trust in the management process, leading to improved health outcomes for patients [97].

Facilitation of Patient Engagement

IoT-enabled pillboxes enable patients to be more engaged in their healthcare, which is a great advantage. For instance, they use personalized feedback, reminders, and connectivity features to encourage participation plus responsibility in medication adherence. This means that connected mobile devices deliver customized reminders; hence, users continuously remember what they are supposed to take, thus enhancing compliance with treatment plans. Nevertheless, these IoT pillboxes provide personal feedback on adherence patterns, thereby giving users the ability to have an insight into their medication-taking habits so as to identify areas that can be improved [98].

The awareness it increases, however, allows users to effectively control their health and medication consumption levels, hence making them more involved in their therapy treatment. IoT pillboxes, on the other hand, enable patients' interaction with clinical doctors, facilitating long-distance monitoring and intervention that help to cure noncompliance or other issues associated with drug usage within a short period. Pills that are equipped with IoT devices enable users to engage more actively in taking care of themselves, thus promoting self-ownership and independence. In general, the increased engagement of patients by IoT-enabled pillboxes improves adherence rates, resulting in better outcomes from treatments and also ensures greater patient-centeredness in healthcare delivery [99].

Cost-Effectiveness

The cost-effective factor is a great benefit of smart pillboxes, which enables them to make financial savings and enhance their health status. These pillboxes simplify medication administration and decrease healthcare service consumption, thus decreasing the likelihood of expensive adverse drug outcomes and eventually saving time for both individuals and medical systems. Internet-based pillboxes prevent people from missing doses or taking excessive amounts, thus reducing visits to the hospital and resulting in huge medical bills [100].

IoT pillboxes have the potential to reduce in-person healthcare visits and costs by allowing for remote monitoring and intervention. Also, IoT pillboxes make it possible to target and optimize efficient treatment interventions by imparting actionable notice about adherence patterns and treatment outcomes, thus helping in resource allocation with less wasteful spending. The economic feasibility of IoT-enabled pill boxes can be traced from their support toward boosting medication adherence, averting adverse events, and upgrading well-being while reducing medical care costs in the long run [101].

CHALLENGES AND LIMITATIONS

To ensure that the integration of IoT-enabled pillboxes in healthcare settings is successful, some significant challenges and limitations have to be addressed. The collection and transmission of sensitive health data present major obstacles to the privacy and security of these entities. Patients and their doctors have serious worries about whether their medical details will be kept secret or reliable, leading to the necessity for strong encryption protocols, access controls, and compliance with regulatory standards like HIPAA for patient privacy protection [102].

Additionally, technological barriers are also an issue as the complexity of device setup, connectivity issues, and interoperability challenges could hinder smooth integration into healthcare IT infrastructure that already exists. Users, especially those with no technical know-how, might experience problems setting up or solving any malfunctions that may arise, making it necessary for such interfaces to be user-friendly and offer training and support materials. Furthermore, there are significant challenges when it comes to user acceptance and adoption since some people fear technology-based healthcare solutions [103].

Cultural parameters, divergences in generations, and socioeconomic gaps might affect the stance people take on embracing technology; therefore, there is a need for specific measures that would help different users accept and use technology. To meet these challenges, a multi-dimensional approach will be needed that prioritizes the protection of privacy, addresses technological obstacles, and cultivates the trustworthiness of stakeholders through transparency and collaboration [104].

FUTURE DIRECTIONS AND INNOVATIONS

The world of IoT-enabled pillboxes is expanding with the promise of future developments and innovations that will change medication management and caregiving to patients. One of the key drivers is connectivity and interoperability, which allow these technologies to be integrated seamlessly with other health devices and general healthcare systems. The progress will allow for a comprehensive medication management system through which pillboxes will be able to share data with electronic health records, pharmacy systems, as well as telehealth platforms that will enhance care coordination while making medication safety more effective [105, 106].

Moreover, combining AI with predictive analytics can enable pillboxes to conduct more efficient analysis of adherence data, pick out trends, and develop personal intervention tactics that suit individual patient requirements. This transition will not only result in higher rates of medication adherence but also better health outcomes for patients. Additionally, smart medicine packaging would be designed and embedded with sensors and RFID/NFC, allowing tracking at the pill level; this technology will prevent mistakes as well as facilitate accurate monitoring, thereby enhancing drug safety and compliance [107, 108].

Voice interface is one of the awe-inspiring frontiers of our world, offering hands-free and intuitive methods of interacting with users. They will also remind patients to take their medications, track adherence, and even allow for refills by voice command, making them more accessible and user-friendly, especially for disabled people. Furthermore, combining IoT-enabled pillboxes with remote patient monitoring and telemedicine platforms will enable healthcare providers to monitor adherence remotely and intervene when necessary to improve access to care and improve patient outcomes [109].

Finally, the utilization of gamification elements and incentive mechanisms within pillbox technology has the potential to motivate users and support positive adherence behaviors. By making medication adherence into a game with challenges, rewards, and interactions with others, pillboxes can make adherence more fun and interesting for users, which in turn influences their motivation and, consequently, long-term adherence [110].

CONCLUSION

In conclusion, IoT-enabled pillbox technology stands at the forefront of revolutionizing medication management and healthcare delivery. IoT-connected medication boxes improve medicine compliance, patient health outcomes, and healthcare processes by enhancing patient experience through connectivity data analysis and creative design. Pillboxes that are IoT-enabled give personalized reminders, monitoring in real-time, and data insights, enabling patients to take charge of their wellness and adhere to their prescriptions better. In addition, IoT-enabled pillboxes enable remote monitoring, integration of telemedicine, and cooperation between patients and those who provide healthcare services, which would make care more accessible and reduce its coordination. In the future, the industry can expect more developments, such as smart drug wrapping materials, voice command interfaces, and games, to improve the ease of use, availability, and impact of IoT-based pill dispensers. The transformational change of the healthcare system towards a patient-centric and technology-oriented direction is evident in how IoT has transformed pillbox technology, which can improve drug administration, optimize healthcare provision, and ultimately improve the standards of living for people all over the world. Therefore, it will be important that more research is done on IoT-enabled pillboxes, investments made in their development, and stakeholders working together toward their realization so as to utilize them fully for better global healthcare.

ACKNOWLEDGEMENTS

Authors are highly thankful to their Universities/Colleges for providing library facilities for the literature survey.

REFERENCES

[1]   B. Jimmy and J. Jose, "Patient medication adherence: Measures in daily practice," *Oman Med. J.*, vol. 26, no. 3, pp. 155–159, Mar. 2011
[http://dx.doi.org/10.5001/omj.2011.38]

[2]   K. Kvarnström, A. Westerholm, M. Airaksinen, and H. Liira, "Factors contributing to medication adherence in patients with a chronic condition: A scoping review of qualitative research", *Pharmaceutics,* vol. 13, no. 7, p. 1100, 2021.
[http://dx.doi.org/10.3390/pharmaceutics13071100] [PMID: 34371791]

[3]   H. Allioui, and Y. Mourdi, "Exploring the Full Potentials of IoT for Better Financial Growth and Stability: A Comprehensive Survey", *Sensors (Basel),* vol. 23, no. 19, p. 8015, 2023.
[http://dx.doi.org/10.3390/s23198015] [PMID: 37836845]

[4]   M. Javaid, A. Haleem, R.P. Singh, S. Rab, M.I. Ul Haq, and A. Raina, "Internet of Things in the global healthcare sector: Significance, applications, and barriers", *Int. J. Intell. Netw.,* vol. 3, pp. 165-175, 2022.
[http://dx.doi.org/10.1016/j.ijin.2022.10.002]

[5]   H. Lin, and N. Bergmann, "IoT privacy and security challenges for smart home environments", *Information (Basel),* vol. 7, no. 3, p. 44, 2016.
[http://dx.doi.org/10.3390/info7030044]

[6]   D. Karagiannis, K. Mitsis, and K.S. Nikita, "Development of a Low-Power IoMT Portable Pillbox for Medication Adherence Improvement and Remote Treatment Adjustment", *Sensors (Basel),* vol. 22, no. 15, p. 5818, 2022.
[http://dx.doi.org/10.3390/s22155818] [PMID: 35957374]

[7]   P. Dayananda, and A.G. Upadhya, *"Development of Smart Pill Expert System Based on IoT,"* Journal of The Institution of Engineers. Series B: India, 2024.
[http://dx.doi.org/10.1007/s40031-023-00956-2]

[8]   E.P.H. Choi, "A pilot study to evaluate the acceptability of using a smart pillbox to enhance medication adherence among primary care patients", *Int. J. Environ. Res. Public Health,* vol. 16, no. 20, p. 3964, 2019.
[http://dx.doi.org/10.3390/ijerph16203964] [PMID: 31627440]

[9]   S. Abdulmalek, A. Nasir, W.A. Jabbar, M.A.M. Almuhaya, A.K. Bairagi, M.A.M. Khan, and S.H. Kee, "IoT-Based Healthcare-Monitoring System towards Improving Quality of Life: A Review", *Healthcare (Basel),* vol. 10, no. 10, p. 1993, 2022.
[http://dx.doi.org/10.3390/healthcare10101993] [PMID: 36292441]

[10] A. Shahani, H.R. Nieva, K. Czado, E. Shannon, R. Gaetani, M. Gresham, J.C. Garcia, H. Ganesan, E. Cerciello, J. Dave, R. Jain, and J.L. Schnipper, "An electronic pillbox intervention designed to improve medication safety during care transitions: challenges and lessons learned regarding implementation and evaluation", *BMC Health Serv. Res.,* vol. 22, no. 1, p. 1304, 2022.
[http://dx.doi.org/10.1186/s12913-022-08702-y] [PMID: 36309744]

[11] K. Wac and S. Wulfovich, Eds., Quantifying Quality of Life: Incorporating Daily Life into Medicine, 1st ed. *Springer Cham*: Switzerland, 2022.

[12]   E.N. Schorr, A.D. Gepner, M.A. Dolansky, D.E. Forman, L.G. Park, K.S. Petersen, C.H. Still, T.Y. Wang, and N.K. Wenger, "Harnessing Mobile Health Technology for Secondary Cardiovascular Disease Prevention in Older Adults: A Scientific Statement From the American Heart Association", *Circ. Cardiovasc. Qual. Outcomes,* vol. 14, no. 5, p. e000103, 2021.
[http://dx.doi.org/10.1161/HCQ.0000000000000103] [PMID: 33793309]

[13]   W. Kanyongo, and A.E. Ezugwu, "Machine learning approaches to medication adherence amongst NCD patients: A systematic literature review", *Informatics in Medicine Unlocked,* vol. 38, p. 101210, 2023.
[http://dx.doi.org/10.1016/j.imu.2023.101210]

[14]   S. A. Wagan, J. Koo, I. F. Siddiqui, M. Attique, D. R. Shin, and N. M. F. Qureshi, "Internet of medical things and trending converged technologies: A comprehensive review on real-time applications," *J. King Saud Univ. Comput. Inf. Sci.*, vol. 34, no. 10, pt. B, pp. 9228–9251, Nov. 2022.
[http://dx.doi.org/10.1016/j.jksuci.2022.09.005]

[15]   M. Alif, I. Azlan, and R. Yahya, "Smart Medicine Pill Box Reminder", *Evol. Electr. Electron. Eng.,* vol. 4, no. 1, pp. 314-320, 2023.
[http://dx.doi.org/10.30880/eeee.2023.04.01.037]

[16]   R.S. Iii, "Gireesh Menta, Thomas Zurales, Dale Dowling, Nabiha Imtiaz, and Arshia Khan,-Evolution of Smart Pillbox: History and Reasons for a Need to Design a Smart Pillbox," |", *Int. Res. J. Adv. Eng. Sci.,* vol. 6, no. 3, pp. 421-429, 2021.

[17]   C. Merlo, "Proposal of a User-Centred Approach for CPS Design", *Pillbox Case Study,* vol. 51, no. 34, pp. 196-201, 2018.
[http://dx.doi.org/10.1016/j.ifacol.2019.01.065ï]

[18]   M.T. Brown, J. Bussell, S. Dutta, K. Davis, S. Strong, and S. Mathew, "Medication Adherence: Truth and Consequences", *Am. J. Med. Sci.,* vol. 351, no. 4, pp. 387-399, 2016.
[http://dx.doi.org/10.1016/j.amjms.2016.01.010] [PMID: 27079345]

[19]   N. Solanki, and D.R. Zope, "Smart pill box health care system", *International Research Journal of Engineering and Technology (IRJET),* vol. 5, no. 7, 2018.

[20]   P. Thangsuk, K. Pinyopornpanish, W. Jiraporncharoen, N. Buawangpong, and C. Angkurawaranon, "Is the association between herbal use and blood-pressure control mediated by medication adherence? A cross-sectional study in primary care", *Int. J. Environ. Res. Public Health,* vol. 18, no. 24, p. 12916, 2021.
[http://dx.doi.org/10.3390/ijerph182412916] [PMID: 34948526]

[21]   J.M. Polinski, A.S. Kesselheim, J.P. Frolkis, P. Wescott, C. Allen-Coleman, and M.A. Fischer, "A matter of trust: patient barriers to primary medication adherence", *Health Education Research,* vol. 29, no. 5, pp. 755-63, 2014.

[22]   B. Petrovska, "Historical review of medicinal plants' usage", *Pharmacogn. Rev.,* vol. 6, no. 11, pp. 1-5, 2012.
[http://dx.doi.org/10.4103/0973-7847.95849] [PMID: 22654398]

[23]   K. Allaham, M.B. Feyasa, R.D. Govender, A. Musa, A.J. AlKaabi, I. ElBarazi, S.D. AlSheryani, R.J. Al Falasi, and M.A.B. Khan, "Medication Adherence Among Patients with Multimorbidity in the United Arab Emirates", *Patient Prefer. Adherence,* vol. 16, pp. 1187-1200, 2022.
[http://dx.doi.org/10.2147/PPA.S355891] [PMID: 35572810]

[24]   W. Polonsky, and R. Henry, "Poor medication adherence in type 2 diabetes: recognizing the scope of the problem and its key contributors", *Patient Prefer. Adherence,* vol. 10, pp. 1299-1307, 2016.
[http://dx.doi.org/10.2147/PPA.S106821] [PMID: 27524885]

[25]   H. Kalantarian, B. Motamed, N. Alshurafa, and M. Sarrafzadeh, "A wearable sensor system for medication adherence prediction", *Artif. Intell. Med.,* vol. 69, pp. 43-52, 2016.
[http://dx.doi.org/10.1016/j.artmed.2016.03.004] [PMID: 27068873]

[26]   L.L. Marengo, and S. Barberato-Filho, "Involvement of Human Volunteers in the Development and Evaluation of Wearable Devices Designed to Improve Medication Adherence: A Scoping Review", *Sensors (Basel),* vol. 23, no. 7, p. 3597, 2023.
[http://dx.doi.org/10.3390/s23073597] [PMID: 37050659]

[27]   M. T. Brown and J. K. Bussell, "Medication adherence: WHO cares?" *Mayo Clin. Proc.*, vol. 86, no. 4, pp. 304–314, Apr. 2011.
[http://dx.doi.org/10.4065/mcp.2010.0575]

[28]   N. Pagès-Puigdemont, M.A. Mangues, M. Masip, G. Gabriele, L. Fernández-Maldonado, S. Blancafort, and L. Tuneu, "Patients' Perspective of Medication Adherence in Chronic Conditions: A Qualitative Study", *Adv. Ther.,* vol. 33, no. 10, pp. 1740-1754, 2016.
[http://dx.doi.org/10.1007/s12325-016-0394-6] [PMID: 27503082]

[29]   A.L. Stangl, V.A. Earnshaw, C.H. Logie, W. van Brakel, L. C Simbayi, I. Barré, and J.F. Dovidio, "The Health Stigma and Discrimination Framework: a global, crosscutting framework to inform research, intervention development, and policy on health-related stigmas", *BMC Med.,* vol. 17, no. 1, p. 31, 2019.
[http://dx.doi.org/10.1186/s12916-019-1271-3] [PMID: 30764826]

[30]   R. Horne, J. Weinman, and M. Barber, "Concordance, Adherence and Compliance in Medicine Taking", A Report for the National Co-ordinating Centre for NHS Service Delivery and Organisation R & D (NCCSDO), Dec. 2005.

[31]   C. Yang, S. Zhu, Z. Hui, and Y. Mo, "Psychosocial factors associated with medication burden among community-dwelling older people with multimorbidity", *BMC Geriatr.,* vol. 23, no. 1, p. 741, 2023.
[http://dx.doi.org/10.1186/s12877-023-04444-6] [PMID: 37964196]

[32]   K. Thomas, E. Nilsson, K. Festin, P. Henriksson, M. Lowén, M. Löf, and M. Kristenson, "Associations of psychosocial factors with multiple health behaviors: A population-based study of middle-aged men and women", *Int. J. Environ. Res. Public Health,* vol. 17, no. 4, p. 1239, 2020.
[http://dx.doi.org/10.3390/ijerph17041239] [PMID: 32075162]

[33]   M. Blusi, and J.C. Nieves, "Feasibility and acceptability of smart augmented reality assisting patients with medication pillbox self-management", In: *Studies in Health Technology and Informatics.* IOS Press, 2019, pp. 521-525.
[http://dx.doi.org/10.3233/SHTI190277]

[34]   H.-J. Hu, "An innovative pillbox design based on the experiences of senior citizens," 2014.

[35]   W. V. Solís, P. Cedillo, J. Parra, A. Guevara, and J. Ortiz, "Intelligent Pillbox: Evaluating the User Perceptions of Elderly People," 2017.

[36]   S. Faisal, J. Ivo, and T. Patel, "A review of features and characteristics of smart medication adherence products", *Can. Pharm. J.,* vol. 154, no. 5, pp. 312-323, 2021.
[http://dx.doi.org/10.1177/17151635211034198] [PMID: 34484481]

[37]   M. Aldeer, M. Javanmard, and R. Martin, "A review of medication adherence monitoring technologies", *Applied System Innovation,* vol. 1, no. 2, p. 14, 2018.
[http://dx.doi.org/10.3390/asi1020014]

[38]   J. Joy, S. Vahab, G. Vinayakan, M.V. Prasad, and S. Rakesh, "SIMoP box - A smart, intelligent mobile pill box", In: *Materials Today: Proceedings.* Elsevier Ltd, 2020, pp. 3610-3619.
[http://dx.doi.org/10.1016/j.matpr.2020.09.829]

[39]   S. Park, I. Sentissi, S.J. Gil, W.S. Park, B. Oh, A.R. Son, Y.J. Kong, S. Park, E. Paek, Y.J. Park, and S.H. Lee, "Medication event monitoring system for infectious tuberculosis treatment in Morocco: A retrospective cohort study", *Int. J. Environ. Res. Public Health,* vol. 16, no. 3, p. 412, 2019.
[http://dx.doi.org/10.3390/ijerph16030412] [PMID: 30709029]

[40]   W. V. Solís, P. Cedillo, J. Parra, A. Guevara, and J. Ortiz, "Journal of Information and Organizational Sciences- Microsoft Word Template," 2017.

[41] A. Naditz, "Medication compliance--helping patients through technology: modern "smart" pillboxes keep memory-short patients on their medical regimen", *Telemed. J. E Health,* vol. 14, no. 9, pp. 875-880, 2008.
[http://dx.doi.org/10.1089/tmj.2008.8476] [PMID: 19062349]

[42] J. Jia, J. Yu, R. S. Hanumesh, S. Xia, P. Wei, H. Choi, and X. Jiang, "Intelligent and privacy-preserving medication adherence system", *Smart Health,* vol. 9–10, pp. 250-264, 2018.
[http://dx.doi.org/10.1016/j.smhl.2018.07.012]

[43] N. Solanki and D. P. H. Zope, "Smart Pill Box Health Care System," International Research Journal of Engineering and Technology (IRJET) Factor, 2008, [Online]. Available from: www.irjet.net

[44] R. Parker, C Frampton, A Blackwood, A. Shannon, and G. Moore, "An electronic medication reminder, supported by a monitoring service, to improve medication compliance for elderly people living independently", *Journal of telemedicine and telecare,* vol. 18, no. 3, pp. 156-8, 2012.

[45] P. Pal, S. Sambhakar, V. Dave, S.K. Paliwal, S. Paliwal, M. Sharma, A. Kumar, and N. Dhama, "A review on emerging smart technological innovations in healthcare sector for increasing patient's medication adherence", *Global Health Journal,* vol. 5, no. 4, pp. 183-189, 2021.
[http://dx.doi.org/10.1016/j.glohj.2021.11.006]

[46] J.K. Schwartz, "Pillbox use, satisfaction, and effectiveness among persons with chronic health conditions", *Assistive Technology,* vol. 29, no. 4, pp. 181-7, 2017.

[47] Q. Wu, Z. Zeng, J. Lin, and Y. Chen, "AI empowered context-aware smart system for medication adherence", *International Journal of Crowd Science,* vol. 1, no. 2, pp. 102-109, 2017.
[http://dx.doi.org/10.1108/IJCS-07-2017-0006]

[48] Y. S. Lee, J. Tullio, N. Narasimhan, P. Kaushik, J. R. Engelsma, and S. Basapur, "Investigating the Potential of In-Home Devices for Improving Medication Adherence," 2009,
[http://dx.doi.org/10.4108/ICST.PERVASIVEHEALTH2009.6025]

[49] J. Lundell, T.L. Hayes, S. Vurgun, U Ozertem, J Kimel, J Kaye, F Guilak, and M. Pavel, "Continuous activity monitoring and intelligent contextual prompting to improve medication adherence", In: *2007 29th Annu. Int. Conf. IEEE Eng. Med. Biol. Soc.* vol. 22. IEEE, 2007, pp. 6286-6289.

[50] S. Thompson, and Walker, "Use of modern technology as an aid to medication adherence: an overview", *Patient Intell.,* no. Jun, p. 49, 2011.
[http://dx.doi.org/10.2147/PI.S8485]

[51] M. Vervloet, A.J. Linn, J.C.M. van Weert, D.H. de Bakker, M.L. Bouvy, and L. van Dijk, "The effectiveness of interventions using electronic reminders to improve adherence to chronic medication: a systematic review of the literature", *J. Am. Med. Inform. Assoc.,* vol. 19, no. 5, pp. 696-704, 2012.
[http://dx.doi.org/10.1136/amiajnl-2011-000748] [PMID: 22534082]

[52] X-Y. Zhang, M.R. Birtwistle, and J.M. Gallo, "A General Network Pharmacodynamic Model–Based Design Pipeline for Customized Cancer Therapy Applied to the VEGFR Pathway", *CPT Pharmacometrics Syst. Pharmacol.,* vol. 3, no. 1, pp. 1-9, 2014.
[http://dx.doi.org/10.1038/psp.2013.65] [PMID: 24429593]

[53] J. Kim, C. Hu, C. Moufawad El Achkar, L.E. Black, J. Douville, A. Larson, M.K. Pendergast, S.F. Goldkind, E.A. Lee, A. Kuniholm, A. Soucy, J. Vaze, N.R. Belur, K. Fredriksen, I. Stojkovska, A. Tsytsykova, M. Armant, R.L. DiDonato, J. Choi, L. Cornelissen, L.M. Pereira, E.F. Augustine, C.A. Genetti, K. Dies, B. Barton, L. Williams, B.D. Goodlett, B.L. Riley, A. Pasternak, E.R. Berry, K.A. Pflock, S. Chu, C. Reed, K. Tyndall, P.B. Agrawal, A.H. Beggs, P.E. Grant, D.K. Urion, R.O. Snyder, S.E. Waisbren, A. Poduri, P.J. Park, A. Patterson, A. Biffi, J.R. Mazzulli, O. Bodamer, C.B. Berde, and T.W. Yu, "Patient-Customized Oligonucleotide Therapy for a Rare Genetic Disease", *N. Engl. J. Med.,* vol. 381, no. 17, pp. 1644-1652, 2019.
[http://dx.doi.org/10.1056/NEJMoa1813279] [PMID: 31597037]

[54] J.M. Gallo, and M.R. Birtwistle, "Network pharmacodynamic models for customized cancer therapy",

Wiley Interdiscip. Rev. Syst. Biol. Med., vol. 7, no. 4, pp. 243-251, 2015.
[http://dx.doi.org/10.1002/wsbm.1300] [PMID: 25914386]

[55] E. Chatelut, J.J.M.A. Hendrikx, J. Martin, J. Ciccolini, and D.J.A.R. Moes, "Unraveling the complexity of therapeutic drug monitoring for monoclonal antibody therapies to individualize dose in oncology", *Pharmacol. Res. Perspect.,* vol. 9, no. 2, p. e00757, 2021.
[http://dx.doi.org/10.1002/prp2.757] [PMID: 33745217]

[56] Figueiro MG, Gonzales K, Pedler D. Designing with circadian stimulus. Lighting Design Application. 2016 Oct;46(10):30-4.
[http://dx.doi.org/10.1177/036063251604601009]

[57] D. Barbolosi, J. Ciccolini, B. Lacarelle, F. Barlési, and N. André, "Computational oncology — mathematical modelling of drug regimens for precision medicine", *Nat. Rev. Clin. Oncol.,* vol. 13, no. 4, pp. 242-254, 2016.
[http://dx.doi.org/10.1038/nrclinonc.2015.204] [PMID: 26598946]

[58] G. Sadigh, J.L. Meisel, K. Byers, A. Robles, L. Serrano, O.S. Jung, D. Coleman, K.A. Yeager, and I. Graetz, "Improving palbociclib adherence among women with metastatic breast cancer using a CONnected CUstomized Treatment Platform: A pilot study", *J. Oncol. Pharm. Pract.,* vol. 29, no. 8, pp. 1957-1964, 2023.
[http://dx.doi.org/10.1177/10781552231161823] [PMID: 36883245]

[59] G. Renaud, R. Lazzari, C. Revenant, A. Barbier, M. Noblet, O. Ulrich, F. Leroy, J. Jupille, Y. Borensztein, C. R. Henry, J.-P. Deville, F. Scheurer, J. Mane-Mane, and O. Fruchart, "Real-Time Monitoring of Growing Nanoparticles," *Science,* vol. 300, no. 5624, pp. 1416–1419, May 2003.

[60] N. Vijayakumar and R. Ramya, "The Real-Time Monitoring of Water Quality in IoT Environment," 2013. Available from: www.ijsr.net
[http://dx.doi.org/10.1109/ICIIECS.2015.7193080]

[61] S. E. Chodrow, F. Jahanian, and M. Donner, "Run-time monitoring of real-time systems", *Proceedings of the Real-Time Systems Symposium,* IEEE, pp. 74-83, 1991.
[http://dx.doi.org/10.1109/REAL.1991.160360]

[62] D. B. Kell, G. H. Markx, C. L. Davey, and R. W. Todd, "Real-time monitoring of cellular biomass: methods and applications," Trends in Analytical Chemistry, vol. 9, no. 6, pp. 190–194, 1990.

[63] G. Coviello, G. Avitabile, and A. Florio, "The Importance of Data Synchronization in Multiboard Acquisition Systems", *20th IEEE Mediterranean Electrotechnical Conference, MELECON 2020 - Proceedings,* Institute of Electrical and Electronics Engineers Inc., pp. 293-297, 2020.
[http://dx.doi.org/10.1109/MELECON48756.2020.9140622]

[64] S. Suzuki, and M. Harrison, "Data Synchronization Specification", *Auto-ID Labs, AEROID-CAM-007,* 2006.

[65] N. Kaempchen, and K. C. J. Dietmayer, "Data synchronization strategies for multi-sensor fusion", In: *Proc. 10th World Congress on Intelligent Transport Systems and Services (ITS 2003)* Madrid, Spain, 2003.

[66] E.P. Csirmaz, and L. Csirmaz, "Data Synchronization: A Complete Theoretical Solution for Filesystems", *Future Internet,* vol. 14, no. 11, p. 344, 2022.
[http://dx.doi.org/10.3390/fi14110344]

[67] B.B. Granger, and H.B. Bosworth, "Medication adherence: emerging use of technology", *Curr. Opin. Cardiol.,* vol. 26, no. 4, pp. 279-287, 2011.
[http://dx.doi.org/10.1097/HCO.0b013e328347c150] [PMID: 21597368]

[68] S. Faisal, J. Ivo, S. Abu Fadaleh, and T. Patel, "Exploring the Value of Real-Time Medication Adherence Monitoring: A Qualitative Study", *Pharmacy (Basel),* vol. 11, no. 1, p. 18, 2023.
[http://dx.doi.org/10.3390/pharmacy11010018] [PMID: 36827656]

[69] J. Car, W.S. Tan, Z. Huang, P. Sloot, and B.D. Franklin, "eHealth in the future of medications

management: personalisation, monitoring and adherence", *BMC Med.,* vol. 15, no. 1, p. 73, 2017.
[http://dx.doi.org/10.1186/s12916-017-0838-0] [PMID: 28376771]

[70]　A. Haleem, M. Javaid, R. Pratap Singh, and R. Suman, "Medical 4.0 technologies for healthcare: Features, capabilities, and applications", *Internet of Things and Cyber-Physical Systems,* vol. 2, pp. 12-30, 2022.
[http://dx.doi.org/10.1016/j.iotcps.2022.04.001]

[71]　E.M. Shannon, S.K. Mueller, and J.L. Schnipper, "Patient, caregiver, and clinician experience with a technologically enabled pillbox: a qualitative study", *ACI Open,* vol. 7, no. 2, pp. e61-70, 2023.

[72]　N. Bashi, M. Karunanithi, F. Fatehi, H. Ding, and D. Walters, "Remote monitoring of patients with heart failure: An overview of systematic reviews", *J. Med. Internet Res.,* vol. 19, no. 1, p. e18, 2017.
[http://dx.doi.org/10.2196/jmir.6571] [PMID: 28108430]

[73]　A.R. Watson, R. Wah, and R. Thamman, "The value of remote monitoring for the COVID-19 pandemic", *Telemed. J. E Health,* vol. 26, no. 9, pp. 1110-1112, 2020.
[http://dx.doi.org/10.1089/tmj.2020.0134] [PMID: 32384251]

[74]　M. Osman, B.D. Glass, Z. Hola, and S. Stollewerk, "Reward and Feedback in the Control over Dynamic Events", *Psychology (Irvine),* vol. 8, no. 7, pp. 1063-1089, 2017.
[http://dx.doi.org/10.4236/psych.2017.87070]

[75]　H. J. Arnold, "Effects of Performance Feedback and Extrinsic Reward upon High Intrinsic Motivation," 1976.
[http://dx.doi.org/10.1016/0030-5073(76)90067-2]

[76]　J. Sheehan, K. Laver, A. Bhopti, M. Rahja, T. Usherwood, L. Clemson, and N.A. Lannin, "Methods and effectiveness of communication between hospital allied health and primary care practitioners: A systematic narrative review", *J. Multidiscip. Healthc.,* vol. 14, pp. 493-511, 2021.
[http://dx.doi.org/10.2147/JMDH.S295549] [PMID: 33654406]

[77]　D.I. Velligan, and S.H. Kamil, "Enhancing patient adherence: introducing smart pill devices", *Ther. Deliv.,* vol. 5, no. 6, pp. 611-613, 2014.
[http://dx.doi.org/10.4155/tde.14.33] [PMID: 25090273]

[78]　A.W. Tadesse, M. Cusinato, G.T. Weldemichael, T. Abdurhman, D. Assefa, H. Yazew, D. Gadissa, A. Shiferaw, M. Belachew, M. Sahile, J. van Rest, A. Bedru, N. Foster, D. Jerene, and K.L. Fielding, "Risk factors for poor engagement with a smart pillbox adherence intervention among persons on tuberculosis treatment in Ethiopia", *BMC Public Health,* vol. 23, no. 1, p. 2006, 2023.
[http://dx.doi.org/10.1186/s12889-023-16905-z] [PMID: 37838677]

[79]　H. Pratiwi, S.A. Kristina, A.W. Widayanti, Y.S. Prabandari, and I.Y. Kusuma, "A Systematic Review of Compensation and Technology-Mediated Strategies to Maintain Older Adults' Medication Adherence", *Int. J. Environ. Res. Public Health,* vol. 20, no. 1, p. 803, 2023.
[http://dx.doi.org/10.3390/ijerph20010803] [PMID: 36613130]

[80]　C. Piquer-Martinez, A. Urionagüena, S.I. Benrimoj, B. Calvo, S. Dineen-Griffin, V. Garcia-Cardenas, F. Fernandez-Llimos, F. Martinez-Martinez, and M.A. Gastelurrutia, "Theories, models and frameworks for health systems integration. A scoping review", *Health Policy,* vol. 141, p. 104997, 2024.
[http://dx.doi.org/10.1016/j.healthpol.2024.104997] [PMID: 38246048]

[81]　G. D. Armitage, E. Suter, N. D. Oelke, and C. E. Adair, "Health systems integration: state of the evidence," 2009. Available from: http://www.ijic.org/
[http://dx.doi.org/10.5334/ijic.316]

[82]　J.F.J. Vos, A. Boonstra, A. Kooistra, M. Seelen, and M. van Offenbeek, "The influence of electronic health record use on collaboration among medical specialties", *BMC Health Serv. Res.,* vol. 20, no. 1, p. 676, 2020.
[http://dx.doi.org/10.1186/s12913-020-05542-6] [PMID: 32698807]

[83] R.R. Aguirre, O. Suarez, M. Fuentes, and M.A. Sanchez-Gonzalez, "Electronic Health Record Implementation: A Review of Resources and Tools", *Cureus,* vol. 11, no. 9, p. e5649, 2019.
[http://dx.doi.org/10.7759/cureus.5649] [PMID: 31700751]

[84] M.A. Arain, A. Ahmad, V. Chiu, and L. Kembel, "Medication adherence support of an in-home electronic medication dispensing system for individuals living with chronic conditions: a pilot randomized controlled trial", *BMC Geriatr.,* vol. 21, no. 1, p. 56, 2021.
[http://dx.doi.org/10.1186/s12877-020-01979-w] [PMID: 33446126]

[85] N. Sultan, "Making use of cloud computing for healthcare provision: Opportunities and challenges", *Int. J. Inf. Manage.,* vol. 34, no. 2, pp. 177-184, 2014.
[http://dx.doi.org/10.1016/j.ijinfomgt.2013.12.011]

[86] G. Elwyn, D. Frosch, R. Thomson, N. Joseph-Williams, A. Lloyd, P. Kinnersley, E. Cording, D. Tomson, C. Dodd, S. Rollnick, A. Edwards, and M. Barry, "Shared decision making: a model for clinical practice", *J. Gen. Intern. Med.,* vol. 27, no. 10, pp. 1361-1367, 2012.
[http://dx.doi.org/10.1007/s11606-012-2077-6] [PMID: 22618581]

[87] O. Ommen, S. Thuem, H. Pfaff, and C. Janssen, "The relationship between social support, shared decision-making and patient's trust in doctors: a cross-sectional survey of 2,197 inpatients using the Cologne Patient Questionnaire", *Int. J. Public Health,* vol. 56, no. 3, pp. 319-327, 2011.
[http://dx.doi.org/10.1007/s00038-010-0212-x] [PMID: 21076932]

[88] S. Iranpak, A. Shahbahrami, and H. Shakeri, "Remote patient monitoring and classifying using the internet of things platform combined with cloud computing", *J. Big Data,* vol. 8, no. 1, p. 120, 2021.
[http://dx.doi.org/10.1186/s40537-021-00507-w]

[89] Z. Khan, D. Ludlow, R. McClatchey, and A. Anjum, "An architecture for integrated intelligence in urban management using cloud computing", *J. Cloud Comput. (Heidelb.),* vol. 1, no. 1, pp. 1-14, 2012.
[http://dx.doi.org/10.1186/2192-113X-1-1]

[90] M. V. V. P. Kantipudi, C. J. Moses, R. Aluvalu, and S. Kumar, "Remote patient monitoring using IoT, cloud computing and AI", In: *in Hybrid Artificial Intelligence and IoT in Healthcare* vol. 209. A. Kumar Bhoi, P. K. Mallick, M. Narayana Mohanty, and V. H. C. de Albuquerque, Eds., Intelligent Systems Reference Library, Singapore: Springer, 2021, pp. 51-74.
[http://dx.doi.org/10.1007/978-981-16-2972-3_3]

[91] W. Qi, M. Sun, and S. R. A. Hosseini, "Facilitating big-data management in modern business and organizations using cloud computing: A comprehensive study", *J. Manag. & Organ.,* vol. 29, no. 4, pp. 697-723, 2023.
[http://dx.doi.org/10.1017/jmo.2022.17]

[92] S. Mohapatra and K. S. Rekha, "Sensor-Cloud: A Hybrid Framework for Remote Patient Monitoring," *Inter. J. Comp. App.,* vol. 55, no. 2, pp. 7–12, Oct. 2012.
[http://dx.doi.org/10.5120/8725-2296]

[93] E. Costa, S. Pecorelli, A. Giardini, M. Savin, E. Menditto, E. Lehane, O. Laosa, A. Monaco, and A. Marengoni, "Interventional tools to improve medication adherence: review of literature", *Patient Prefer. Adherence,* vol. 9, pp. 1303-1314, 2015.
[http://dx.doi.org/10.2147/PPA.S87551] [PMID: 26396502]

[94] M. Papus, A.L. Dima, M Viprey, A.M. Schott, M.P. Schneider, and T. Novais, "Motivational interviewing to support medication adherence in adults with chronic conditions: systematic review of randomized controlled trials", *Patient Education and Counseling,* vol. 105, no. 11, pp. 3186-203, 2022.

[95] P. A. M, "Meta-analysis of trials of interventions to improve medication adherence," 2017. Available from: www.tcpdf.org

[96] A. Palacio, D. Garay, B. Langer, J. Taylor, B.A. Wood, and L. Tamariz, "Motivational Interviewing Improves Medication Adherence: a Systematic Review and Meta-analysis", *J. Gen. Intern. Med.,* vol.

31, no. 8, pp. 929-940, 2016.
[http://dx.doi.org/10.1007/s11606-016-3685-3] [PMID: 27160414]

[97] E. B. Fortescue, R. Kaushal, C. P. Landrigan, K. J. McKenna, M. D. Clapp, F. Federico, D. A. Goldmann, and D. W. Bates, "Prioritizing strategies for preventing medication errors and adverse drug events in pediatric inpatients", *Pediatrics,* vol. 111, 2003no. 4, pp. 722-729.
[http://dx.doi.org/10.1542/peds.111.4.722]

[98] M. Garrouste-Orgeas, F. Philippart, C. Bruel, A. Max, N. Lau, and B. Misset, "Overview of medical errors and adverse events", *Ann. Intensive Care,* vol. 2, no. 1, p. 2, 2012.
[http://dx.doi.org/10.1186/2110-5820-2-2] [PMID: 22339769]

[99] C.U. Lehmann, and G.R. Kim, "Prevention of medication errors", *Clin. Perinatol.,* vol. 32, no. 1, pp. 107-123, vii, 2005.
[http://dx.doi.org/10.1016/j.clp.2004.10.003] [PMID: 15777824]

[100] P. A. M, "Meta-analysis of trials of interventions to improve medication adherence," 2017. Available from: www.tcpdf.org

[101] M. Waleed, T. Kamal, T.W. Um, A. Hafeez, B. Habib, and K.E. Skouby, "Unlocking Insights in IoT-Based Patient Monitoring: Methods for Encompassing Large-Data Challenges", *Sensors (Basel),* vol. 23, no. 15, p. 6760, 2023.
[http://dx.doi.org/10.3390/s23156760] [PMID: 37571543]

[102] M.T. Ghozali, "Implementation of the IoT-Based Technology on Patient Medication Adherence: A Comprehensive Bibliometric and Systematic Review", *J. Inf. Commun. Technol.,* vol. 22, no. 4, pp. 503-544, 2023.
[http://dx.doi.org/10.32890/jict2023.22.4.1]

[103] A.I. Stoumpos, F. Kitsios, and M.A. Talias, "Digital Transformation in Healthcare: Technology Acceptance and Its Applications", *Int. J. Environ. Res. Public Health,* vol. 20, no. 4, p. 3407, 2023.
[http://dx.doi.org/10.3390/ijerph20043407] [PMID: 36834105]

[104] P. Carayon, A.S. Hundt, and P. Hoonakker, "Technology barriers and strategies in coordinating care for chronically ill patients", *Appl. Ergon.,* vol. 78, pp. 240-247, 2019.
[http://dx.doi.org/10.1016/j.apergo.2019.03.009] [PMID: 31046955]

[105] B.R. International, "Retracted: A Permissioned Blockchain-Based Clinical Trial Service Platform to Improve Trial Data Transparency", *BioMed Res. Int.,* vol. 2024, p. 1, 2024.
[http://dx.doi.org/10.1155/2024/9753878] [PMID: 38550214]

[106] E. B. Michans, "Development of an IoT Network for Elderly Healthcare," 2021.

[107] K. Sagdic, I. Eş, M. Sitti, and F. Inci, "Smart materials: rational design in biosystems via artificial intelligence", *Trends Biotechnol.,* vol. 40, no. 8, pp. 987-1003, 2022.
[http://dx.doi.org/10.1016/j.tibtech.2022.01.005] [PMID: 35241311]

[108] C. Chen, S. Ding, and J. Wang, "Digital health for aging populations", *Nat. Med.,* vol. 29, no. 7, pp. 1623-1630, 2023.
[http://dx.doi.org/10.1038/s41591-023-02391-8] [PMID: 37464029]

[109] D. Krishnan, and S. Singh, "Medical IoT: Opportunities, issues in security and privacy - a comprehensive review", In: *Smart and Secure Internet of Healthcare Things.* CRC Press, 2022, pp. 91-112.
[http://dx.doi.org/10.1201/9781003239895-6]

[110] R.S. Alsawaier, "The effect of gamification on motivation and engagement", *International Journal of Information and Learning Technology,* vol. 35, no. 1, pp. 56-79, 2018.
[http://dx.doi.org/10.1108/IJILT-02-2017-0009]

CHAPTER 7

Personalized Medicine: AI-Driven Prescription Plans

Neeraj Kumar Fuloria[1], **Akhil Sharma**[2], **Ashish Verma**[3], **S. Ananda Kumar**[4] and **Shaweta Sharma**[5,*]

[1] *Department of Pharmaceutical Chemistry, Faculty of Pharmacy, AIMST University Semeling Campus, Bedong, Kedah, Malaysia*

[2] *R.J. College of Pharmacy, Raipur, Gharbara, Tappal, Khair, Uttar Pradesh, India*

[3] *Mangalmay Pharmacy College, Plot No. 9, Knowledge Park II, Greater Noida, Uttar Pradesh, India*

[4] *Department of Civil Engineering, Aditya University, Surampalem, India*

[5] *School of Medical and Allied Sciences, Galgotias University Plot No. 2, Yamuna Expy, Opposite Buddha International Circuit, Sector 17A, Greater Noida, Uttar Pradesh, India*

Abstract: In healthcare, personal medicine has changed dramatically through AI growth. This chapter explores the link between personalized medicine and AI prescription plans, outlining the current status, challenges faced, and future implications of these systems. This approach is essentially based on a personalized medicine system where therapies are adjusted to suit individuality traits like genetic makeup, lifestyles, and environmental factors. The traditional approach of one size fits all used in the field of health may not be comprehensive enough to fit all the patients' needs. However, personalized medicine utilizes AI to analyze huge amounts of patient data and produce individualized plans that enhance treatment efficiency and reduce unfavorable reactions. AI assists in precision oncology, drug discovery, and treatment optimization with notable initiatives like IBM Watson for Drug Discovery, AiCure for medication adherence, and Pillo Health for patient engagement demonstrating its promise. AI makes patients feel more empowered and involved in healthcare decisions using patient-centric tools, such as shared decision-making platforms, personalized educational content, and support communities. Various sources of data are integrated and combined with AI-driven decision support systems that provide accurate diagnoses, risk predictions, and personalized care plans. Implementing these innovations depends on economic and societal implications, such as cost-effectiveness and equitable access to humanized personalized treatments. To unleash the full potential of AI, data privacy, algorithmic transparency, how it will fit into the overall health market ecosystem, and other challenges must be addressed. Looking ahead, AI integration in personalized medicine has better patient outcomes, generates real-world evidence, and paves the way for a more efficient and focused patient healthcare system.

* **Corresponding author Shaweta Sharma:** School of Medical and Allied Sciences, Galgotias University Plot No. 2, Yamuna Expy, Opposite Buddha International Circuit, Sector 17A, Greater Noida, Uttar Pradesh, India; E-mail: shawetasharma@galgotiasuniversity.edu.in

Akhil Sharma, Neeraj Kumar Fuloria, Pankaj Kumar Singh & Shaweta Sharma (Eds.)

This chapter outlines the fundamentals of the transformative effect of AI, including its modality-specific applications, advantages, and prospective trends of development in personalized medicine.

Keywords: Artificial intelligence, Google deep variant, Genomic data, Health, IBM Watson, Medicine, Medication, Patient, Personalized, Treatment.

INTRODUCTION

Personalized medicine, also known as precision or individualized medicine is a new healthcare approach that involves customizing medical treatments and prevention strategies to individual patients. The fact that individuals react differently to medicines, treatments, and intercessions is acknowledged by this approach. This may be due to genetic constitution, lifestyle choices, environmental exposures, or other personal attributes [1, 2].

The ultimate goal of personalized medicine is to achieve maximum effectiveness with minimum harm by focusing on the specific biological, genetic, and environmental factors that affect a person's health and disease risks. Modern technologies such as genomics, proteomics, metabolomics, and bioinformatics are exploited in the effort to identify biomarkers and genetic variants that contribute towards disease progressions, treatment responses, as well as risk [3, 4].

A treatment plan, or prescription plan, is a fundamental part of healthcare delivery that explains the steps to be taken in managing an illness or health condition. Prescription plans mean that the right medicine is prescribed at the right dose for an individual patient's diagnosis and medical history. This ensures that appropriate pharmacotherapy is administered to reach therapeutic targets. A prescription plan gives a complete approach to handling the patient's condition, thereby facilitating collaborative care among healthcare givers by outlining this approach. As such it may entail multidisciplinary collaboration, referral of patients to consultants, or integration of other services such as physiotherapy or counseling [5].

Patients are given instructions about drug use, changes in lifestyle, and how to manage themselves under prescription plans. By giving patients the necessary information and tools, these plans make sure that they adhere to medication as well as participate actively in their own care which is fundamental for effective treatment. Prescription plans are fluid documents that need to be reviewed periodically and adjusted according to a patient's response to therapy, change in health status, or new clinical guidelines. This will ensure that interventions continue to be relevant and useful by making it possible for the regimen to be modified on a routine basis depending on the changing needs of the patient [6].

Integration of AI in the tailoring of treatment plans is helping to make personalized medicine more accurate and impactful through the use of advanced analytics and decision support tools. Prescription plans are crucial in turning individualized treatment recommendations into workable strategies that are aimed at optimizing patient outcomes and improving overall treatment effectiveness [7, 8].

GOALS OF PERSONALIZED MEDICINE

The basic principles, objectives, and application of personalized medicine in the larger healthcare setting must be well understood. These aims of personalized medical services are focused on different directions that should change traditional ways of giving out health care to become more patient-centered [9, 10]. The primary goals of personalized medicine are elaborated below and summarized in Fig. (**1**).

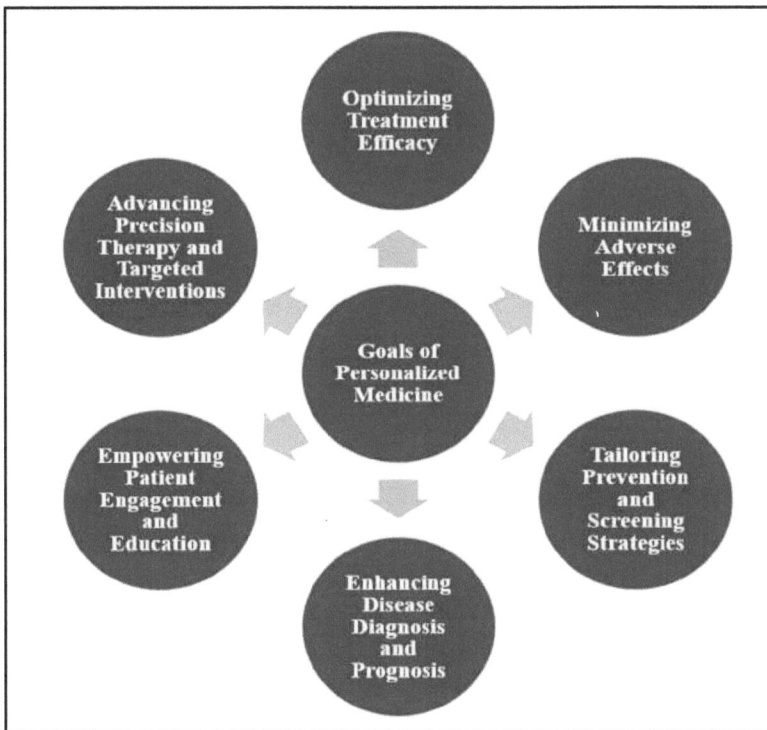

Fig. (1). Primary goals of personalized medicine.

Optimizing Treatment Efficacy

In order to make the most of medical procedures, personalized medicine is aimed at individualizing treatment plans according to the specific attributes and needs of each patient. Patient's genetic makeup, biomarker profiles, and disease subtypes can be used to develop personalized treatment strategies that target underlying disease mechanisms better than conventional approaches bringing forth more improved outcomes [11, 12].

Minimizing Adverse Effects

The second goal of personalized medicine is to minimize the chance of adverse drug reactions as well as other complications connected with treatment. This will involve identifying genetic variations and other factors that affect how an individual reacts to medication so that healthcare providers can choose therapies likely to be safe and effective for each patient, thus reducing the likelihood of such events [13, 14].

Enhancing Patient Safety

The personalized medicine approach is aimed at improving patient safety by providing customized interventions that consider differences in drug metabolism, drug interactions, and susceptibility to side effects on individual patients. Personalized medicine makes medication errors and treatment-related complications less likely by optimizing treatments for every patient's unique biology and context [15, 16].

Improving Patient Outcomes

The underlying aim of personalized medicine is to enhance patient outcomes for a variety of different ailments. Personalized medicine may improve overall health results, including better management of diseases, control over symptoms, and increased quality of life by tailoring treatment plans to meet the special requirements and characteristics of each patient [17, 18].

Empowering Patients

The main objective of personalized medicine is to enable patients to actively participate in their healthcare through the provision of personalized information, education, and resources. It also involves the patient in treatment decisions and making them care partners, thereby facilitating shared decision-making, adherence to treatment plans, and self-management of health conditions [19, 20].

Advancing Scientific Knowledge

Personalized medicine is the source of scientific knowledge that enhances our understanding of what causes disease, and how people respond to treatment. Personalized medicine enables the discovery of new biomarkers, molecular targets or treatment regimens by conducting research and collecting data on individual patient characteristics and outcomes thereby resulting in constant improvements in healthcare delivery [21, 22].

LIMITATIONS OF TRADITIONAL APPROACHES

Traditional healthcare, though the backbone, most often does not meet the complex and varied requirements of patients due to various inherent restrictions. The major disadvantage of conventional healthcare is that it tends to gravitate towards a 'one-size-fits-all' system. In this regard, standardized treatment protocols are useful for handling large numbers of patients; however, such plans disregard patient-specific differences in terms of local environment lifestyles and genetic makeup whose influence on outcomes can be significant. Consequently, sub-optimally suited interventions may be administered to people which may have negative consequences and instead worsen the state of health [23 - 25].

Traditional healthcare normally depends on a trial-and-error treatment method in which healthcare professionals prescribe drugs or therapies based on general rules but tune them according to patient feedback. This method could be time-consuming, and expensive and may cause additional agony to the patients who have to go through several ineffective rounds of medication before getting one that is effective. It can also lead to patient disappointment and erode confidence in healthcare institutions as patients may perceive the process as non-caring for their own needs and choices [26, 27].

Another limitation of traditional healthcare is that it depends on the use of usual ways to diagnose illnesses. These methods do not have sufficient predictive power that can accurately foretell disease progression or treatment response. Diagnostic tools often focus on identifying symptoms and medical histories provided by patients, but this approach does not help capture slight variations and early signs of diseases. Therefore, some diseases may go unnoticed, or get falsely diagnosed resulting in a delay in starting a treatment process and exacerbating the situation for patients [28, 29].

Traditional healthcare settings are known for fragmented data and limited communication between medical caregivers. Frequently, patient records are kept in separate systems that may not be linked together or easily accessible hence making it difficult for physicians to get a complete view of their patients' health status. This disconnectedness impairs continuity of care among different health-care providers who might have incomplete clinical information on the same patients. Consequently, diagnosis mistakes as well as treatment errors can occur along with disruptions in the delivery of care [30 - 32].

Moreover, conventional healthcare systems are generally more reactive than proactive. In most cases, their main focus is on curing diseases that have already shown themselves instead of preventing them from occurring in the first place. This method could miss early interventions and preventative strategies thus resulting in poor long-term health outcomes and an increase in healthcare expenses to manage chronic illnesses that could otherwise have been avoided or curtailed with timely intervention [33, 34].

Traditional healthcare systems can lead to inefficiency in resource allocation because sometimes the resources are diverted towards patients who do not need the most. This results in the wastage of resources and an increase in the costs of health care without corresponding improvements in patient outcomes. Besides, emphasis on treating diseases instead of ensuring wellness may continue the cycle of illness and reliance on medical interventions rather than enabling individuals to manage their health [35].

THE ROLE OF AI IN PERSONALIZED MEDICINE

There are various methods and techniques in AI that enable computers to perform tasks such as those requiring human intelligence. Machine learning and Natural Language Processing (NLP) are two prominent AI techniques, wherein each of them has its applications. It is a process consisting of algorithms that can learn from data, identify patterns, and make decisions or predictions without being explicitly programmed. This approach relies on the idea of training models using large datasets in order to detect relationships and gain knowledge leading to better results [36].

The models learn from labeled data, where the algorithm learns to map input features to corresponding output labels. This method is often employed for classification and regression tasks. By working with unlabeled data, the models learn to identify hidden patterns or structures in it. Clustering and dimensionality reduction are usual examples of unsupervised learning. Algorithms learn the best actions while interacting with an environment and getting feedback as rewards or penalties. Applications using this technique include game-playing and robotics [37].

NLP puts its emphasis on computers getting to understand human language and interpreting and generating it. It is an area that involves working on techniques for processing text data as well as analyzing it in order to derive meaningful information and facilitate communication among humans, machines, *etc*. There are practices like tokenization, stemming, and lemmatization applied before textual data can be analyzed. NLP algorithms extract structured information from unstructured text, including entities, relationships, and events [38].

Sentiment or opinion can be determined by NLP models that analyze text, allowing for such applications as social media monitoring and customer feedback analysis. To translate text across languages, NLP techniques are utilized in machine translation systems which facilitate cross-lingual communication [39].

Foundational components in the development of intelligent systems across various domains such as healthcare, finance, transportation, and entertainment are these AI techniques. The use of machine learning and NLP allows computers to do tasks automatically, learn from data, and communicate with people in a more human way thereby resulting in greater efficacy, precision, and user experience. In shaping the future of technology and society, these technologies will become increasingly important as AI progresses [40].

Integration of AI with Genomic Data

Thus, the integration of AI into genomics provides a great opportunity to change the practice of personalized medicine and increase our knowledge about genetics and diseases. This fusion necessitates using AI methods when carrying out analysis on genomic data sets which are huge in size, recognizing regularities from them, and extracting useful information that can be used in making clinical decisions as well as medical treatment procedures [41]. The integration of AI with genomic data is described below and shown in Fig. (**2**).

Data Analysis and Interpretation

Genomic data (including DNA sequencing, gene expression profiles, and genetic variations) provide valuable information about an individual's genetic makeup and its implications for health and disease. AI methods such as machine learning and deep learning are used to study genomic data, identify genetic variations related to diseases, and forecast individuals' risk of illness. These algorithms can sift through large genomic datasets, detect patterns, and prioritize genetic variants that are most relevant to specific diseases or conditions [42, 43].

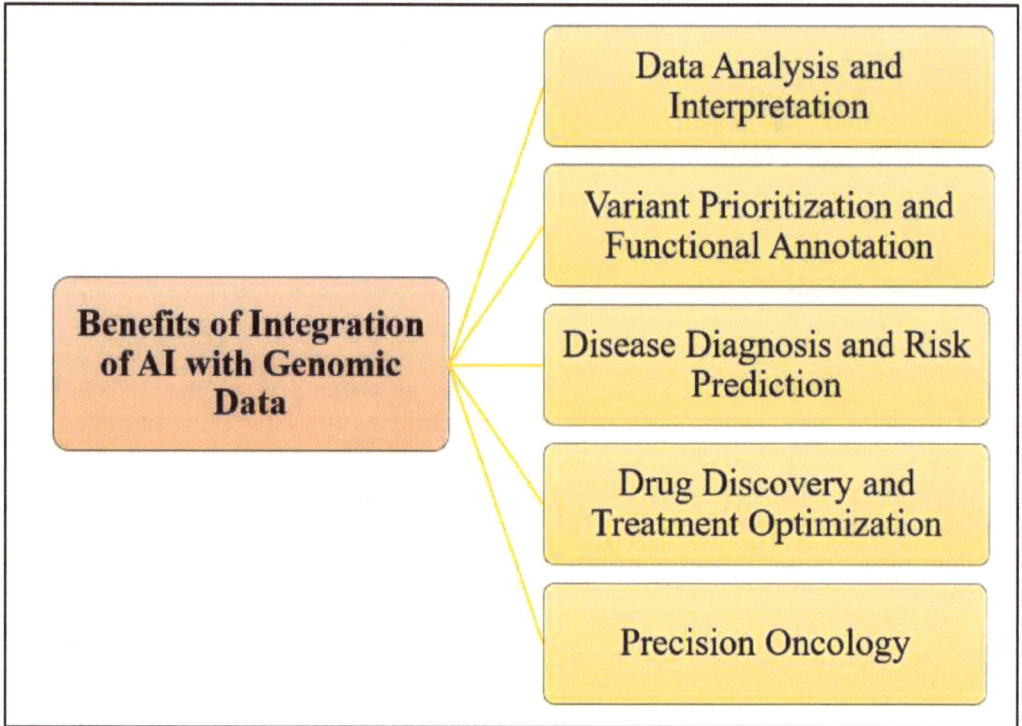

Fig. (2). Benefits of integration of AI with genomic data.

Variant Prioritization and Functional Annotation

AI algorithms may rank genetic variants on their level of functional impact, disease relevance, and occurrence in population databases. It is also possible to predict the functional effects of a given genetic variant such as its effect on protein structure and function with machine learning techniques using functional annotation tools. AI can combine genomic and functional annotation data to prioritize variants that are most likely to play a role in disease susceptibility or treatment response, thereby pointing out areas for further investigation and validation [36, 44].

Disease Diagnosis and Risk Prediction

The use of AI techniques in analyzing genetic data is a valuable tool for disease diagnosis and prediction. Genetic variants and other clinical features can be analyzed by machine learning algorithms to identify patterns that are linked to specific diseases or phenotypes. This can help in formulating predictive models that use genomic information to assess the likelihood that certain diseases or conditions will develop, allowing early treatment and individualized preventive approaches. For instance, AI-based risk-prediction models may detect people prone to inherited ailments like cancers and heart complications thus aiding focused screening programs and preventive measures [45, 46].

Drug Discovery and Treatment Optimization

A combination of genomics and other omics data (such as transcriptomics, proteomics, and metabolomics) is increasingly being used in drug discovery and development. Genomic data can be analyzed by AI algorithms to determine drug targets, predict responses to drugs based on genetic variants, and tailor treatment options for patients. Personalized medicine utilizes AI to identify the most suitable treatments for patients with different genetic profiles thereby reducing adverse effects as well as improving therapeutic outcomes [47, 48].

Precision Oncology

Cancer centers are looking forward to AI-driven genomic data integration. Using AI algorithms in the analysis of tumor genomic profiles can recognize driver mutations, predict treatment responses, and provide guidance for personalized cancer therapy. By examining the molecular properties of tumors AI is able to recommend targeted therapies, immunotherapies, or clinical trials that may be most effective for specific cancer patients leading to better outcomes and patient results [49].

The integration of AI with genomic data holds tremendous potential to transform healthcare by enabling more precise diagnosis, personalized treatment, and preventive interventions tailored to individual genetic profiles. As AI technologies continue to advance, we can expect further innovations in genomic medicine and personalized healthcare, leading to improved patient care and outcomes [50].

Successful AI-Driven Initiatives

AI-based interventions for prescription schemes apply AI methodologies to fine-tune the drug diversity, dosage, and personalized treatment approaches of individual patients. These efforts employ various machine learning algorithms alongside NLP and data analytics in reviewing patient information, clinical protocols, and medical literature in order to offer customized suggestions for healthcare providers [51]. AI-driven initiatives for prescription plans are described below.

IBM Watson for Drug Discovery and Healthcare

Drug discovery and healthcare solutions with AI are offered by IBM Watson Health. These include Watson for Oncology and Watson for Drug Discovery. Watson for Drug Discovery utilizes the knowledge of a humongous amount of scientific articles, clinical trials, and drug databases to identify promising molecules that serve as potential drugs while forecasting their interactions with targets thereby speeding up the development of new drugs. For cancer patients' personal treatment recommendations based on their medical records, genomic data, and the latest medical literature, oncologists normally use Watson for Oncology. Through analyzing patient data against clinical guidelines, this system provides evidence-based treatment options that fit an individual patient's characteristics and preferences [52, 53].

Suki AI for Clinical Documentation and Prescription Assistance

Suki AI is an AI-powered virtual assistant built to automate clinical paperwork and support medical staff in prescribing medication. Through the application of NLP, Suki AI listens to physician-patient conversations and gives instant clinical notes reducing documentation time, among other administrative duties. Suki AI also helps healthcare practitioners with drug prescription tasks by providing related information on drug interactions, dosages, and alternative treatment options. The system enhances medication safety and adherence to clinical guidelines for better patient outcomes [54, 55].

AiCure for Medication Adherence and Monitoring

AiCure is a computer vision and machine learning-driven platform that uses AI to monitor patient behavior and medication adherence. The platform employs smartphone cameras to confirm visually if the patients have taken their medications as prescribed in real-time. Its AI algorithms scrutinize the behavior and medication compliance patterns of a patient in search of any lapse in adherence for personalized interventions to be made to improve compliance. The goal of AiCure is to boost treatment efficacy, decrease healthcare expenditure, and optimize patient outcomes by enhancing drug adherence levels [56 - 58].

Pillo Health for Medication Management and Patient Engagement

Pillo Health is a companion that incorporates AI for home care. It helps patients manage their medication, deal with chronic diseases, and facilitate healthcare communication. The device employs machine learning algorithms as well as NLP to interact with patients, remind them about taking medications, and respond to questions about their medical conditions or therapy regimens. On top of that, Pillo Health collects patient data, analyses it, and offers personalized health recommendations and insights to the patients themselves and caregivers thereby encouraging patient involvement and self-empowerment [59].

These AI-empowered plans concerning prescriptions show the possibility of AI for medication control, enhancing treatment compliance, and giving a personal touch to healthcare provision. Using Artificial Intelligence (AI) techniques, healthcare practitioners can better design patients' medications, doses, and monitoring with regard to individual patient's interests. This would lead to improved patient outcomes as well as better quality care [60, 61].

DATA INTEGRATION AND SOURCES

Data integration is a crucial aspect of AI-driven initiatives for prescription plans, as it involves combining and harmonizing data from various sources to provide comprehensive and actionable insights for healthcare providers [62].

Genomic Databases

In personalized medicine, genomic databases are the pioneers because they offer critical gene-storing information that is necessary for AI-based prescription plans. The genomic databases include volumes of genomic data like DNA sequences, genetic variations, gene expression profiles, and related phenotypic data. These act as useful materials for healthcare providers and researchers who want to know about the genetics of diseases, predict treatment responses, or design interventions based on individual patient characteristics [63, 64].

Combining genomics databases with AI-driven prescription plans is opening up unprecedented possibilities for precision medicine. For example, AI algorithms exploit genetic data to detect genomic factors that affect disease risk, drug response, and metabolism. In addition, *via* other clinical data in the EHRs and medical literature, AI-driven prescription plans optimize therapy options and dosage hence providing personalized interventions leading to better patient outcomes with minimal side-effects [65, 66].

For personalized medicine, one of the main benefits of genomic databases is their potential to pinpoint genetic variation associated with particular diseases or drug reactions. AI algorithms can detect even rare or common variants across diverse populations that contribute to disease susceptibility, pharmacokinetics, and therapeutic response by querying large amounts of genomic data stored in these databases. With the aid of such a wealth of information about genes, AI-driven prescription plans could then be used for treatment that is tailored to individual patients on the basis of their unique genetic profiles resulting in improved healthcare outcomes characterized by enhanced efficacy and personalization [67 - 69].

The use of Artificial Intelligence (AI) analysis in genomic databases also supports the identification of new therapeutic targets and biomarkers. Scientists can identify genetic variations or RNA profiles indicative of chronic diseases or treatment outcomes using machine learning techniques. This, in turn, can result in targeted therapies, pharmacogenomics interventions, and precision medicine approaches based on individual patient's traits. The merging of genomic data with AI-driven prescribing schemes quickens the translation from genomics to healthcare practice opening up novel personalized treatment strategies [70 - 72].

Genomic databases also contribute significantly to pharmacogenomics, the research that examines how drug responses are influenced by genetic variations. Genomic databases hold pharmacogenetic data, which explains the impact of genetic variants on drugs' metabolism and efficacy as well as toxicity. In light of such information, AI algorithms can predict individual patient response to drugs, and determine an optimal dosage while minimizing adverse effects connected with medicines. Artificial intelligence-based techniques bring about improved medication safety and efficiency in personalized medicine through the integration of pharmacogenomics into the prescription planning process [73 - 75].

Genomic databases are also useful in facilitating the identification of actionable genetic variants for disease risk assessment and prevention besides pharmacogenomics. AI algorithms scrutinize genomic data to put patients into risk groups according to their predisposition to some diseases which are genetically determined. The AI-based prescription plans can advise on personalized preventive measures, screening protocols, and lifestyle interventions that are appropriate for individuals at high risk of certain conditions. This proactive approach to personalized medicine focuses on preventing diseases and intervening early, resulting in better health outcomes and lower healthcare expenses [76 - 78].

Additionally, collaborative research and data sharing are also made possible by the presence of genomic databases in healthcare institutions, researchers, and pharmaceutical companies. These databases facilitate knowledge sharing, data harmonization, and collaborative research initiatives for advancing personalized medicine through central access to genomic data from diverse populations. Researchers can use AI-driven approaches to analyze large-scale genomic datasets, recognize novel genetic associations, confirm predictive biomarkers, as well as develop innovative treatment strategies that suit each patient's requirements [79, 80].

AI ALGORITHMS AND DECISION SUPPORT SYSTEMS

AI algorithms and decision support systems play a crucial role in healthcare by leveraging advanced technologies such as machine learning models and NLP to assist healthcare providers in making informed decisions [81, 82].

Machine learning models are algorithms that enable computers to learn from and make predictions or decisions based on data. In healthcare, machine learning models can be utilized for various tasks such as disease diagnosis, patient risk prediction, treatment recommendation, and personalized medicine. Examples of machine learning algorithms commonly used in healthcare include logistic regression, decision trees, random forests, support vector machines, neural networks, and deep learning models such as Convolutional Neural Networks (CNNs) and Recurrent Neural Networks (RNNs). Consequently, these models need a lot of training on big datasets in order to study patterns carefully hence making accurate predictions [83 - 85].

NLP techniques can be applied in healthcare to examine unstructured textual data such as medical records, clinical notes, research articles, and patient feedback. NLP can get useful information from textual data like symptoms, diagnoses, treatments, and outcomes enabling it to make decisions easily by the medical practitioners. Healthcare commonly involves various Natural Language Processing tasks that include text classification, Named Entity Recognition (NER), sentiment analysis, topic modeling, and language translation [86].

Healthcare Decision Support Systems (DSS) are computer-based decision-making aid tools used by healthcare providers to recommend data and advice based on patient information and medical knowledge. DSS could incorporate machine learning models, clinical guidelines, NLP techniques, expert systems, and medical databases in order to make decisions. These can help in patient care for diagnostic purposes, medication choices during treatment planning, risk analysis as well as overall disease management. They can also be used for the purpose of quality improvement in healthcare delivery systems or even optimize resource utilization as it relates to patient outcomes and decrease medical errors in the process [84, 87].

AI algorithms, machine learning models, and natural language processing techniques are all crucial elements of decision support systems used by healthcare providers. These technologies allow health data to be analyzed, insights drawn from unstructured text, and clinical decision-making supported with a view to improving patient care [88 - 90].

PATIENT ENGAGEMENT AND EMPOWERMENT

Patient engagement and empowerment are facilitated by various tools and mechanisms designed to involve patients actively in their healthcare journey which is described below and summarized in Fig. (**3**) [91].

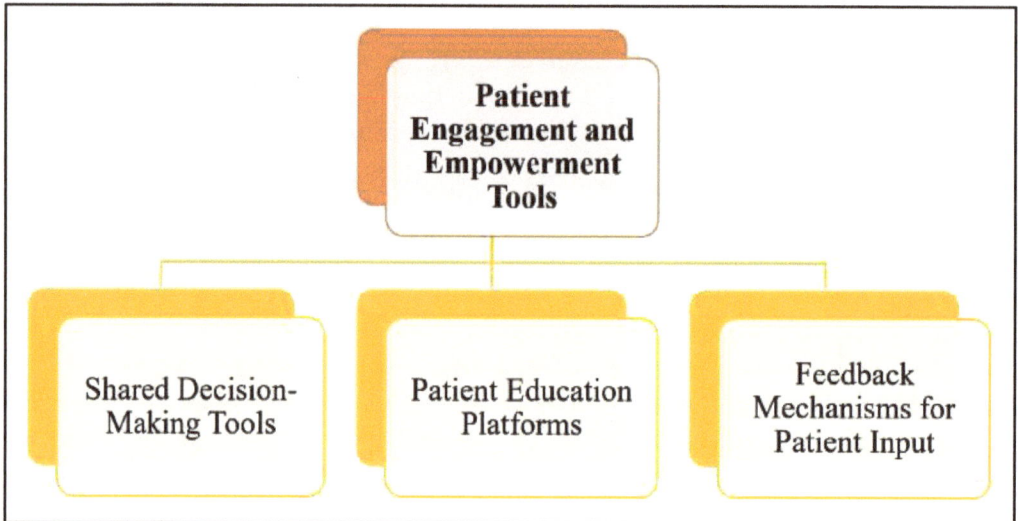

Fig. (3). Patient engagement and empowerment tools.

Shared Decision-Making Tools

Tools, which are called shared decision-making tools, can be used to facilitate collaborative decision-making processes between patients and healthcare providers. This empowers the individuals involved to play an active role in their healthcare journey. Such tools have become very important in promoting autonomy, informed choice, and patient satisfaction in the current era of patient-centered care [92].

Shared decision-making is basically a process that requires collaboration between patients and doctors in order to reach a common decision about treatment choices that fit with the patient's preferences, values, and goals. These tools are supplementary during shared decision-making as they provide organized, evidential information regarding different treatment options, possible results of each alternative, hazards, and benefits. In this way, these tools enable patients to comprehend their healthcare options better and therefore engage in fruitful talks with their healthcare providers by presenting the information in an understandable manner [93].

Another type of shared decision-making tool is called aids to decision-making. Such aids come in the form of brochures, films, internet courses, or interactive websites. These tools are designed based on clinical evidence and guidelines, providing information on treatment options in a balanced way that is unbiased. Decision aids mostly have visual features like option grids or decision trees that enable patients to compare various treatment modalities based on their individual preferences and situations [94].

The purpose of decision aids is to improve patients' comprehension of their medical problems and the various forms of treatment that are available to them so that they can make choices based on full information that aligns with their preferences. Decision aids promote patient autonomy, reduce decisional conflict, and decrease anxiety and uncertainty by involving patients in the process [95].

Additionally, decision aids improve the communication between providers and patients by facilitating treatment options discussions, exploring patients' fears and desires as well as resolving any misconceptions. By using shared decision-making enhanced by decision aids, patients and professionals can engage in a mutual process of developing individual patient-specific treatment plans leading to increased patient satisfaction and involvement [96].

In addition to decision aids, technology-based shared decision-making tools have cropped up as invaluable resources in healthcare. Mobile applications, web-based platforms, and electronic health record systems can give patients access to decision-support tools and educational resources so that they can participate in a shared decision-making dialogue away from the clinical encounter. These digital tools may include features like personalized risk calculators, interactive decision trees, and multimedia presentations to improve patients' comprehension of their healthcare options enabling them to participate in shared decision discussions [97].

Additionally, shared decision tools have the potential to help healthcare providers standardize decision-making and at the same time lead to an increase in patient contentment and compliance towards treatment programs while reducing the chances of provision of services that are not parallel with patients' choices or beliefs. Routine clinical practices should incorporate these shared tools in order to foster patient-centered care culture within healthcare institutions as well as improve the general quality of service delivery [98].

Patient Education Platforms

Digital tools that offer patients information and knowledge regarding their health status, treatment options, and ways of managing it are called patient education platforms. They can be used as valuable tools to promote good health conditions, enhance the participation of patients in their own care, and improve the outcomes [99].

Accessible Information

Many educational platforms for patients display a variety of health problems in a language understandable to individuals with different literacy levels, therefore making it a useful tool for everyone. They also provide information about various diseases or medical conditions as well as their treatment or prevention strategies that are personalized to meet the needs and wants of patients [100].

Multimedia Content

Patient education platforms encompass various multimedia tools such as articles, videos, infographics, animations, and interactive tools to render information in visually captivating and engaging formats. Using multimedia like this one makes it easier to understand the key concepts of health and remember complex medical pieces that have been made more digestible and memorable for patients [101].

Tailored Content

Some patient education platforms offer personalized content based on the patient's specific health conditions, treatment plans, and individual preferences several of these forums improve relevance as well as efficiency in that they are patient-centric and therefore gear up the chances of such knowledge being used by the patients in their management of health [102].

Self-paced Learning

Patient education systems allow patients to receive information for their personal use and understanding, giving them an opportunity to manage their own health education. This makes it possible for patients to access educational resources through computers, mobile devices such as smartphones, or any other internet-connected device resulting in continual learning and reinforcement of medical knowledge [103].

Empowerment through Self-management

Patient education platforms provide useful information on ways to self-manage, take medications, monitor the symptoms, and make changes in lifestyle. These platforms empower patients to manage their health better by providing them with the requisite skills and resources hence promoting self-efficacy as well as autonomy in healthcare decision-making [104].

Integration with Healthcare Providers

Seamless integration between some of the patient education platforms with EHR systems or patient portals can allow healthcare providers to prescribe certain educational resources and keep track of how patients interact with them. Patient-doctor partnership, continuity of care, and treatment adherence are all supported by its combination with health care systems [105].

Supportive Communities

Various patient teaching programs include the provision of online discussions, clubs, or even a social media infrastructure so as to enable patients to reach out to each other and share stories plus emotional support from people with the same health conditions. Supportive communities promote a feeling of inclusion and self-determination, thereby motivating patients to actively participate in their healthcare process [106].

Evidence-based Information

Patient education platforms aim to provide evidence-based information that comes from reliable medical literature, clinical guidelines, and healthcare professionals. Such platforms give patients confidence by allowing them to make informed choices about their health and treatment options as they can therefore trust the information provided on them [107].

One of the major functions of patient education platforms is to increase people's health literacy, boost their participation in healthcare issues, and help them take up an active role in their personal care. Hence, through the provision of information that can be easily accessed by patients, tailored to suit personal needs as well as drawn from the evident base, this will enable patients to make more informed choices about their health status, and consequently adopt effective management styles and behaviors all aimed at positively impacting on health outcomes [107].

Feedback Mechanisms for Patient Input

For healthcare systems, feedback systems by patients are indispensable as they provide a platform for expressing opinions, sharing experiences, and making suggestions about the medical treatment received. These mechanisms facilitate patient-centered care by enabling healthcare organizations to understand patients' needs, preferences, and concerns, ultimately improving the quality of care delivery [108].

Patient Satisfaction Surveys

Patient satisfaction surveys are often used as a way to collect feedback from patients about their experiences with healthcare services. These surveys generally focus on different dimensions of the patient experience including communication with healthcare professionals, waiting times, cleanliness of the facility, and overall satisfaction with the care provided. Lastly, healthcare organizations use both quantitative and qualitative data to help them know where they should fix or improve in order to make targeted interventions that will improve the patient experience [109].

Comment Boxes and Suggestion Forms

Patient feedback and suggestions can be given to healthcare providers or administrators through comment boxes and suggestion forms. People can use either electronic or paper formats to provide their thoughts anonymously, thus encouraging openness and frankness in their statements. As a result of reviewing comments from such sources as comment boxes and suggestion forms, specific cases will be addressed, and alterations implemented with the aim of responding to patients [110].

Online Feedback Forms

Online feedback forms can be described as an easy and accessible platform for patients to send a response about the health-based services they have had. They can be combined with hospital websites, patient portals, or mobile applications so that the patients can provide feedback at any time and place. Additional components of online feedback forms may involve fixed questions and free text areas where patients will be required to give more detail on what they are saying. Healthcare organizations can study data from online feedback forms to find out trends, patterns, and areas for improvement [111].

Focus Groups and Patient Advisory Councils

In order to consistently improve the quality and efficiency of health care, focus groups as well as patient advisory councils are created. Patients can take part in these forums to give suggestions, raise issues, or share advice with those who are responsible for their health care. Through this process of involving patients in decision-making, focus groups and patient advisory councils make sure that the viewpoints of patients are taken into account while formulating guidelines, programs, and operations [112].

Patient Advocacy Forums

Patient advocacy forums facilitate collective patient, caregiver, and advocacy organizations meetings where they discuss issues concerning patient care, health care access, and health policies. In these forums, patients get a chance to advocate for their rights, narrate their own experiences in the healthcare system, and work together towards improving patient-oriented healthcare systems. These platforms enable patients to address collective systemic problems, create awareness of medical matters, and run campaigns for positive transformations in health care [113].

Social Media and Online Reviews

Social media sites and online review forums allow patients to broadcast their experiences of health care. Patients are able to post their reviews, comments, or ratings on healthcare providers, facilities, and services, thereby giving valuable insights to other patients and healthcare organizations. But despite the broad reach and real-time feedback of social media platforms and online reviews, healthcare organizations should keep monitoring the feedback actively in order to address concerns, manage reputational risks, and maintain patient trust.

Patient input feedback systems are essential to foster patient-centeredness in care, enhance the quality of delivery, and improve patient satisfaction. When healthcare organizations seek and include input from patients, they show that they value hearing from them, meeting their needs, and constantly improving the healthcare experience provided for such patients. Through efficient feedback mechanisms, patients can contribute to shaping their health journeys resulting in transformative changes in healthcare systems [114].

ECONOMIC AND SOCIETAL IMPLICATIONS

The economic and societal implications of integrating AI algorithms, decision support systems, and patient engagement tools into healthcare are profound as they impact spending on healthcare, where resources are allocated, cost-effectiveness, and personalized treatment accessibility.

Impact on Healthcare Spending

AI algorithms and decision support systems hold the potential for health optimization by enhancing the efficiency of care delivery. These technologies can enable healthcare providers to find low-expense treatment alternatives, improve administrative processes, reduce medical errors, and eliminate unnecessary hospitalizations or readmissions. By applying predictive analytics and machine learning models, healthcare organizations may enhance resource allocation, intervention prioritization, and targeting of interventions towards high-risk patient populations thereby reducing healthcare costs associated with preventable complications and adverse events. Additionally, tools for involving patients such as telemedicine platforms, mobile health applications, and remote monitoring devices facilitate early intervention in chronic diseases, and self-care among patients that result in better health outcomes and thus lower healthcare utilization [115].

Resource Allocation and Cost-Effectiveness

Healthcare providers are able to make decisions on resource allocation and treatment plans using decision support systems that provide evidence. They can analyse large volumes of patient data, clinical guidelines, and medical literature to suggest the most suitable and cost-effective interventions. By integrating cost-effectiveness analysis into clinical decision-making, healthcare providers will be able to focus on the interventions that offer greater improvements in outcomes relative to costs incurred. This method guarantees that such limited resources of healthcare get allocated to interventions, which are most effective in delivering health gains to patients and populations. In addition, AI-powered predictive modeling tools can estimate future resource needs for healthcare hence enabling the anticipation of the demand, optimization of staffing levels and proactive allocation of resources to meet patient needs while minimizing inefficiencies and waste [116].

Societal Implications and Access to Personalized Treatments

AI algorithms and decision support systems are being used in healthcare to bring personalized treatments as well as precision medicine within the reach of all. They can delve into individual patient information, gene data, and biomarkers to make treatment plans specifically for each person based on their uniqueness and requirements. AI-driven decision-support tools offer doctors useful recommendations and prescriptions, thus making it easier for them to decide on the right course of action when diagnosing, choosing a therapy or monitoring their patient's responses. This strategy is very effective because it helps improve patient outcomes as well as reduce the chances of side effects from drugs, treatment failures or unnecessary interventions [117].

Nevertheless, guaranteeing equal access to personalized therapeutic strategies requires tackling digital disparities, healthcare barriers, and socioeconomic variances. Therefore, healthcare institutions must prioritize the achievement of health equity, which implies dealing with social determinants and inequality in population access to medical care as well as its outcomes.

The economic and social implications of the integration of AI algorithms, decision support systems, and patient engagement tools, have significant effects on how healthcare is spending its money, using resources, its cost-effectiveness as well as access to personalized therapies. Through the appropriate and responsible use of these technologies, healthcare providers can improve service delivery in terms of quality, efficiency, and equity which will result in better health for individuals and populations [118].

PATIENT OUTCOMES AND REAL-WORLD EVIDENCE

Patient Outcomes and Real-World Evidence are crucial components in understanding the effectiveness and impact of healthcare interventions. Table **1** summarizes the impact of patient outcomes and real-world evidence in healthcare.

Table 1. Summary of the impact of patient outcomes and real-world evidence in healthcare.

Aspect	Description
Patient Outcomes	The term "patient outcomes" refers to the effect on a patient's health status and general well-being after undergoing healthcare interventions. These may consist of clinical measures like lowering blood pressure, and reduction in symptom severity; functional outputs such as the ability to carry out daily exercises, and patients' self-reports for example the level of quality of life and satisfaction with care. The central aim of any intervention by health workers is to improve patient outcomes due to better care provided by them. This would indicate that care is efficient and of good quality [119].
Real-World Evidence (RWE)	RWE means data collected from actual settings like EHRs, registries, databases of claims, and patient-generated data. RWE gives more information on healthcare intervention efficacy, safety, and value in everyday medical practice than the evidence that comes out from clinical trials. On the other hand, traditional clinical trials are not able to compare with RWE when it comes to broader patient populations, varied treatment patterns as well as long-term outcomes that reflect real-world diversity and variability [120].
Impact on Healthcare	It is very important that healthcare decision-making, clinical practice guidelines, as well as policy development, are based on RWE and patient outcomes. RWE along with patient outcomes assists healthcare stakeholders in evaluating the cost-effectiveness, safety, and comparative effectiveness of interventions. Identifying evidence gaps, guiding resource allocation to interventions that offer the greatest benefits to patients, and informing clinical decision support tools are among the many ways through which RWE can be useful. Healthcare organizations can use patient outcomes and real-world evidence (RWE) to improve care quality, optimize treatment pathways, and enhance patient-centered outcomes. Incorporating patient-reported outcomes in RWE improves patient engagement and captures the most important outcomes for patients while ensuring interventions align with their preferences and priorities [121, 122].

CHALLENGES AND CONSIDERATIONS

Numerous challenges and considerations are involved in addressing the introduction of AI algorithms, decision support systems, and patient engagement tools into healthcare settings. These include ethical issues, integration complexities, and the need for transparency and accountability. Ethical concerns like privacy and bias are central to the responsible deployment of these technologies. As health-related information is sensitive, it is important to ensure that patient privacy as well as data security is protected. Healthcare companies have to establish rigorous data management policies and encryption methods that will protect patient information and observe regulations. Also, ensuring fairness in AI algorithms is important to avoid biased outcomes and healthcare inequalities. Healthcare facilities must guarantee inclusivity in training datasets and the use of equality-conscious algorithms for fair health service provision [123].

The combination of these AI technologies with healthcare systems creates technical and organizational difficulties, such as interoperability problems and workflow disturbances. The development of interoperability standards and data exchange protocols is necessary that allow seamless integration into the current health IT infrastructure while incorporating user-centered design principles and conducting workflow analysis are important to ensure the customization of AI solutions for the specific needs of health professionals. Sufficient training and education for healthcare providers are also vital in ensuring the proper application and interpretation of AI-enabled tools within clinical practice.

Transparency and accountability are key pillars in establishing trust, responsible AI deployment, and patient safety as well as autonomy. The algorithms' performance can also be evaluated through the use of monitoring and auditing systems to ensure that they adhere to ethical and regulatory standards. To ensure accountability and keep up with the integrity of AI-enabled systems, audits should be conducted on a regular basis alongside continuous monitoring for compliance with ethical and regulatory requirements. Further, stakeholders must also be obligated to ethical behavior, good data management, and patient outcomes through clear management structures and regulatory mechanisms. The algorithms of AI should provide details on the constraints, prejudices as well as risks that enable clients to take charge of their decisions and maintain their principles in healthcare delivery [124].

Responsible integration of AI algorithms, decision support systems, and patient engagement tools into healthcare systems hinges on ethics, seamless integration, transparency, and accountability. For this reason, adherence to ethical principles, promoting interoperability, and encouraging transparency and accountability in healthcare organizations can help harness the transformative potential of AI technologies for improved patient outcomes, better healthcare delivery as well as the advancement of the patient-centered care principle [125].

FUTURE DIRECTIONS AND IMPLICATIONS

Emerging trends like wearables and mobile health technologies are shaping the future of healthcare, which could revamp patient care, enhance results, and change the role of doctors. Devices that can be worn by individuals such as wristbands or watches that can track our physical fitness levels have become more common. To add to this, there has been an increase in mobile health apps that provide patients with convenient access to their health information, help them track their symptoms over time, give them reminders concerning medications, and support telemedicine consultations. Patients will have more control over their own well-being through active participation in taking care of themselves [126].

These current happenings in the field of medicine have big consequences for health care outcomes, costs, and satisfaction of patients. With wearables and mobile health technologies, healthcare providers can get important data on the health of patients as well as how they behave thereby enabling early recognition of diseases, intervention, and customized treatment methods. These include wearable devices and mobile health apps that enable remote patient monitoring; managing chronic conditions; and preventing illness; thus improving clinical outcomes and reducing hospitalization rates, which correlates with better patient engagement and adherence to recommended care. Additionally, patient empowerment- where individuals are driven to self-manage their conditions while gaining access to information along with other pertinent resources and technologies in addition to mobile health presents improved satisfaction levels among patients as well as enhanced overall quality of care [126].

However, the widespread acceptance of wearables and mobile health technologies also poses challenges and implications for healthcare practitioners. As a result, professionals in the medical field must adapt to this changing scenario of digital health by including these devices in their practice to provide patient-centered care effectively. Medical practitioners need to be up-to-date with recent technological advancements, know how much they can do and what they can't do, and use them in the treatment plans and decision-making process. Moreover, doctors have to deal with ethical issues involving patient privacy, data protection, and informed consent associated with the use of wearables or mobile healthcare applications [127].

The growing dependence on wearable devices and mobile healthcare technology is forcing healthcare providers to rethink their role from episodic carers to proactive health coaches and coordinators. This means doctors will have to become more collaborative, patient-centered caregivers who interpret information emanating from wearables as well as mobile health applications, guide patients in making informed decisions about their health, and engage them in this process. In order to effectively use wearables and mobile health technologies in patient care, medical professionals should be given continuous education and training that equips them with the required competencies in digital health literacy, data interpretation as well as communication [128].

CONCLUSION

In conclusion, the application of artificial intelligence algorithms that depend on machine learning techniques to assess substantial quantities of patient data such as medical history, genetic information, and lifestyle elements has facilitated the customization of treatment options for patients by doctors in the health sector. This approach is different from the usual one-size-fits-all treatments and it has a chance of providing better custom-made interventions that cater to each individual's personal characteristics and nature. The adoption of AI-driven prescription plans shows a significant pledge to advancing patient results, enhancing drug adherence, as well as optimizing medical resource use. Artificial intelligent driven prescription plans can minimize side effects, reduce the possibility of treatment failure, and improve patient satisfaction by selecting appropriate treatments and doses based on individual patient profiles. In addition, these plans have the ability to change patient-centered care delivery by facilitating more streamlined clinical decision-making that gives healthcare providers data-driven insights. However, there are also concerns and thoughts about the widespread adoption of AI-driven prescription plans. Maintaining patient trust and complying with regulatory standards necessitates safeguarding data privacy and transparency. Furthermore, medical practitioners require appropriate training and assistance that would facilitate the successful integration of AI-aided prescription plans into their daily practice as well as interpreting the analytics provided by such algorithms correctly. Personalized medicine driven by AI prescriptions is a revolutionary system for healthcare delivery, which may change how we diagnose, treat, and manage diseases. Medical practitioners can improve patient outcomes, enhance medication safety, and ultimately revolutionize the way medicine is practiced by tailoring treatments to individual patients through artificial intelligence. The future of personalized medicine has much promise for bettering the health and well-being of people globally as we continue to innovate and refine these technologies.

ACKNOWLEDGEMENTS

Authors are highly thankful to their Universities/Colleges for providing library facilities for the literature survey.

REFERENCES

[1]   S. Qiu, Y. Cai, H. Yao, C. Lin, Y. Xie, S. Tang, and A. Zhang, "Small molecule metabolites: discovery of biomarkers and therapeutic targets", *Signal Transduction and Targeted Therapy,* vol. 8, no. 1, p. 132, 2023.
[http://dx.doi.org/10.1038/s41392-023-01399-3]

[2]   G. Pravettoni, and S. Triberti, P5 eHealth:, *An Agenda for the Health Technologies of the Future,* Cham, Switzerland: Springer, 2020.
[http://dx.doi.org/10.1007/978-3-030-27994-3]

[3]   L. Marques, B. Costa, M. Pereira, A. Silva, J. Santos, L. Saldanha, I. Silva, P. Magalhães, S. Schmidt, and N. Vale, "Advancing Precision Medicine: A Review of Innovative In Silico Approaches for Drug Development, Clinical Pharmacology and Personalized Healthcare", *Pharmaceutics,* vol. 16, no. 3, p. 332, 2024.
[http://dx.doi.org/10.3390/pharmaceutics16030332] [PMID: 38543226]

[4]   H. Fröhlich, R. Balling, N. Beerenwinkel, O. Kohlbacher, S. Kumar, T. Lengauer, M.H. Maathuis, Y. Moreau, S.A. Murphy, T.M. Przytycka, M. Rebhan, H. Röst, A. Schuppert, M. Schwab, R. Spang, D. Stekhoven, J. Sun, A. Weber, D. Ziemek, and B. Zupan, "From hype to reality: data science enabling personalized medicine", *BMC Med.,* vol. 16, no. 1, p. 150, 2018.
[http://dx.doi.org/10.1186/s12916-018-1122-7] [PMID: 30145981]

[5]   C.L. Overby, and P. Tarczy-Hornoch, "Personalized medicine: challenges and opportunities for translational bioinformatics", *Per. Med.,* vol. 10, no. 5, pp. 453-462, 2013.
[http://dx.doi.org/10.2217/pme.13.30] [PMID: 24039624]

[6]   L.H. Goetz, and N.J. Schork, "Personalized medicine: motivation, challenges, and progress", *Fertil. Steril.,* vol. 109, no. 6, pp. 952-963, 2018.
[http://dx.doi.org/10.1016/j.fertnstert.2018.05.006] [PMID: 29935653]

[7]   L.H. Goetz, and N.J. Schork, "Personalized medicine: motivation, challenges, and progress", *Fertil. Steril.,* vol. 109, no. 6, pp. 952-963, 2018.
[http://dx.doi.org/10.1016/j.fertnstert.2018.05.006] [PMID: 29935653]

[8]   M.C. Roberts, A.E. Fohner, L. Landry, D.L. Olstad, A.K. Smit, E. Turbitt, and C.G. Allen, "Advancing precision public health using human genomics: examples from the field and future research opportunities", *Genome Med.,* vol. 13, no. 1, p. 97, 2021.
[http://dx.doi.org/10.1186/s13073-021-00911-0] [PMID: 34074326]

[9]   W.K. Redekop, and D. Mladsi, "The faces of personalized medicine: a framework for understanding its meaning and scope", *Value Health,* vol. 16, no. 6, suppl. Suppl., pp. S4-S9, 2013.
[http://dx.doi.org/10.1016/j.jval.2013.06.005] [PMID: 24034312]

[10]   A. Blasiak, J. Khong, and T. Kee, "CURATE.AI: Optimizing Personalized Medicine with Artificial Intelligence", *SLAS Technol.,* vol. 25, no. 2, pp. 95-105, 2020.
[http://dx.doi.org/10.1177/2472630319890316] [PMID: 31771394]

[11]   S.R. Gajare, A.S. Deshmukh, and C.K. Shinde, "Personalized Medicine: A Review", *Int. J. Pharm. Sci. Rev. Res.,* vol. 69, no. 1, 2021.
[http://dx.doi.org/10.47583/ijpsrr.2021.v69i01.023]

[12]   M.J. Sorich, and R.A. McKinnon, "Personalized medicine: potential, barriers and contemporary issues", *Curr. Drug Metab.,* vol. 13, no. 7, pp. 1000-1006, 2012.
[http://dx.doi.org/10.2174/138920012802138615] [PMID: 22591350]

[13]   R.C. Wang, and Z. Wang, "Precision Medicine: Disease Subtyping and Tailored Treatment", *Cancers (Basel),* vol. 15, no. 15, p. 3837, 2023.
[http://dx.doi.org/10.3390/cancers15153837] [PMID: 37568653]

[14]   L. Silva, T. Pacheco, E. Araújo, R.J. Duarte, I. Ribeiro-Vaz, and R. Ferreira-da-Silva, *Unveiling the future: precision pharmacovigilance in the era of personalized medicine.* International Journal of Clinical Pharmacy. Springer Science and Business Media Deutschland GmbH, 2024.
[http://dx.doi.org/10.1007/s11096-024-01709-x]

[15]   D. Alemayehu, and J.C. Cappelleri, *Conceptual and Analytical Considerations toward the Use of Patient-reported Outcomes in Personalized Medicine,* 2012. Available from: www.AHDBonline.com

[16]   P.H. Roth, and T. Bruni, *Participation, Empowerment, and Evidence in the Current Discourse on Personalized Medicine-A Critique of 'Democratizing Healthcare,',* 2021. Available from: https://www.researchgate.net/publication/351437129

[17]   D.E. Pritchard, F. Moeckel, M.S. Villa, L.T. Housman, C.A. McCarty, and H.L. McLeod, "Strategies for integrating personalized medicine into healthcare practice", *Per. Med.,* vol. 14, no. 2, pp. 141-152, 2017.
[http://dx.doi.org/10.2217/pme-2016-0064] [PMID: 29754553]

[18]   J. de Leon, "Evidence-based medicine *versus* personalized medicine: are they enemies?", *J. Clin. Psychopharmacol.,* vol. 32, no. 2, pp. 153-164, 2012.
[http://dx.doi.org/10.1097/JCP.0b013e3182491383] [PMID: 22367661]

[19]   G. Zhang, and D.W. Nebert, "Personalized medicine: Genetic risk prediction of drug response", *Pharmacol. Ther.,* vol. 175, pp. 75-90, 2017.
[http://dx.doi.org/10.1016/j.pharmthera.2017.02.036] [PMID: 28213088]

[20]   V. Mishra, P. Chanda, M.M. Tambuwala, and A. Suttee, "Personalized medicine: An overview", *International Journal of Pharmaceutical Quality Assurance,* vol. 10, no. 2, pp. 290-294, 2019.
[http://dx.doi.org/10.25258/ijpqa.10.2.13]

[21]   J. Kinkorová, "Biobanks in the era of personalized medicine: objectives, challenges, and innovation", *EPMA J.,* vol. 7, no. 1, p. 4, 2015.
[http://dx.doi.org/10.1186/s13167-016-0053-7] [PMID: 26904153]

[22]   S. McGrath, and D. Ghersi, "Building towards precision medicine: empowering medical professionals for the next revolution", *BMC Med. Genomics,* vol. 9, no. 1, p. 23, 2016.
[http://dx.doi.org/10.1186/s12920-016-0183-8] [PMID: 27160306]

[23]   G. S. Ginsburg and H. F. Willard, "Genomic and personalized medicine: foundations and applications," *Transl. Res.,* vol. 154, no. 6, pp. 277–287, Dec. 2009.
[http://dx.doi.org/10.1016/j.trsl.2009.09.005]

[24]   K. Cornetta and C. G. Brown, "Balancing personalized medicine and personalized care," *Acad. Med.,* vol. 88, no. 3, pp. 309–313, Mar. 2013.
[http://dx.doi.org/10.1097/ACM.0b013e3182806345]

[25]   A. Zhavoronkov, and C.R. Cantor, "From personalized medicine to personalized science: uniting science and medicine for patient-driven, goal-oriented research", *Rejuvenation Res.,* vol. 16, no. 5, pp. 414-418, 2013.
[http://dx.doi.org/10.1089/rej.2013.1471] [PMID: 23889730]

[26]   Available from: http://www.future-medicine.co.uk

[27]   H. Fröhlich, R. Balling, N. Beerenwinkel, O. Kohlbacher, S Kumar, T Lengauer, M.H. Maathuis, Y. Moreau, S.A. Murphy, T.M. Przytycka, and M. Rebhan, "From hype to reality: data science enabling personalized medicine", *BMC medicine,* vol. 16, pp. 1-5, 2018.

[28]   M. Cassotta, F. Pistollato, and M. Battino, "Rheumatoid arthritis research in the 21st century: limitations of traditional models, new technologies, and opportunities for a human biology-based

approach", *Altern. Anim. Exp.,* vol. 37, no. 2, pp. 223-242, 2019.
[http://dx.doi.org/10.14573/altex.1910011] [PMID: 31854453]

[29]   A. Alyass, M. Turcotte, and D. Meyre, "From big data analysis to personalized medicine for all: challenges and opportunities", *BMC Med. Genomics,* vol. 8, no. 1, p. 33, 2015.
[http://dx.doi.org/10.1186/s12920-015-0108-y] [PMID: 26112054]

[30]   K. Offit, "Personalized medicine: new genomics, old lessons", *Hum. Genet.,* vol. 130, no. 1, pp. 3-14, 2011.
[http://dx.doi.org/10.1007/s00439-011-1028-3] [PMID: 21706342]

[31]   N.J. Schork, "Artificial intelligence and personalized medicine", *in Precision Medicine in Cancer Therapy,* vol. 178, D. Von Hoff and H. Han, Eds., Cancer Treatment and Research. Cham, Switzerland: Springer, pp. 265-283, 2019.
[http://dx.doi.org/10.1007/978-3-030-16391-4_11]

[32]   J.M. Anaya, C. Duarte-Rey, J.C. Sarmiento-Monroy, D. Bardey, J. Castiblanco, and A. Rojas-Villarraga, "Personalized medicine. Closing the gap between knowledge and clinical practice", *Autoimmun. Rev.,* vol. 15, no. 8, pp. 833-842, 2016.
[http://dx.doi.org/10.1016/j.autrev.2016.06.005] [PMID: 27302209]

[33]   C. Savoia, M. Volpe, G. Grassi, C. Borghi, E.A. Rossi, and R.M. Touyz, *Personalized medicine - A modern approach for the diagnosis and management of hypertension,* 2017.
[http://dx.doi.org/10.1042/CS20160407]

[34]   E. Drucker, and K. Krapfenbauer, *Pitfalls and limitations in translation from biomarker discovery to clinical utility in predictive and personalized medicine,* 2013.
[http://dx.doi.org/10.1186/1878-5085-4-7]

[35]   M.S. Lee, A.J. Flammer, L.O. Lerman, and A. Lerman, "Personalized medicine in cardiovascular diseases", *Korean Circ. J.,* vol. 42, no. 9, pp. 583-591, 2012.
[http://dx.doi.org/10.4070/kcj.2012.42.9.583] [PMID: 23091501]

[36]   B. Mesko, "The role of artificial intelligence in precision medicine," *Expert Rev. Precis. Med. Drug Dev.,* vol. 2, no. 5, pp. 239–241, 2017.
[http://dx.doi.org/10.1080/23808993.2017.1380516]

[37]   D. Ho, S.R. Quake, E.R.B. McCabe, W.J. Chng, E.K. Chow, X. Ding, B.D. Gelb, G.S. Ginsburg, J. Hassenstab, C.M. Ho, W.C. Mobley, G.P. Nolan, S.T. Rosen, P. Tan, Y. Yen, and A. Zarrinpar, "Enabling Technologies for Personalized and Precision Medicine", *Trends Biotechnol.,* vol. 38, no. 5, pp. 497-518, 2020.
[http://dx.doi.org/10.1016/j.tibtech.2019.12.021] [PMID: 31980301]

[38]   S. Rezayi, S. R. Niakan Kalhori, and S. Saeedi, "Effectiveness of artificial intelligence for personalized medicine in neoplasms: A systematic review", In: *Biomed Res Int* vol. 2022. , 2022.
[http://dx.doi.org/10.1155/2022/7842566]

[39]   H. Sotoudeh, O. Shafaat, J. D. Bernstock, M. D. Brooks, G. A. Elsayed, J. A. Chen, P. Szerip, G. Chagoya, F. Gessler, E. Sotoudeh, A. Shafaat, and G. K. Friedman, "Artificial intelligence in the management of glioma: Era of personalized medicine", In: *Front Oncol* vol. 9. , 2019, p. 768.
[http://dx.doi.org/10.3389/fonc.2019.00768]

[40]   J. Awwalu, A.G. Garba, A. Ghazvini, and R. Atuah, "Artificial Intelligence in Personalized Medicine Application of AI Algorithms in Solving Personalized Medicine Problems", *International Journal of Computer Theory and Engineering,* vol. 7, no. 6, pp. 439-443, 2015.
[http://dx.doi.org/10.7763/IJCTE.2015.V7.999]

[41]   C. Caudai, A. Galizia, F. Geraci, L. Le Pera, V. Morea, E. Salerno, A. Via, and T. Colombo, "AI applications in functional genomics", *Comput. Struct. Biotechnol. J.,* vol. 19, pp. 5762-5790, 2021.
[http://dx.doi.org/10.1016/j.csbj.2021.10.009] [PMID: 34765093]

[42]   J. Lipkova, R.J. Chen, B. Chen, M.Y. Lu, M. Barbieri, D. Shao, A.J. Vaidya, C. Chen, L. Zhuang,

D.F.K. Williamson, M. Shaban, T.Y. Chen, and F. Mahmood, "Artificial intelligence for multimodal data integration in oncology", *Cancer Cell,* vol. 40, no. 10, pp. 1095-1110, 2022.
[http://dx.doi.org/10.1016/j.ccell.2022.09.012] [PMID: 36220072]

[43]   J.C. Restrepo, D. Dueñas, Z. Corredor, and Y. Liscano, "Advances in Genomic Data and Biomarkers: Revolutionizing NSCLC Diagnosis and Treatment", *Cancers (Basel),* vol. 15, no. 13, p. 3474, 2023.
[http://dx.doi.org/10.3390/cancers15133474] [PMID: 37444584]

[44]   B. Louie, P. Mork, F. Martin-Sanchez, A. Halevy, and P. Tarczy-Hornoch, "Data integration and genomic medicine", *J. Biomed. Inform.,* vol. 40, no. 1, pp. 5-16, 2007.
[http://dx.doi.org/10.1016/j.jbi.2006.02.007] [PMID: 16574494]

[45]   G. Abraham, and M. Inouye, "Genomic risk prediction of complex human disease and its clinical application", *Curr. Opin. Genet. Dev.,* vol. 33, pp. 10-16, 2015.
[http://dx.doi.org/10.1016/j.gde.2015.06.005] [PMID: 26210231]

[46]   L. Jostins, and J.C. Barrett, "Genetic risk prediction in complex disease", *Hum. Mol. Genet.,* vol. 20, no. R2, pp. R182-R188, 2011.
[http://dx.doi.org/10.1093/hmg/ddr378] [PMID: 21873261]

[47]   D. Prada-Gracia, S. Huerta-Yépez, and L.M. Moreno-Vargas, "Aplicación de métodos computacionales para el descubrimiento, diseño y optimización de fármacos contra el cáncer", *Bol. Méd. Hosp. Infant. México,* vol. 73, no. 6, pp. 411-423, 2016.
[http://dx.doi.org/10.1016/j.bmhimx.2016.10.006] [PMID: 29421286]

[48]   Graham A. Showell and John S. Mills, "The challenge for medicinal chemists," 2003. [Online]. Available: http://www.merck.com Available from: http://www.merck.com

[49]   L. K. Vestergaard, D. N. P. Oliveira, C. K. Høgdall, and E. V. Høgdall, "Next generation sequencing technology in the clinic and its challenges," *Cancers (Basel)*, vol. 13, no. 8, p. 1751, Apr. 2021.

[50]   L.A. Garraway, J. Verweij, and K.V. Ballman, "Precision oncology: an overview", *J. Clin. Oncol.,* vol. 31, no. 15, pp. 1803-1805, 2013.
[http://dx.doi.org/10.1200/JCO.2013.49.4799] [PMID: 23589545]

[51]   D. Sjödin, V. Parida, M. Palmié, and J. Wincent, "How AI capabilities enable business model innovation: Scaling AI through co-evolutionary processes and feedback loops", *J. Bus. Res.,* vol. 134, pp. 574-587, 2021.
[http://dx.doi.org/10.1016/j.jbusres.2021.05.009]

[52]   J. Bosch, H. H. Olsson, and I. Crnkovic, "It takes three to tango: Requirement, outcome/data, and AI-driven development," In: *Proc. 1st Int. Workshop on Software-Intensive Business: Start-Ups, Ecosystems and Platforms (SiBW 2018)*, Espoo: Finland, 2018, vol. 2305, pp. 177–192.

[53]   T. Fountaine, B. McCarthy, and T. Saleh, "Building the AI-powered organization: Technology isn't the biggest challenge. Culture is," *Harv. Bus. Rev.*, vol. 96, no. 4, pp. 62–73, 2019.

[54]   Ullah H, Manickam S, Obaidat M, Laghari SU, Uddin M. "Exploring the potential of metaverse technology in healthcare: Applications, challenges, and future directions". *IEEE Access.* 2023 Jun 15;11:69686-707.

[55]   J.C. Quiroz, L. Laranjo, A.B. Kocaballi, S. Berkovsky, D. Rezazadegan, and E. Coiera, "Challenges of developing a digital scribe to reduce clinical documentation burden", *NPJ Digit. Med.,* vol. 2, no. 1, p. 114, 2019.
[http://dx.doi.org/10.1038/s41746-019-0190-1] [PMID: 31799422]

[56]   V. Koesmahargyo, A. Abbas, L. Zhang, L. Guan, S. Feng, V. Yadav, and I.R. Galatzer-Levy, "Accuracy of machine learning-based prediction of medication adherence in clinical research", *Psychiatry Res.,* vol. 294, p. 113558, 2020.
[http://dx.doi.org/10.1016/j.psychres.2020.113558] [PMID: 33242836]

[57]   P. Boehme, P. Wienand, M. Herrmann, H. Truebel, and T. Mondritzki, "New digital adherence devices could prevent millions of strokes from atrial fibrillation by the end of the next century", *Med.*

Hypotheses, vol. 108, pp. 46-50, 2017.
[http://dx.doi.org/10.1016/j.mehy.2017.07.034] [PMID: 29055399]

[58]   D. Roy, Z. Zhu, L. Guan, S. Feng, K. Daniels, and M. Sand, "AI-based adherence prediction for patients: Leveraging a mobile application to improve clinical trials", *J Clin Psychopharmacol,* vol. 43, no. 4, pp. 456-463, 2023.
[http://dx.doi.org/10.1017/S1092852923001438]

[59]   J. Hanley, J. Ure, C. Pagliari, A. Sheikh, and B. Mckinstry, "Experiences of patients and professionals participating in the HITS home blood pressure telemonitoring trial: a qualitative study", *BMJ Open,* vol. 3, no. 5, p. e002671, 2013.
[http://dx.doi.org/10.1136/bmjopen-2013-002671]

[60]   C. Hudon, M.C. Chouinard, M. Lambert, F. Diadiou, D. Bouliane, and J. Beaudin, "Key factors of case management interventions for frequent users of healthcare services: a thematic analysis review", *BMJ Open,* vol. 7, no. 10, p. e017762, 2017.
[http://dx.doi.org/10.1136/bmjopen-2017-017762] [PMID: 29061623]

[61]   M. Orebaugh, "Instigating and Influencing Patient Engagement: A Hospital Library's Contributions to Patient Health and Organizational Success", *J. Hosp. Librariansh.,* vol. 14, no. 2, pp. 109-119, 2014.
[http://dx.doi.org/10.1080/15323269.2014.888511]

[62]   E. Kim, S.M. Rubinstein, K.T. Nead, A.P. Wojcieszynski, P.E. Gabriel, and J.L. Warner, "The Evolving Use of Electronic Health Records (EHR) for Research", *Semin. Radiat. Oncol.,* vol. 29, no. 4, pp. 354-361, 2019.
[http://dx.doi.org/10.1016/j.semradonc.2019.05.010] [PMID: 31472738]

[63]   R. S. Lunetta, R. G. Congalton, L. K. Fenstermaker, J. R. Jensen, K. C. McGwire, and L. R. Tinney, "Remote sensing and geographic information system data integration: error sources and research issues", *Photogramm Eng Remote Sens,* vol. 57, no. 6, pp. 677-687, 1991. . Available from: https://www.asprs.org/wp-content/uploads/pers/1991journal/jun/1991_jun_677-687.pdf

[64]   A. Ailamaki, Ed., Advances in Database Technology: EDBT 2011: 14th International Conference on Extending Database Technology, Uppsala, Sweden, March 22–24, 2011: *Proceedings*, New York, NY, USA: Association for Computing Machinery, 2011. [Online]
[http://dx.doi.org/10.1145/1951365]

[65]   A. Doan, P. Domingos, and A. Levy, "Learning source descriptions for data integration", *Proc Int Workshop WebDB,* Dallas, TX, USA, pp. 81-86, 2000. Available from: https://homes.cs.washington.edu/~pedrod/papers/webdb00.pdf

[66]   S. Ajami, and R. ArabChadegani, "Barriers to implement Electronic Health Records (EHRs)", *Mater. Sociomed.,* vol. 25, no. 3, pp. 213-215, 2013.
[http://dx.doi.org/10.5455/msm.2013.25.213-215] [PMID: 24167440]

[67]   M. Lenzerini, "Data integration: a theoretical perspective," In: *Proc. 21st ACM SIGMOD-SIGAC--SIGART Symp. Principles of Database Systems (PODS '02)*, Madison, WI, USA, 2002, pp. 233–246.
[http://dx.doi.org/10.1145/543613.543644]

[68]   N.M. Lorenzi, A. Kouroubali, D.E. Detmer, and M. Bloomrosen, "How to successfully select and implement electronic health records (EHR) in small ambulatory practice settings", *BMC Med. Inform. Decis. Mak.,* vol. 9, no. 1, p. 15, 2009.
[http://dx.doi.org/10.1186/1472-6947-9-15] [PMID: 19236705]

[69]   H. E. Williams, and J. Zobel, "Indexing and retrieval for genomic databases", *IEEE Trans Knowl Data Eng,* vol. 14, no. 1, pp. 63-78, 2002.
[http://dx.doi.org/10.1109/69.979973]

[70]   B.M. Knoppers, M.H. Abdul-Rahman, and K. Bédard, "Genomic Databases and International Collaboration", *Kings Law J.,* vol. 18, no. 2, pp. 291-311, 2007.
[http://dx.doi.org/10.1080/09615768.2007.11427678]

[71]   B.D. Solomon, A.D. Nguyen, K.A. Bear, and T.G. Wolfsberg, "Clinical genomic database", *Proc. Natl. Acad. Sci. USA,* vol. 110, no. 24, pp. 9851-9855, 2013.
[http://dx.doi.org/10.1073/pnas.1302575110] [PMID: 23696674]

[72]   M. Fernandez, M. Villasana, and D. Streja, "The minimal model of glucose disappearance in type I diabetes", *Studies in Computational Intelligence,* vol. 224, pp. 295-315, 2009.
[http://dx.doi.org/10.1007/978-3-642-02193-0_13]

[73]   C.J. Bult, J.A. Blake, C.L. Smith, J.A. Kadin, J.E. Richardson, A. Anagnostopoulos, R. Asabor, R.M. Baldarelli, J.S. Beal, S.M. Bello, O. Blodgett, N.E. Butler, K.R. Christie, L.E. Corbani, J. Creelman, M.E. Dolan, H.J. Drabkin, S.L. Giannatto, P. Hale, D.P. Hill, M. Law, A. Mendoza, M. McAndrews, D. Miers, H. Motenko, L. Ni, H. Onda, M. Perry, J.M. Recla, B. Richards-Smith, D. Sitnikov, M. Tomczuk, G. Tonorio, L. Wilming, and Y. Zhu, "Mouse Genome Database (MGD) 2019", *Nucleic Acids Res.,* vol. 47, no. D1, pp. D801-D806, 2019.
[http://dx.doi.org/10.1093/nar/gky1056] [PMID: 30407599]

[74]   M.D. Gale, and K.M. Devos, *32, j. L. Bennetzen, personal communication. 33. K. M. Devos, unpublished data,* 1971. Available from: www.sciencernag.org

[75]   P.D. Karp, M. Riley, M. Saier, I.T. Paulsen, S.M. Paley, and A. Pellegrini-Toole, *The EcoCyc and MetaCyc databases,* 2000. Available from: http://ecocyc.PangeaSystems.com:1555/ECOLI/
[http://dx.doi.org/10.1093/nar/28.1.56]

[76]   A. Shehab, A. Ismail, L. Osman, M. Elhoseny, and I.M. El-Henawy, *"Quantified self-using IoT wearable devices,"* in *Advances in Intelligent Systems and Computing.* Springer Verlag, 2018, pp. 820-831.
[http://dx.doi.org/10.1007/978-3-319-64861-3_77]

[77]   T.G. Stavropoulos, A. Papastergiou, L. Mpaltadoros, S. Nikolopoulos, and I. Kompatsiaris, "Iot wearable sensors and devices in elderly care: A literature review", *Sensors (Basel),* vol. 20, no. 10, p. 2826, 2020.
[http://dx.doi.org/10.3390/s20102826] [PMID: 32429331]

[78]   S. Mukhopadhyay, N. Suryadevara, and A. Nag, "Wearable sensors and systems in the IoT", *Sensors (Basel),* vol. 21, no. 23, p. 7880, 2021.
[http://dx.doi.org/10.3390/s21237880] [PMID: 34883879]

[79]   R.S. Bisht, S. Jain, and N. Tewari, "Study of Wearable IoT devices in 2021: Analysis Future Prospects", *Proceedings of 2021 2nd International Conference on Intelligent Engineering and Management, ICIEM 2021,* Institute of Electrical and Electronics Engineers Inc., pp. 577-581, 2021.
[http://dx.doi.org/10.1109/ICIEM51511.2021.9445334]

[80]   N. Surantha, and P. Atmaja, *David, and M. Wicaksono, "A Review of Wearable Internet-of-Things Device for Healthcare,"* in *Procedia Computer Science.* Elsevier B.V., 2021, pp. 939-943.
[http://dx.doi.org/10.1016/j.procs.2021.01.083]

[81]   P. Narindrarangkura, M.S. Kim, and S.A. Boren, "A Scoping Review of Artificial Intelligence Algorithms in Clinical Decision Support Systems for Internal Medicine Subspecialties", *ACI Open,* vol. 5, no. 2, pp. e67-e79, 2021.
[http://dx.doi.org/10.1055/s-0041-1735470]

[82]   A. Mosavi, P. Ozturk, and K. Chau, "Flood prediction using machine learning models: Literature review", *Water,* vol. 10, no. 11, p. 1536, 2018.
[http://dx.doi.org/10.3390/w10111536]

[83]   C. Song, T. Ristenpart, and V. Shmatikov, "Machine learning models that remember too much", *Proceedings of the ACM Conference on Computer and Communications Security,* Association for Computing Machinery, pp. 587-601, 2017.
[http://dx.doi.org/10.1145/3133956.3134077]

[84]   E. Sullivan, "Understanding from machine learning models", *Br J Philos Sci,* vol. 73, no. 1, pp. 109-

133, 2022.
[http://dx.doi.org/10.1093/bjps/axz035]

[85] J.T. Kim, "Application of Machine and Deep Learning Algorithms in Intelligent Clinical Decision Support Systems in Healthcare", *J. Health Med. Inform.,* vol. 9, no. 5, 2018.
[http://dx.doi.org/10.4172/2157-7420.1000321]

[86] R. Egger, and E. Gokce, *"Natural Language Processing (NLP): An Introduction: Making Sense of Textual Data,"* in *Tourism on the Verge, vol. Part F1051.* Springer Nature, 2022, pp. 307-334.
[http://dx.doi.org/10.1007/978-3-030-88389-8_15]

[87] N. van Berkel, M. Bellio, M.B. Skov, and A. Blandford, "Measurements, Algorithms, and Presentations of Reality: Framing Interactions with AI-Enabled Decision Support", *ACM Trans. Comput. Hum. Interact.,* vol. 30, no. 2, pp. 1-33, 2023.
[http://dx.doi.org/10.1145/3571815]

[88] F. S. Gharehchopogh, and Z. A. Khalifelu, "Analysis and evaluation of unstructured data: text mining versus natural language processing", *Proc 5th Int Conf Appl Inf Commun Technol (AICT),* Baku, Azerbaijan, pp. 1-4, 2011.
[http://dx.doi.org/10.1109/ICAICT.2011.6111017]

[89] A. Ranerup, L. Norén, and C. Sparud-Lundin, "Decision support systems for choosing a primary health care provider in Sweden", *Patient Educ. Couns.,* vol. 86, no. 3, pp. 342-347, 2012.
[http://dx.doi.org/10.1016/j.pec.2011.06.013] [PMID: 21778027]

[90] P. D. Clayton and G. Hripcsak, "Decision support in healthcare," *Int. J. Bio-Med. Comput.,* vol. 39, no. 1, pp. 59–66, Apr. 1995.
[http://dx.doi.org/10.1016/0020-7101(94)01080-K]

[91] J.F. Stichler, and L.R. Pelletier, "Psychometric testing of a patient empowerment, engagement, and activation survey", *J. Nurs. Care Qual.,* vol. 35, no. 4, pp. E49-E57, 2020.
[http://dx.doi.org/10.1097/NCQ.0000000000000452] [PMID: 31821184]

[92] N. Wickramasekera, S.K. Taylor, E. Lumley, T. Gray, E. Wilson, and S. Radley, "Can electronic assessment tools improve the process of shared decision-making? A systematic review", *HIM J.,* 2020.
[http://dx.doi.org/10.1177/1833358320954385] [PMID: 33016126]

[93] N. Bouniols, B. Leclère, and L. Moret, "Evaluating the quality of shared decision making during the patient-carer encounter: a systematic review of tools", *BMC Res. Notes,* vol. 9, no. 1, p. 382, 2016.
[http://dx.doi.org/10.1186/s13104-016-2164-6] [PMID: 27485434]

[94] I. Spronk, J.S. Burgers, F.G. Schellevis, L.M. van Vliet, and J.C. Korevaar, "The availability and effectiveness of tools supporting shared decision making in metastatic breast cancer care: a review", *BMC Palliat. Care,* vol. 17, no. 1, p. 74, 2018.
[http://dx.doi.org/10.1186/s12904-018-0330-4] [PMID: 29747628]

[95] K.R. Sepucha, M. Breslin, C. Graffeo, C.R. Carpenter, and E.P. Hess, "State of the Science: Tools and Measurement for Shared Decision Making", *Acad. Emerg. Med.,* vol. 23, no. 12, pp. 1325-1331, 2016.
[http://dx.doi.org/10.1111/acem.13071] [PMID: 27770488]

[96] A.F. Heen, P.O. Vandvik, L. Brandt, V.M. Montori, L. Lytvyn, G. Guyatt, C. Quinlan, and T. Agoritsas, "A framework for practical issues was developed to inform shared decision-making tools and clinical guidelines", *J. Clin. Epidemiol.,* vol. 129, pp. 104-113, 2021.
[http://dx.doi.org/10.1016/j.jclinepi.2020.10.002] [PMID: 33049326]

[97] C.A. Austin, D. Mohottige, R.L. Sudore, A.K. Smith, and L.C. Hanson, "Tools to promote shared decision making in serious illness: A systematic review", *JAMA Intern. Med.,* vol. 175, no. 7, pp. 1213-1221, 2015.
[http://dx.doi.org/10.1001/jamainternmed.2015.1679] [PMID: 25985438]

[98] D.D. Matlock, and E.S. Spatz, "Design and testing of tools for shared decision making", *Circ. Cardiovasc. Qual. Outcomes,* vol. 7, no. 3, pp. 487-492, 2014.

[http://dx.doi.org/10.1161/CIRCOUTCOMES.113.000289] [PMID: 24714602]

[99]   J.B. Schulz, P. Dubrowski, E. Blomain, L. Million, Y. Qian, C. Marquez, and A.S. Yu, "An Affordable Platform for Virtual Reality–Based Patient Education in Radiation Therapy", *Pract. Radiat. Oncol.,* vol. 13, no. 6, pp. e475-e483, 2023.
[http://dx.doi.org/10.1016/j.prro.2023.06.008] [PMID: 37482182]

[100]   K. Baxter, C. Glendinning, and S. Clarke, "Making informed choices in social care: the importance of accessible information", *Health Soc. Care Community,* vol. 16, no. 2, pp. 197-207, 2008.
[http://dx.doi.org/10.1111/j.1365-2524.2007.00742.x] [PMID: 18290984]

[101]   Y. Deldjoo, M. Schedl, P. Cremonesi, and G. Pasi, "Recommender Systems Leveraging Multimedia Content", *ACM Comput. Surv.,* vol. 53, no. 5, pp. 1-38, 2021.
[http://dx.doi.org/10.1145/3407190]

[102]   A. Summerville, M. Guzdial, M. Mateas, and M. Riedl, "Learning Player Tailored Content From Observation: Platformer Level Generation from Video Traces using LSTMs," In: *Proc. Workshops of the Twelfth AAAI Conf. Artif. Intell. Interact. Digit. Entertain.,* vol. 12, no. 2, 2016.

[103]   M. P. Kumar, B. Packer, and D. Koller, "Self-paced learning for latent variable models", *Adv Neural Inf Process Syst,* vol. 23, Vancouver, Canada, pp. 1189-1197, 2010. Available from: https://papers.nips.cc/paper/3923-self-paced-learning-for-latent-variable-models

[104]   M. Pulvirenti, J. McMillan, and S. Lawn, "Empowerment, patient centred care and self-management", *Health Expect.,* vol. 17, no. 3, pp. 303-310, 2014.
[http://dx.doi.org/10.1111/j.1369-7625.2011.00757.x] [PMID: 22212306]

[105]   I. Sheiman, and V. Shevsky, "Concentration of health care providers: does it contribute to integration of service delivery?", *Risk Manag. Healthc. Policy,* vol. 12, pp. 153-166, 2019.
[http://dx.doi.org/10.2147/RMHP.S205905] [PMID: 31496851]

[106]   A.-M. Séguin and G. Divay, Urban Poverty: Fostering Sustainable and Supportive Communities. Ottawa, ON, Canada: Canadian Policy Research Networks, Dec. 2002.

[107]   A.K. Ghosh, "On the challenges of using evidence-based information: The role of clinical uncertainty", *J. Lab. Clin. Med.,* vol. 144, no. 2, pp. 60-64, 2004.
[http://dx.doi.org/10.1016/j.lab.2004.05.013] [PMID: 15322499]

[108]   D.E. Iakovakis, F.A. Papadopoulou, and L.J. Hadjileontiadis, "Fuzzy logic-based risk of fall estimation using smartwatch data as a means to form an assistive feedback mechanism in everyday living activities", *Healthc. Technol. Lett.,* vol. 3, no. 4, pp. 263-268, 2016.
[http://dx.doi.org/10.1049/htl.2016.0064] [PMID: 28008361]

[109]   S. F. Gray, I. C. Spencer, P. G. Spry, S. T. Brookes, I. A. Baker, T. J. Peters, J. M. Sparrow, and D. L. Easty, "The Bristol shared care glaucoma study—validity of measurements and patient satisfaction", *J Public Health Med,* vol. 19, 1997no. 4, pp. 431-436.
[http://dx.doi.org/10.1093/oxfordjournals.pubmed.a024673]

[110]   C. G. Madamombe, "Automatic classification of complaints and/or suggestions using a mobile-based suggestion box system", *Int J Comput Sci Eng,* vol. 7, no. 3, pp. 75-83, 2018. Available from: https://www.ijcse.net/docs/IJCSE18-07-03-009.pdf

[111]   T. Hatziapostolou, and I. Paraskakis, "Enhancing the Impact of Formative Feedback on Student Learning through an Online Feedback System", *Electron. J. e-Learn.,* vol. 8, pp. 111-122, 2010. [Online]. [. Available: www.ejel.org].

[112]   A.E. Sharma, R. Willard-Grace, A. Willis, O. Zieve, K. Dubé, C. Parker, and M.B. Potter, "'How can we talk about patient-centered care without patients at the table?' Lessons learned from patient advisory councils", *J. Am. Board Fam. Med.,* vol. 29, no. 6, pp. 775-784, 2016.
[http://dx.doi.org/10.3122/jabfm.2016.06.150380] [PMID: 28076261]

[113]   F. Mazanderani, B. O'Neill, and J. Powell, ""People power" or "pester power"? YouTube as a forum for the generation of evidence and patient advocacy", *Patient Educ. Couns.,* vol. 93, no. 3, pp. 420-

425, 2013.
[http://dx.doi.org/10.1016/j.pec.2013.06.006] [PMID: 23830239]

[114]   L.J. Wang, B Casto, J.Y. Luh, and S.J. Wang, "Virtual reality-based education for patients undergoing radiation therapy", *Journal of Cancer Education,* vol. 37, no. 3, pp. 694-700, 2022.

[115]   S. Harper, "Economic and social implications of aging societies", *Science,* vol. 346, no. 6209, pp. 587-591, 2014.
[http://dx.doi.org/10.1126/science.1254405] [PMID: 25359967]

[116]   J.T. King Jr, J. Tsevat, J.R. Lave, and M.S. Roberts, "Willingness to pay for a quality-adjusted life year: implications for societal health care resource allocation", *Med. Decis. Making,* vol. 25, no. 6, pp. 667-677, 2005.
[http://dx.doi.org/10.1177/0272989X05282640] [PMID: 16282217]

[117]   E. Faulkner, L. Annemans, L. Garrison, M. Helfand, A.P. Holtorf, J. Hornberger, D. Hughes, T. Li, D. Malone, K. Payne, U. Siebert, A. Towse, D. Veenstra, and J. Watkins, "Challenges in the development and reimbursement of personalized medicine-payer and manufacturer perspectives and implications for health economics and outcomes research: a report of the ISPOR personalized medicine special interest group", *Value Health,* vol. 15, no. 8, pp. 1162-1171, 2012.
[http://dx.doi.org/10.1016/j.jval.2012.05.006] [PMID: 23244820]

[118]   I. Akhmetov, and R.V. Bubnov, "Assessing value of innovative molecular diagnostic tests in the concept of predictive, preventive, and personalized medicine", *EPMA J.,* vol. 6, no. 1, p. 19, 2015.
[http://dx.doi.org/10.1186/s13167-015-0041-3] [PMID: 26425215]

[119]   M.E. Porter, S. Larsson, and T.H. Lee, "Standardizing Patient Outcomes Measurement", *N. Engl. J. Med.,* vol. 374, no. 6, pp. 504-506, 2016.
[http://dx.doi.org/10.1056/NEJMp1511701] [PMID: 26863351]

[120]   A. Dang, "Real-World Evidence: A Primer", *Pharmaceut. Med.,* vol. 37, no. 1, pp. 25-36, 2023.
[http://dx.doi.org/10.1007/s40290-022-00456-6] [PMID: 36604368]

[121]   S. Cruz Rivera, D.G. Kyte, O.L. Aiyegbusi, T.J. Keeley, and M.J. Calvert, "Assessing the impact of healthcare research: A systematic review of methodological frameworks", *PLoS Med.,* vol. 14, no. 8, p. e1002370, 2017.
[http://dx.doi.org/10.1371/journal.pmed.1002370] [PMID: 28792957]

[122]   R.J. Piscotty Jr, B. Kalisch, and A. Gracey-Thomas, "Impact of Healthcare Information Technology on Nursing Practice", *J. Nurs. Scholarsh.,* vol. 47, no. 4, pp. 287-293, 2015.
[http://dx.doi.org/10.1111/jnu.12138] [PMID: 25950795]

[123]   N.G. Chamba, K.C. Byashalira, D.L. Christensen, K.L. Ramaiya, E.P. Kapyolo, P.J. Shayo, T. Lillebaek, N.E. Ntinginya, B.T. Mmbaga, I.C. Bygbjerg, S.G. Mpagama, and R.N. Manongi, "Experiences and perceptions of participants on the pathway towards clinical management of dual tuberculosis and diabetes mellitus in Tanzania", *Glob. Health Action,* vol. 15, no. 1, p. 2143044, 2022.
[http://dx.doi.org/10.1080/16549716.2022.2143044] [PMID: 36441076]

[124]   D. King and M. Knapp, "Patterns of, and factors associated with, atypical and typical antipsychotic prescribing by general practitioners in the UK during the 1990s," *J. Ment. Health,* vol. 15, no. 3, pp. 269–278, 2006.

[125]   R. Wesche, S.E. Claxton, E.S. Lefkowitz, and M.H.M. van Dulmen, "Evaluations and Future Plans After Casual Sexual Experiences: Differences Across Partner Type", *J. Sex Res.,* vol. 55, no. 9, pp. 1180-1191, 2018.
[http://dx.doi.org/10.1080/00224499.2017.1298714] [PMID: 28339298]

[126]   S. Erikainen, and S. Chan, "Contested futures: envisioning "Personalized," "Stratified," and "Precision" medicine", *New Genet. Soc.,* vol. 38, no. 3, pp. 308-330, 2019.
[http://dx.doi.org/10.1080/14636778.2019.1637720] [PMID: 31708685]

[127]   K.B. Johnson, W.Q. Wei, D. Weeraratne, M.E. Frisse, K. Misulis, K. Rhee, J. Zhao, and J.L.

Snowdon, "Precision Medicine, AI, and the Future of Personalized Health Care", *Clin. Transl. Sci.,* vol. 14, no. 1, pp. 86-93, 2021.
[http://dx.doi.org/10.1111/cts.12884] [PMID: 32961010]

[128] M. Raparthi, "AI-driven decision support systems for precision medicine: Examining the development and implementation of AI-driven decision support systems in precision medicine", *J Artif Intell Res,* vol. 1, no. 1, pp. 11-20, 2021. Available from: https://thesciencebrigade.com/JAIR/article/view/126

CHAPTER 8

Real-Time Tracking with IoT Sensors Revolutionizing Healthcare System

Shivkanya Fuloria[1], Akhil Sharma[2], Akanksha Sharma[2], B. Rama Mohana Reddy[3] and Shaweta Sharma[4,*]

[1] *Department of Pharmaceutical Chemistry, Faculty of Pharmacy, AIMST University Semeling Campus, Bedong, Kedah, Malaysia*

[2] *R.J. College of Pharmacy, Raipur, Gharbara, Tappal, Khair, Uttar Pradesh, India*

[3] *Department of Civil Engineering, Aditya University, Surampalem, India*

[4] *School of Medical and Allied Sciences, Galgotias University Plot No. 2, Yamuna Expy, Opposite Buddha International Circuit, Sector 17A, Greater Noida, Uttar Pradesh, India*

Abstract: A transformative revolution has been triggered by the inclusion of Internet of Things (IoT) sensors in healthcare's real-time tracking capabilities. Recent advancements in miniaturization and low-power designs, wireless connectivity, and sensor fusion (integration of information from multiple sensors) continue to have a profound impact on the monitoring of health. Intelligent embeddability and superior sensing capabilities facilitate seamless patient data tracking, and strong security protects data against breaches. The role of IoT sensors in healthcare is to connect devices, such as biometric and temperature sensors or imaging and environmental sensors. IoT sensors are used in multiple applications such as fitness and vital signs tracking information, and patient care in smart healthcare facilities. Such technologies enable IoT-based medication adherence systems so that patients follow prescribed treatments, thus improving outcomes and reducing the possibility of hospital readmissions. Compared to regular monitoring devices, IoT sensors provide continuous data capture, increased accuracy, improved patient mobility and personalized healthcare solutions. Healthcare IoT adoption faces challenges in data privacy, regulation, and the complexity of technical integration of healthcare IoT in existing infrastructures. Ethical considerations must also be addressed to ensure equitable access and unbiased use of IoT technology. However, despite these obstacles, the future of IoT-based healthcare technologies remains an attractive proposition with continuous technology evolution likely to improve the quality of care, optimal resource allocation, and decision-making in real-time. This chapter explores the evolution of healthcare monitoring through IoT sensors, detailing their technological mechanisms, applications, benefits, and the potential for transforming the healthcare landscape.

---

* **Corresponding author Shaweta Sharma:** School of Medical and Allied Sciences, Galgotias University Plot No. 2, Yamuna Expy, Opposite Buddha International Circuit, Sector 17A, Greater Noida, Uttar Pradesh, India; E-mail: shawetasharma@galgotiasuniversity.edu.in

Keywords: Abnormality, Blood pressure, Disease, Heart rate, Healthcare, Implant, Internet of things, Patient, Real-time, Remote, Sensor, Technology, Wearable.

INTRODUCTION

The Internet of Things (IoT) is a system where devices are connected to each other, and they can communicate among themselves. It is a huge step towards the creation of smart environments. In healthcare, IoT has many implications, like enabling real-time health monitoring and data access which eventually results in better patient health experience and improved healthcare operations [1, 2].

Simultaneous report and monitoring, data collection and analysis, and end-to-end connection can be improved by IoT in healthcare. Examples of medical devices that are based on IoT include remote patient monitoring, smart inhalers, swallowable sensors, mood tracking, sugar level tracking, heart rate watching; smart contact lenses; robot surgery, and Parkinson's disease identification [3, 4].

Real-time health monitoring, data access, and enhanced healthcare operations are some of the major ways in which IoT could transform patient care. Remote monitoring *via* IoT sensor technologies can help improve medication management and enhance operational efficiency. However, ethical guidelines must be put in place by healthcare providers and policymakers to deal with challenges such as cost, usability, and data security so that this potential can be fully utilized [5, 6].

Real-time healthcare monitoring is a concept that requires the use of IoT devices like wearables and other wirelessly connected devices in order to collect patient health data constantly. The information can range from physical conditions such as blood pressure, heartbeat rate, and glucose levels as well as sleeping patterns. In summary, this type of monitoring enables medical staff to monitor patients' health status for quick response to any abnormality detected that may lead to better treatment outcomes and lower healthcare costs in the end [7, 8].

The idea behind real-time healthcare monitoring is that it uses Health Monitoring Systems (HMS) that take physiological measurements using biosensors, get important attributes and measures from the output, and analyze records right away. Therefore, the main intent of HMSs is to observe the patient's health condition and identify abnormalities timely in advance leading to an intervention beforehand and enhancing patient welfare. This makes IoT-based healthcare monitoring systems very useful because they allow secure, real-time remote patient monitoring, thereby making it easy for doctors to obtain real-time data [9, 10].

These systems can monitor various parameters such as heart rate, blood pressure, blood glucose levels, and sleep patterns so that real-time data can be analyzed for informed patient care decision-making by health workers. Smart real-time healthcare monitoring and tracking systems using GSM and GPS technologies can provide an effective system model that tracks, traces, and monitors patient vital readings in order to offer efficient healthcare services [11].

Such systems can facilitate real-time monitoring of the health status of patients by healthcare providers, early detection of anomalies, and intervention in a timely manner, thus improving patient outcomes while reducing healthcare costs. Real-time sickness detection and constant monitoring of patients' health state are some of the benefits associated with Remote Patient Monitoring Systems (RPMS). Quick medical attention can be provided by the RPMS in case death that would occur untimely is detected making its performance in treatment better. RPMS also assists in the management of chronic diseases, enhancement of medicine administration as well as minimizing rates at which patients revisit hospitals [12].

These devices, such as wearable and connected medical devices use IoT to collect real-time health data, which can inform timely interventions in chronic diseases like COPD, asthma, or heart failure. By using IoT technology, healthcare providers will develop a more effective, patient-focused, and integrated healthcare system [13].

Additionally, IoT makes it possible to collect and analyze data in real time, thus giving medical service providers a wide range of information on the condition of patients. The approach based on this data can be the basis for personalized care plans and timely interventions. Besides, having more information will enable physicians and other healthcare professionals to get a better understanding of patients' behavior, preferences and patterns hence making care given to patients more individual [14].

One other significant advantage of IoT in healthcare is that it fosters smoother workflows and operational efficiency. For instance, there are smart beds and asset tracking systems linked through the internet that will optimize resource utilization, minimize errors, and automatically perform routine duties. This leads to savings on costs by healthcare facilities, as well as improved output by the staff and more efficient delivery of health services [15].

Preventive and predictive healthcare is also facilitated by IoT through continuous monitoring of patient data, recognizing early warning signs, and enabling proactive interventions for better healthcare decision-making. Additionally, medication management and adherence are improved through IoT-enabled smart pill bottle dispensers, medication tracking systems, and wearable reminders [16].

The IoT also augments telehealth and telemedicine services. In fact, remote consultations, virtual monitoring, and telehealth interventions are empowered by IoT-enabled RPM devices and wearables. Besides, especially in rural or underserved places, it enables patients to connect with healthcare providers thus allowing them access to important care when needed. This reduces the pressure on traditional health facilities [17].

The healthcare facility has the potential to be revolutionized with IoT sensing technologies that enable real-time data sharing, remote patient monitoring, and individualized care plans. By using the power of IoT, providers can establish a more effective, patient-oriented, and connected healthcare system that improves patient outcomes as well as enhances the general quality of care. Implementing and maintaining IoT infrastructure in healthcare facilities can be expensive; but, the usability of IoT devices is one major factor that has a direct impact on their adoption and effectiveness. Despite this, the potential of IoT in healthcare is huge, and constant progressions and innovations being made in IoT technology have created a prospect for revolutionizing healthcare delivery systems with better patient outcomes and improved quality of care [18, 19].

EVOLUTION OF HEALTHCARE MONITORING

The historical background and emergence of the IoT in healthcare can be traced back to the convergence of various technological advancements and healthcare needs over the past few decades, which is summarized in Table **1.**

Technological Advancements Driving IoT Sensor Development

Technological advancements have been pivotal in driving the development of IoT sensor technologies, enabling them to become smaller, more efficient, and more versatile. Technological advancements driving IoT sensor development are discussed below.

Miniaturization of Components

It is essential to reduce the dimensions of electronic parts, such as microprocessors, memory modules, and the sensors themselves. This trend leads to sensors that can be built into smaller devices as well as working with many other objects and places [27].

Low-Power Design

IoT sensors require energy efficiency especially those that operate in far-flung areas and remote locations. With improvements in low-power design techniques like using ultra-low-power microcontrollers and optimizing sensor operation modes, sensors' battery life has increased and the need for frequent replacement of batteries has decreased [28].

Table 1. Evolution of healthcare monitoring.

Milestone	Description
Early Development of IoT Concepts	The emergence of the concept of connecting physical devices to the Internet was first seen towards the end of the 20th century. The establishment of technologies like RFID (Radio Frequency Identification) formed the basis [20, 21].
Advancements in Sensor Technology	- Smaller sensor technology and low power consumption, high-performance sensors for medicine. Sensors that can measure human body functions including heart rate, blood pressure, and temperature [22].
Rise of Wearable Devices	- The popularity of consumer wearables has led to an increased interest in applying similar techniques to medicine by using remote patient monitoring [23].
Advancements in Connectivity	- Development of wireless technologies such as Bluetooth, Wi-Fi, and cellular networks. Seamless data transmission and remote monitoring are enabled, which are important for IoT applications in healthcare [24].
Shift towards Value-Based Care	- The healthcare industry is focused on improving patient outcomes and reducing costs, which is driving the demand for innovation. The emergence of IoT as a promising technology has facilitated proactive and personalized healthcare delivery [25].
Regulatory and Technological Advances	- The establishment of guidelines and regulations for medical devices by regulatory bodies such as the FDA and EMA. To build trust in IoT-enabled healthcare solutions, there have been advances in cybersecurity and data privacy [26].

Wireless Connectivity

Fundamental to IoT sensors have the ability to wirelessly transport data. Developments in wireless communication technologies, Bluetooth Low Energy (BLE), Wi-Fi, Zigbee, and cellular networks (4G LTE, 5G), have made it easy for IoT sensors to communicate with other devices and connect them to the internet without being physically connected [29].

Sensor Fusion and Integration

Fusing sensors refer to the combining of data from different sensors to give a better understanding of the environment or object under observation. The incorporation of different sensors into one device ensures that measurements are more precise, and dependable and can record various types of data at once [30].

Embedded Intelligence

IoT sensors are now integrating embedded intelligence like microcontrollers with on-board processing capacities and machine learning algorithms. Thus, the sensors can carry out local data processing and analysis rather than having to constantly communicate with remote servers, thus improving their real-time decision-making capabilities [31].

Enhanced Sensing Capabilities

The sensor technology has made tremendous strides in improving sensing capabilities such as sensitivity, resolution, accuracy, and reliability. This is apparent for imaging sensors that have advanced to high-resolution medical imaging devices while environmental sensors are now capable of accurately monitoring air quality, temperature, and humidity [32].

Security and Privacy Measures

IoT sensor data protection from unauthorized access and tampering is a matter that requires the application of security measures like encryption, authentication protocols, and secure boot mechanisms. Given the rapid increase in the number of IoT devices as well as concerns about cybersecurity and data privacy, there are so many benefits that come with having better measures to ensure that such security lapses do not happen [33, 34].

The development and adoption of IoT sensor technologies have been driven by these technological advancements, enabling them to play a transformative role across various sectors such as healthcare, agriculture, manufacturing, transportation, and smart cities [23].

Integration of IoT Sensors into Healthcare Systems

In order to carry out the seamless integration of these sensing technologies in various aspects of healthcare delivery, such as patient monitoring and operational management, some healthcare systems are incorporating IoT sensors. The role of integration of IoT sensors into healthcare systems is summarized in Fig. (**1**).

IOT SENSOR TECHNOLOGIES IN HEALTHCARE

IoT Sensor Technologies Mechanisms in Healthcare Monitoring

The combination of data collection, transmission, and processing enables IoT sensor technologies to gather valuable information from the physical world, leading to enhanced efficiency, productivity, and decision-making across various domains, which are discussed below [35].

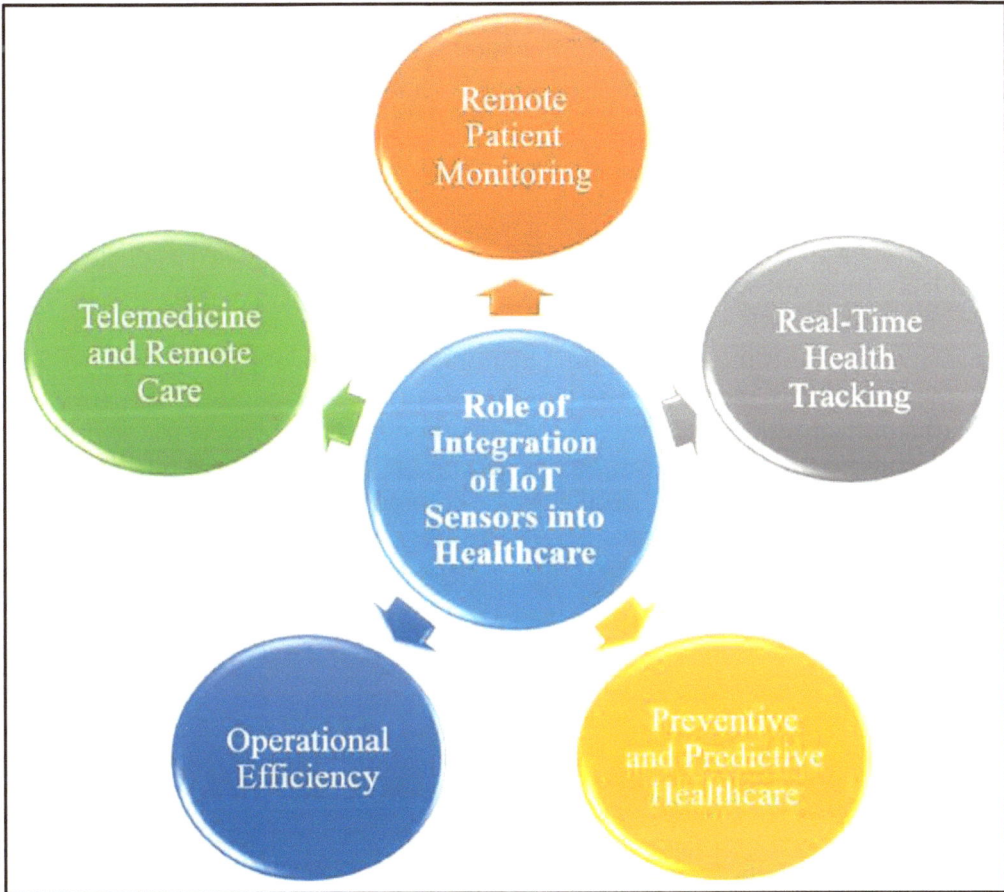

Fig. (1). Role of integration of IoT sensors into healthcare systems.

Most IoT sensors are built to directly measure physical quantities like temperature, humidity, pressure, light intensity, motion, and others. They change the measured physical quantities into electrical signals for further processing and analysis. The physical presence or absence of items or persons within a specific boundary can be detected using proximity sensors. Proximity or touch is detected using technologies such as ultrasonic, infrared, or capacitive sensing in these sensors. In some cases, like in healthcare and agriculture, IoT sensors may interface with biological tissues to collect data. Biosensors, for instance, determine blood glucose levels, while plant health monitoring relies on soil moisture content measurement [36].

Data collected by sensors must be sent to centralized databases or cloud platforms so that further processing and analysis can be done. Wi-Fi, Bluetooth, Zigbee, and cellular networks are some of the wireless communication protocols commonly used for data transmission in IoT systems. This is good for Local Area Network (LAN) over short distances with high-speed data transmission. Mostly useful for IoT devices' powered short-range communication with smartphones or any other nearby devices. More specifically, it is suitable for low-power applications, such as smart lighting for homes, and automation industries, such as industrial control systems [37].

It is important to mention that the first stage of processing involves cleaning and organizing the transmitted information. The latter may involve activities like data filtering, normalization, or aggregation. From there, raw sensor data is analyzed using several algorithms and machine learning methods that provide a deeper look into the data. They include statistical analysis, predictive modeling, clustering, classification as well as anomaly detection among others. It is instructive to note that the main aim of processing and analysis of data is to generate actionable insights for decision-making processes or automation triggers. For instance, by analyzing such information in a smart building system, it can be revealed how energy usage can be optimized to improve efficiency in HVAC systems [35].

Various Types of IoT Sensors Used in Healthcare Applications

IoT sensors have found wide applications in healthcare, enabling remote monitoring, improving patient care, and enhancing healthcare delivery. Various types of IoT sensors used in healthcare applications are summarized in Fig. (2) and discussed below.

Biometric Sensors

In healthcare, biometric sensors are very important in various applications that enhance patient care, ensure security, and simplify processes. These devices, such as palm or fingerprint scanners, are used for patient identification and authentication to ensure that the appropriate person is receiving suitable medical treatment. They can also support continuous biometric patient monitoring through wearable devices to record vital signs such as heart rate and blood pressure in real-time, allowing intervention measures before they escalate into major problems. Additionally, these devices help with medication management by confirming the identity of patients before administering drugs, thus making them safer and reducing blunders. Moreover, hospitals use these gadgets to control access to restricted areas while providing safety and privacy for their patients. Generally, there are several uses of biometric sensors within healthcare settings that enhance the security of patients, facilitate conformity with regulatory requirements, and promote efficiency in delivering health services [38].

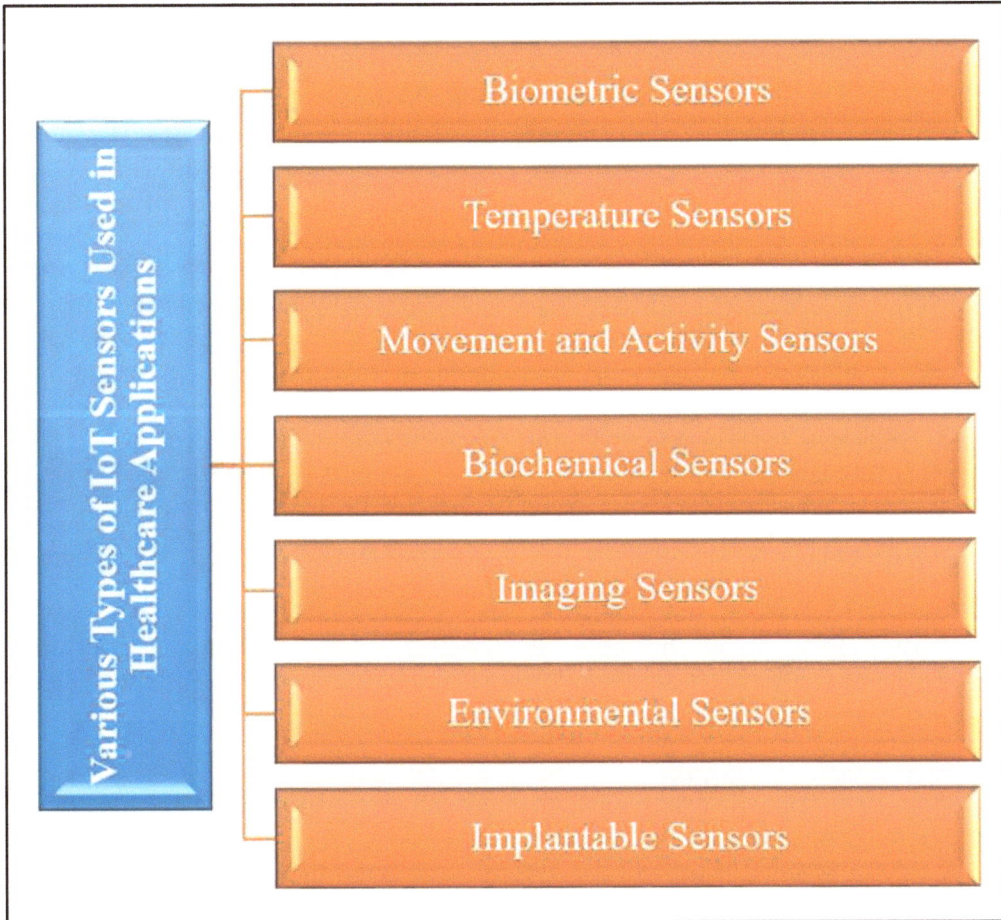

Fig. (2). Various types of IoT sensors used in healthcare applications.

Temperature Sensors

In healthcare, there exist a number of applications in which temperature sensors are used, and they perform a very important role in enabling exact and dependable readings of temperature for various uses. These sensors can be found in both in-vitro and in-vivo senses that facilitate medical operations, diagnostic tools, and patient monitoring. This is why, within the field of health care, temperature measurement represents an extensive range of situations, from cryogenic applications such as drug formulation or vaccine storage to high-temperature situations inside autoclaves and sterilizers [39].

A crucial point about temperature sensing in healthcare is that it is a crucial aspect of pH measurement. Temperature has a significant influence on the pH measurement results, and accurate temperature compensation is, therefore, necessary for precise pH measurement. These help to accurately measure temperature using Pt RTDs (Platinum Resistance Temperature Detectors) that provide pH measurements with perfect temperature compensation, ensuring correct readings. Modernized pH meters incorporate miniaturized Pt RTDs, which prevent the need for an extra separate temperature probe, resulting in real-time error-free instantaneous readings [39].

Furthermore, temperature sensors matter a lot in autoclaves and sterilizers used by the medical industry to recycle surgical instruments as well as other medical apparatus. Pt RTDs ensure high precision and low measurement drift, which guarantee conformity with sterilization standards and autoclaving throughout the device's service life. Accurate temperature measurement is important to curb disease transmission and preserve sterility during sterilization procedures [40].

In addition, wearable temperature detectors for healthcare have their peculiarities, which allow their use in patient monitoring, post-operation care, and fever monitoring. These are the sensors that are attached to the skin of a person to help maintain temperature at a certain level and so quickly alert those who care when the wearer reaches this temperature. For compactness and conformability, these wearables employ flexible printed electronics, hence increasing patients' comfort and usage [41].

Movement and Activity Sensors

Healthcare employ movement and activity sensors, which are used to track and monitor the movements and actions of a patient. These are now being employed more frequently in remote patient monitoring systems so that healthcare professionals can follow up on their patients' movements and activity even while they are very far from them. There are examples such as accelerometer sensors that can monitor the patient's movements and activities, thus enabling healthcare givers to make informed decisions about patient care [42].

In the healthcare industry, there is a wide range of applications for movement and activity sensors, which include but are not limited to patient monitoring in hospitals and clinics, home healthcare, rehabilitation, and physical therapy, medical research and clinical trials, ambulances and emergency medical services, medical devices and implants as well as wearable healthcare devices. They provide crucial data needed for monitoring, diagnosis, treatment, and research, thus enabling healthcare practitioners to give evidence-based care [43].

Healthcare applications are becoming increasingly popular for wearable sensors, specifically. These sensors can gather data consistently during ordinary walking activities and thereby provide useful information about movement patterns and activity levels of patients. By utilizing the cheapness and widespread availability of wearable sensors, healthcare providers can conduct a few trials on new approaches to using this sensor to estimate propulsion function along with common clinical metrics like walking speed in individuals with gait disorder [44].

The use of motion and activity sensors in healthcare can change the ways healthcare providers receive real-time information about a patient's movements and activities. It is important to identify these mobility problems early enough, monitor how rehabilitation and physical therapy are progressing, and provide individualized care for patients. Patient outcomes, healthcare costs, and overall quality of care can be improved by adopting the most recent sensor technology advancements in this field [45].

Biochemical Sensors

Biochemical sensors are used in healthcare, and they are analytical tools with living compounds that help regulate biochemical reactions. The latter is a group of sensors that change the ligand-receptor interaction to an optical, spectral, or electrochemical signal proportional to the concentration of an analyte. The development of biosensors began more than fifty years ago; these were the first devices designed to determine relatively simple biomolecules such as glucose, cholesterol, urea, myoglobin, and prothrombin [46].

The healthcare sector widely uses biochemical sensors for various applications, including monitoring the glucose levels of patients through home-use glucometers. The biosensing part of these devices is made up of enzymes such as glucose oxidase or glucose dehydrogenase that are immobilized on the surface of an electrode and break down glucose. The physicochemical signal is formed from products for enzymatic reactions. For example, in recent years, there has been a widespread exploration of the concept of biosensing after combining nanoelectronics and biochemistry. The different types of transducers include optical, micromechanical, and interferometric, among others, used by many biosensors depending on their type in order to detect quantitatively some biomarkers characteristic of infectious processes using a variety of biological materials [47].

Biochemical sensors are used in different applications such as monitoring patients at hospitals and clinics, home healthcare, rehabilitation therapy, medical research, clinical trials, ambulances, emergency medical services, medical devices, as well as implants and wearable health care. These sensors provide crucial information that would be relevant for observing, diagnosing, treating, and researching, hence enabling healthcare providers to render this kind of care that is supported by evidence. Biochemical sensors in health care facilitate accurate biochemical measurement in various medical procedures, diagnostic tools, and patient monitoring. They play a role in ensuring the safety of the patient during treatment, resulting in improved treatment outcomes, thus leading to better quality of care [45].

Imaging Sensors

Medical and life science applications benefit greatly from imaging sensors as they enable them to capture high-resolution images with more detailed precision and faster than before. All these types of sensors are used in different applications, including digital X-ray systems, CT scans, microscopy, and imaging of biological samples. Two categories that are available for imaging sensors include Charge Coupled Devices (CCD) or Complementary Metal Oxide Semiconductor (CMOS) arrays. A lower noise level of CCD sensors, higher single-shot dynamic range, and uniform response to light across the entire sensor have been their hallmarks. CMOS sensors have become popular because they use less power in terms of energy consumed per area, are smaller in size, and are cheaper compared to CCDs [48].

Imaging sensors are used in medical and life science applications to capture high-resolution pictures of the human body, thereby enabling doctors to identify and diagnose ailments with greater precision. Besides, they are also useful for microscopy analysis and biological sample imaging, which allows scientists to take high-resolution images of targeted portions of cells or even tissues. Imaging sensors can also be used in low-light situations, such as fluorescence microscopy, where the sample is photophobic. Large sensor cameras can produce low-light pictures of high quality, hence being vital for applications that require very sensitized samples [49].

In medical and life science applications, imaging sensors are very critical as they help capture high-resolution images with increased details, accuracy, and faster speeds. They are used in various applications, including digital X-ray systems, Computed Tomography (CT) scans, microscopy, and imaging of biological samples. Imaging sensors will remain vital to medical and life science research, facilitating discoveries and understanding of intricate biology and medicine due to continued technological advancements [50].

Environmental Sensors

Healthcare environmental sensors are used to monitor different environmental factors that can have an impact on a patient's health. Air pressure, humidity, ambient temperature, and relative humidity for climate control in smart homes can be measured by these sensors. Moreover, they are capable of measuring gas levels to ensure air quality monitoring and enhance the welfare of individuals. Environmental sensors are applied for indoor navigation as well as altitude stabilization [51].

Real-time monitoring of health for the wearer and the environments surrounding them can be carried out by integrating environmental sensors into wearable gadgets. The accuracy of wearable biosensors can greatly benefit from these sensors. In order to provide long-term reliability on-body, strong anti-pollution surface protection is required, and dynamic calibration techniques such as multi-mode, multimarker sensing, and drift correction are necessary [52].

The practical deployment of these sensing devices is characterized by hardware, providing power, and communication difficulties. The components that make up the hardware must be interconnected with biosensor platforms and customized to suit the needs of a specific application. Wireless platforms often use printed wireless circuit boards that have full-featured microcontrollers [53].

There are numerous applications of environmental sensors in healthcare, such as patient monitoring in hospitals and clinics, home healthcare, rehabilitation and physical therapy, medical research and clinical trials, ambulances and emergency medical services, medical devices and implants, and wearable healthcare devices. Such sensors provide critical information for monitoring, diagnosis, treatment, and research that enables health professionals to deliver evidence-based care [54].

Healthcare has seen a great revolution in the use of implanted sensors that allow for simultaneous monitoring of various biophysical and biochemical parameters. The concept of Healthcare 5.0 is also in line with these devices, which are driven by smart disease control and detection, virtual care, intelligent health management, smart monitoring, and decision-making. Biophysical and bioelectrical parameters, along with specific biomarkers like ions, neurotransmitters, hormones, and volatile organic compounds, can be accurately measured by implantable sensors, thus contributing to early diagnosis and prevention for a variety of diseases, including limb ischemia, stroke, myocardial infarction, *etc* [55].

Precise recording of physiology and closed-loop therapy are the drivers behind the development of implantable sensors. These sensors can be as small as 1 inch and weigh less than 15 grams, thereby enabling the use of minimally invasive techniques during their implantation. Medical professionals have employed implantable sensors in many areas, such as cardiology, pulmonology, neurology, gastroenterology, urology, orthopedics, and otolaryngology, proving that they are versatile and can have a wide scope of influence on healthcare in general [56].

Even though implantable sensors can greatly improve health care, they are faced with major hurdles, including long-term performance, biocompatibility, power sources, and translational gaps. Calibration, power dissipation, thermal stress, data security, and patient-related issues like discomfort and social norms are some of the challenges that researchers and designers are struggling with. Embedding these biosensors in medical technologies could enhance care for patients as well as lead to better treatment outcomes and progress in healthcare across different fields [54].

Advantages of IoT Sensors Over Traditional Monitoring Devices

The advent of IoT sensors has transformed everything we know about data acquisition and processing, outperforming traditional monitoring tools in several ways. The real-time monitoring capabilities are among the biggest strengths of these devices. Unlike their traditional counterparts, Internet of Things sensors provide continuous data collection and reporting, meaning that one can instantly follow any process or system through it and will not miss anything on its way. In this regard, real-time monitoring enables swifter decision-making and faster response to arising issues or anomalies, thereby correcting them in a timely manner [57].

IoT sensors have the added advantage of scalability. These sensor networks can expand or contract to suit changing monitoring requirements without heavy-duty infrastructure development. In this regard, more sensors can be placed in the field, while some may be reconfigured as well. They provide considerable long-term cost savings for organizations as their initial set-up costs might be higher when compared to traditional monitoring systems. By doing so, IoT sensors enable companies to optimize resource use and minimize operational costs by streamlining processes, reducing downtime, and preventing costly breakdowns or failures [58, 59].

Integration of the Internet of Things (IoT) sensors with advanced analytics platforms and machine learning algorithms can unlock valuable insights, as well as predictive models. Thus, businesses get better-informed decision-making based on data, optimized operations, and unobserved patterns or trends in traditional monitoring methods. Automation and control capabilities further enhance the advantages of IoT sensors. This helps to automate various processes or systems through these sensors using real-time data inputs and, therefore, promotes efficiency while facilitating proactive implementation of predictive and preventive measures [60, 61].

Besides, there is environmental monitoring where IoT sensors can be utilized, such as for monitoring air quality, water quality, temperatures, and humidity. They help in the continuous monitoring of environmental parameters, which is essential for the early detection of anomalies and potential hazards, leading to compliance with regulatory requirements and ensuring environmental sustainability. When IoT sensors monitor motion temperature or the presence of hazardous gases in real time, it enhances safety and security. If any anomaly or potential risks are noticed immediately, corrective action can be taken to prevent accidents or security breaches from on time [62, 63].

APPLICATIONS OF IOT SENSORS IN REAL-TIME HEALTHCARE MONITORING

Fitness Tracking and Vital Sign Monitoring Devices

Fitness tracking devices, which can be worn on the body and used to monitor vital signs continuously during daily life, are a new technology. The sensors measure more than ten biomarkers such as the heart rate, respiration rate, blood pressure, blood glucose level, capnography as well as Cardiac Implantable Devices (CIDs), skin perspiration, and others. These can be integrated into different gadgets, including smartwatches, fitness trackers, and smartphones, among others, to enable real-time health status checkups of an individual's condition. At all times, when one is exercising, at night while asleep, or just engaging in daily activities that do not require much energy, these have a significant impact on a person's understanding concerning their physical fitness [64].

Stretchable wearable sensors that can be integrated into clothes or worn directly on the skin represent one of the recent advancements in wearable sensors. They could monitor many biomarkers such as blood pressure, heart rate, respiration rate, body temperature, blood oxygen saturation, and glucose levels in blood capnography and motion evaluation cardiac implantable devices. The VitalPatch is actually an instance of a wearable sensor for monitoring vital signs, which measures heart rate, respiratory rates, and temperature while being a patch worn on the chest. The device is meant to gather physiological data in healthcare settings such as hospitals and medical centers, and it has accuracy checks done by several studies [65].

The Fitbit Charge 3 is another example of a wearable sensor for fitness tracking. It is worn on the wrist and is capable of calculating heart rate, footsteps, distance covered, and calories burned. Many studies have been conducted to determine its accuracy and dependability. Thus, it has been certified for use in fitness monitoring and health management. However, there are also some challenges associated with wearable sensors, such as their precision and consistency, power consumption, and user interface. To ensure that wearable sensors are safe, effective, and user-friendly, these challenges must be addressed. Wearable sensors have several advantages over conventional monitoring instruments: they provide real-time data, they are non-invasive, and they can be used while participating in daily activities. These devices can also be integrated into larger health monitoring systems so that healthcare providers can obtain useful information from patients' records [66].

Smart Healthcare Facilities for Enhanced Patient Care

IoT has made it possible for smart health facilities to offer several advantages over conventional healthcare monitoring equipment. These facilities are intended for optimum clinical processes, redesigning, or creating new management systems and infrastructures facilitated through digitized networks. By exploiting technology such as IoT, AI, telemedicine, and data analytics, smart hospitals can offer their patients care that is more personalized and efficient [67].

Smart hospitals are primarily known for their focus on innovations and technological integrations to improve the efficiency and quality of healthcare delivery. These facilities have hyperconnected, participatory, agile, and high-quality designs. Smart hospitals may make use of cutting-edge technology to enhance the patient's experience as well as to improve the interoperability of medical systems and devices [68].

Investments in smart hospitals include the integration of health information systems to ensure electronic records can easily be accessed and shared by other hospital departments or staff. It enables faster medical care by fostering collaboration with different healthcare professionals and departments [69].

In addition, the Implementation of IoT permits medical tools to talk and communicate with medics, leading to real-time monitoring and quick responses to changes in the health status of a patient. For this reason, patients and healthcare providers benefit greatly, including increased effectiveness, improved medical judgment, decreased mistakes in the field of medicine, and saved money [70].

Beyond older buildings, these institutions may also be found in remote centers that are linked with each other functionally to offer healthcare services. They are situated in other hospitals, clinics, primary health care facilities, ambulatory care sites, and home-based social organizations. There is a decentralization of healthcare access, which necessitates data security and privacy, service quality, interoperability with data and services, and the network and communication infrastructure [71].

The Smart healthcare centers, which are constructed using IoT technology, have several benefits compared to traditional healthcare monitoring devices. They are intended to optimize or redesign existing clinical processes, management systems, and infrastructures facilitated by a network that has gone digital. With advanced technologies such as telemedicine, AI, IoT, and data analytics at their disposal, smart hospitals can offer highly individualized care that is also efficient for patients, enhance medical decision-making, minimize medical errors, and reduce costs [72].

REGULATORY AND ETHICAL CONSIDERATIONS

Legal requirements and industrial standards regulate IoT sensors' use in healthcare through regulatory frameworks and standards. In the United States, the Health Insurance Portability and Accountability Act (HIPAA) sets rules for safeguarding sensitive patient health data. At the same time, the U.S. Food and Drug Administration (FDA) oversees medical devices like some IoT sensors. Furthermore, the General Data Protection Regulation (GDPR) of the European Union provides for personal data processing and protection, including healthcare data [73, 74].

For instance, the International Organization for Standardization (ISO) formulates international standards that give guidelines on quality management systems and information security in medical device production. In healthcare, ethical concerns about the use of IoT sensors revolve around matters like consent, patient privacy, and data ownership. Robust security measures, encryption techniques, and access controls must be implemented to protect sensitive health information gathered by IoT sensors while maintaining patient privacy. The understanding of informed consent is critical so that patients are fully aware and in agreement with the data collection activities linked to IoT sensors. Further, it is important for patients' rights and their control over health information to be respected by clarifying data ownership, thus enabling them to reach change or remove it as necessary. Therefore, these regulatory and ethical concerns must be addressed if trust has to be built in the healthcare systems that utilize IoT and the digital age by protecting patients' rights [75, 76].

CHALLENGES AND CONSIDERATIONS

The healthcare system is about to be completely changed by real-time tracking with IoT sensors, but there are some problems to overcome. The most important thing that should be kept in mind is the security and privacy of sensitive patient data; it should be encrypted strongly, and companies have to comply with some regulations such as HIPAA and GDPR. A barrier to interoperability needs to be recognized, and the standardization of data formats and communication protocols must be enforced to enable it to integrate smoothly into existing healthcare IT systems [77].

To manage the increase in data, scalability is key, requiring scalable infrastructure and advanced analytic platforms. For informed decision-making, accurate sensor data and reliability are crucial; hence, strict calibration and maintenance procedures are necessary. Ensuring patients' rights and regulatory compliance would require addressing ethical and legal issues, including patient consent and ownership of data [78].

A complete redesign and training of the staff are required to incorporate real-time tracking information into clinical works. While deploying IoT sensor networks, however, cost and resource constraints must be considered, and initiatives focused on improving patient outcomes must be prioritized first. It is important to comply with regulations such as those provided by HIPAA and FDA to ensure the privacy and security of data. These challenges can only be surmountable through a collective effort from healthcare providers, technology vendors, and regulators, thus enabling the transformative potential of IoT-enabled healthcare systems [79].

FUTURE DIRECTIONS AND IMPLICATIONS

The future of real-time tracking with IoT sensors is full of potential for revolutionizing the healthcare system, but it also presents significant impacts and directions. Sensor technology, data analytics, and artificial intelligence have improved the capabilities of IoT sensors that allow accurate and personalized healthcare interventions. The application of wearable devices, remote monitoring systems, and intelligent healthcare infrastructures will enable a continuous care approach for better patient outcomes at a lower cost [80].

IoT-enabled healthcare can shift from reactive to proactive and personalized by facilitating real-time tracking through IoT sensors that enable early disease detection, predictive analytic measures for preventive care, and remote patient monitoring. Achieving the full potential of IoT-based healthcare delivery, however, requires addressing issues related to data security, interoperability, ethical concerns, and regulatory compliance [81].

To achieve this goal, a combined effort from healthcare providers and developers in the field of technology, together with policymakers and regulatory authorities, is essential in order to navigate these challenges so as to leverage the transformative power of real-time tracking using IoT sensors on steering future health service provision. Over time, integration of IoT in healthcare systems will result in entirely new models for clinical decision-making processes along with patient care workflows, resulting in more efficient access to patients who are now considered a focal point in a healthcare ecosystem, which is much more effective at delivering better outcomes [82, 83].

CONCLUSION

In conclusion, the healthcare system is about to be completely transformed by combining real-time tracking with IoT sensors, providing a number of novel ways to enhance individual patient outcomes, improve clinical decision-making, and optimize healthcare delivery. IoT sensors provide access to continuous monitoring of patient's health parameters, which enables early detection of diseases, prevention strategies, and personalized treatment methods. By enabling the seamless collection and transmission of data, smart healthcare infrastructure, remote monitoring systems, and wearable devices make it possible for patients and healthcare providers to be empowered by real-time decision-making. Additionally, healthcare systems enabled by the Internet of Things can lead to a change in attention from reactive to proactive and preventive care, thereby decreasing the rate of hospital admissions, overall healthcare expenditures, and burden on healthcare resources. Despite that, several challenges must be addressed in order to leverage the full potential of IoT-enabled healthcare, which includes data security, privacy concerns, interoperability issues, ethical considerations, and regulatory compliance. These challenges can only be overcome through concerted efforts among healthcare stakeholders like technology developers, policymakers, and regulatory agencies to navigate the challenges and establish a framework within which IoT sensors can be responsibly and ethically applied in healthcare. The future of healthcare delivery lies in the investment of research, infrastructure development, and continued innovation so as to harness the transformative potential of real-time tracking through IOT sensors. The utilization of the Internet of Things technology can empower healthcare systems to be more efficient, patient-centered, and accessible, hence enhancing the quality of care and improving global health experiences among patients.

REFERENCES

[1]   P. Sethi, and S.R. Sarangi, "Internet of Things: Architectures, Protocols, and Applications", *J. Electr. Comput. Eng.,* vol. 2017, pp. 1-25, 2017.
[http://dx.doi.org/10.1155/2017/9324035]

[2]   S. Kumar, P. Tiwari, and M. Zymbler, "Internet of Things is a revolutionary approach for future technology enhancement: a review", *J. Big Data,* vol. 6, no. 1, p. 111, 2019.
[http://dx.doi.org/10.1186/s40537-019-0268-2]

[3]   T. Magara, and Y. Zhou, "Internet of Things (IoT) of Smart Homes: Privacy and Security", *J. Electr. Comput. Eng.,* vol. 2024, pp. 1-17, 2024.
[http://dx.doi.org/10.1155/2024/7716956]

[4]   K. Potter, and J. Oloyede, "The internet of things: Transforming industries, empowering connectivity, and shaping the future", *J Internet Things,* vol. 2023, 2023pp. 1-10.2023. Available from: https://www.researchgate.net/publication/376784526

[5]   C. Li, and J. Wang, "S. Wang, and Y. Zhang, "A review of IoT applications in healthcare,"", *Neurocomputing,* vol. 565, 2024.
[http://dx.doi.org/10.1016/j.neucom.2023.127017]

[6]   A. Rahman, M.A.H. Wadud, M.J. Islam, D. Kundu, T.M.A.U.H. Bhuiyan, G. Muhammad, and Z. Ali, "Internet of medical things and blockchain-enabled patient-centric agent through SDN for remote patient monitoring in 5G network", *Sci. Rep.,* vol. 14, no. 1, p. 5297, 2024.
[http://dx.doi.org/10.1038/s41598-024-55662-w] [PMID: 38438526]

[7]   A. Rejeb, K. Rejeb, H. Treiblmaier, A. Appolloni, S. Alghamdi, Y. Alhasawi, and M. Iranmanesh, "The Internet of Things (IoT) in healthcare: Taking stock and moving forward," *Inter of Thin,* vol. 22, p. 100721, Jul. 2023.
[http://dx.doi.org/10.1016/j.iot.2023.100721]

[8]   C.L. Stergiou, A.P. Plageras, V.A. Memos, M.P. Koidou, and K.E. Psannis, "Secure Monitoring System for IoT Healthcare Data in the Cloud", *Appl. Sci. (Basel),* vol. 14, no. 1, p. 120, 2023.
[http://dx.doi.org/10.3390/app14010120]

[9]   M. Javaid, and I.H. Khan, "Internet of Things (IoT) enabled healthcare helps to take the challenges of COVID-19 Pandemic", *J. Oral Biol. Craniofac. Res.,* vol. 11, no. 2, pp. 209-214, 2021.
[http://dx.doi.org/10.1016/j.jobcr.2021.01.015] [PMID: 33665069]

[10]   T. Singh Karki, M. Rashid Ansari, A. Kumar, and Y. Kumar, "Wearable Tracking System with Heart Monitoring", 2022. Available from: https://ssrn.com/abstract=4157637
[http://dx.doi.org/10.2139/ssrn.4157637]

[11]   S. Bag, and A. Bhowmick, "Smart Healthcare Monitoring and Tracking System", *International Research Journal of Engineering and Technology,* vol. 4, 2017no. 6, . Available from: www.irjet.net

[12]   L. Gholamhosseini, F. Sadoughi, and A. Safaei, "Hospital real-time location system (A practical approach in healthcare): A narrative review article", *Iran J Public Health,* vol. 48, 2019no. 4, pp. 593-602.
[http://dx.doi.org/10.18502/ijph.v48i4.980]

[13]   W.H. Wang, and W.S. Hsu, "Integrating Artificial Intelligence and Wearable IoT System in Long-Term Care Environments", *Sensors (Basel),* vol. 23, no. 13, p. 5913, 2023.
[http://dx.doi.org/10.3390/s23135913] [PMID: 37447763]

[14]   J. Wan, "Wearable IoT enabled real-time health monitoring system", *EURASIP J. Wirel. Commun. Netw.,* vol. 2018, no. 1, 2018.
[http://dx.doi.org/10.1186/s13638-018-1308-x]

[15]   M. Elahi, S.O. Afolaranmi, J.L. Martinez Lastra, and J.A. Perez Garcia, "A comprehensive literature review of the applications of AI techniques through the lifecycle of industrial equipment", *Discover Artificial Intelligence,* vol. 3, no. 1, p. 43, 2023.
[http://dx.doi.org/10.1007/s44163-023-00089-x]

[16]   M. Soori, B. Arezoo, and R. Dastres, "Internet of things for smart factories in industry 4.0, a review", In: *Internet of Things and Cyber-Physical Systems.* vol. 3. KeAi Communications Co., 2023, pp. 192-204.
[http://dx.doi.org/10.1016/j.iotcps.2023.04.006]

[17]   M. Javaid, A. Haleem, R.P. Singh, S. Rab, M.I. Ul Haq, and A. Raina, "Internet of Things in the global healthcare sector: Significance, applications, and barriers", *Int. J. Intell. Netw.,* vol. 3, pp. 165-175,

2022.
[http://dx.doi.org/10.1016/j.ijin.2022.10.002]

[18]   A. Amjad, P. Kordel, and G. Fernandes, "A Review on Innovation in the Healthcare Sector (Telehealth) through Artificial Intelligence", *Sustainability (Switzerland),* vol. 15, no. 8, 2023.
[http://dx.doi.org/10.3390/su15086655]

[19]   Akoh Atadoga, T.T. Omaghomi, O.A. Elufioye, I.P. Odilibe, A.I. Daraojimba, and O.R. Owolabi, "Internet of Things (IoT) in healthcare: A systematic review of use cases and benefits", *Int. J. Sci. Res. Arch.,* vol. 11, no. 1, pp. 1511-1517, 2024.
[http://dx.doi.org/10.30574/ijsra.2024.11.1.0243]

[20]   M. Shiao, "Risk monitoring of aircraft fatigue damage evolution at critical locations utilizing structural health monitoring", *Encyclopedia of Structural Health Monitoring,* vol. 1, John Wiley & Sons, pp. 1-10, 2009.
[http://dx.doi.org/10.1002/9780470061626.shm185]

[21]   N. K. Mangal, and A. K. Tiwari, "A review of the evolution of scientific literature on technology-assisted approaches using RGB-D sensors for musculoskeletal health monitoring", *Computers in Biology and Medicine,* vol. 132, Elsevier Ltd, 2021.
[http://dx.doi.org/10.1016/j.compbiomed.2021.104316]

[22]   M.U. Tariq, ""Advanced wearable medical devices and their role in transformative remote health monitoring", In: *in Transformative Approaches to Patient Literacy and Healthcare Innovation* M. B. Garcia and R. P. P. de Almeida, Eds. Hershey, PA, USA: IGI Global, 2024, pp. 308-326.
[http://dx.doi.org/10.4018/979-8-3693-3661-8.ch015]

[23]   S. Palanivel Rajan, and T. Dineshkumar, "In hospital and home remote patient monitoring", In: *in Connected e-Health: Integrated IoT and Cloud Computing.,* D. Dutta, N. Jadav, S. Tanwar, H. K. D. Sarma, E. Pricop, Eds., vol. 1021. Singapore: Springer, 2022, pp. 333-347.
[http://dx.doi.org/10.1007/978-3-030-97929-4_15]

[24]   M. Hassanalieragh, "Health monitoring and management using Internet-of-things (IoT) sensing with cloud-based processing: Opportunities and challenges", *Proc IEEE Int Conf Serv Comput (SCC),* New York, NY, USA, pp. 285-292, 2015.
[http://dx.doi.org/10.1109/SCC.2015.47]

[25]   R.S.H. Istepanaian, and Y.T. Zhang, "Guest editorial. Introduction to the special section: 4G Health--the long-term evolution of m-Health", *IEEE Trans. Inf. Technol. Biomed.,* vol. 16, no. 1, pp. 1-5, 2012.
[http://dx.doi.org/10.1109/TITB.2012.2183269] [PMID: 22271836]

[26]   V. Pakrashi, A. O'Connor, and B. Basu, "A bridge-vehicle interaction based experimental investigation of damage evolution", *Struct. Health Monit.,* vol. 9, no. 4, pp. 285-296, 2010.
[http://dx.doi.org/10.1177/1475921709352147]

[27]   M. E. E. Alahi, "Integration of IoT-Enabled Technologies and Artificial Intelligence (AI) for Smart City Scenario: Recent Advancements and Future Trends", *Sensors,* vol. 23, no. 11, 2023.
[http://dx.doi.org/10.3390/s23115206]

[28]   Q. Shi, Y. Yang, Z. Sun, and C. Lee, "Progress of Advanced Devices and Internet of Things Systems as Enabling Technologies for Smart Homes and Health Care", In: *ACS Materials* vol. 2. American Chemical Society, 2022, no. 4, pp. 394-435.
[http://dx.doi.org/10.1021/acsmaterialsau.2c00001]

[29]   O. Arshi, and S. Mondal, "Advancements in sensors and actuators technologies for smart cities: a comprehensive review", *Smart Construction and Sustainable Cities,* vol. 1, no. 1, p. 18, 2023.
[http://dx.doi.org/10.1007/s44268-023-00022-2]

[30]   Y. Perwej, M.A. AbouGhaly, B. Kerim, and H.A. Harb, "An extended review on internet of things (iot) and its promising applications", *Commun. Appl. Electron.,* vol. 7, no. 26, pp. 8-22, 2019.

[31]   R. Chataut, A. Phoummalayvane, and R. Akl, "Unleashing the power of IoT: A comprehensive review of IoT applications and future prospects in healthcare, agriculture, smart homes, smart cities, and Industry 4.0", In: *Sensors* vol. 23. , 2023, no. 16, p. 7194.
[http://dx.doi.org/10.3390/s23167194]

[32]   S.F. Ahmed, M.S.B. Alam, M. Hoque, A. Lameesa, S. Afrin, T. Farah, M. Kabir, G.M. Shafiullah, and S.M. Muyeen, "Industrial Internet of Things enabled technologies, challenges, and future directions", *Comput. Electr. Eng.,* vol. 110, p. 108847, 2023.
[http://dx.doi.org/10.1016/j.compeleceng.2023.108847]

[33]   KC Rath, A Khang, and D. Roy, "The role of Internet of Things (IoT) technology in Industry 4.0 economy", In: *Advanced IoT technologies and applications in the industry 4.0 digital economy* CRC Press, 2024, pp. 1-28.

[34]   M. R. Jahanshahi, S. F. Masri, and G. S. Sukhatme, "Multi-image stitching and scene reconstruction for evaluating defect evolution in structures", *Struct Health Monit,* vol. 10, no. 6, pp. 643-657, 2011.
[http://dx.doi.org/10.1177/1475921710395809]

[35]   S. B. Baker, W. Xiang, and I. Atkinson, "Internet of things for smart healthcare: Technologies, challenges, and opportunities", *IEEE Access,* vol. 5, pp. 26521-26544, 2017.
[http://dx.doi.org/10.1109/ACCESS.2017.2775180]

[36]   M. M. Dhanvijay, and S. C. Patil, "Internet of Things: A survey of enabling technologies in healthcare and its applications", *Computer Networks,* vol. 153, Elsevier B.V., pp. 113-131, 2019.
[http://dx.doi.org/10.1016/j.comnet.2019.03.006]

[37]   G. Gardašević, K. Katzis, D. Bajić, and L. Berbakov, "Emerging wireless sensor networks and internet of things technologies—foundations of smart healthcare", *Sensors (Basel),* vol. 20, no. 13, p. 3619, 2020.
[http://dx.doi.org/10.3390/s20133619] [PMID: 32605071]

[38]   M. H. Kashani, M. Madanipour, M. Nikravan, P. Asghari, and E. Mahdipour, "A systematic review of IoT in healthcare: Applications, techniques, and trends," *J. Netw. Comput. Appl.,* vol. 192, p. 103164, Oct. 2021.
[http://dx.doi.org/10.1016/j.jnca.2021.103164]

[39]   B. Pradhan, S. Bhattacharyya, and K. Pal, "IoT-Based Applications in Healthcare Devices", *J. Healthc. Eng.,* vol. 2021, pp. 1-18, 2021.
[http://dx.doi.org/10.1155/2021/6632599] [PMID: 33791084]

[40]   H. H. Nguyen, F. Mirza, M. A. Naeem, and M. Nguyen, "A review on IoT healthcare monitoring applications and a vision for transforming sensor data into real-time clinical feedback", *Proc IEEE 21st Int Conf Comput Suppt Coop Work Des (CSCWD),* Wellington, New Zealand, pp. 257-262, 2017.
[http://dx.doi.org/10.1109/CSCWD.2017.8066704]

[41]   D. Sehrawat, and N. S. Gill, "Smart sensors: Analysis of different types of IoT sensors", *Proc IEEE 3rd Int Conf Trends Electron Informatics (ICOEI),* pp. 523-528, 2019.
[http://dx.doi.org/10.1109/ICOEI.2019.8862778]

[42]   R. Liu, A.A. Ramli, H. Zhang, E. Henricson, and X. Liu, "An Overview of Human Activity Recognition Using Wearable Sensors", *Healthcare and Artificial Intelligence,* no. Mar, 2021.
[http://dx.doi.org/10.1007/978-3-030-96068-1_1]

[43]   H.H. Mohamad Jawad, Z. Bin Hassan, B.B. Zaidan, F.H. Mohammed Jawad, D.H. Mohamed Jawad, and W.H. Alredany, "A systematic literature review of enabling IoT in healthcare: Motivations, challenges, and recommendations", *Electronics,* vol. 11, no. 19, p. 3223, 2022.

[44]   S.A. Khowaja, A.G. Prabono, F. Setiawan, B.N. Yahya, and S.L. Lee, "Contextual activity based Healthcare Internet of Things, Services, and People (HIoTSP): An architectural framework for healthcare monitoring using wearable sensors", *Comput. Netw.,* vol. 145, pp. 190-206, 2018.
[http://dx.doi.org/10.1016/j.comnet.2018.09.003]

[45]   L. Hickman, and M. Akdere, "Developing intercultural competencies through virtual reality: Internet of things applications in education and learning", In: *Proc IEEE 15th Learn Technol Conf (L&T)* Jeddah, Saudi Arabia, 2018, pp. 24-28.
[http://dx.doi.org/10.1109/LT.2018.8368506]

[46]   J. Qi, P. Yang, A. Waraich, Z. Deng, Y. Zhao, and Y. Yang, "Examining sensor-based physical activity recognition and monitoring for healthcare using Internet of Things: A systematic review", In: *J. Biomed. Inform.* vol. 87. Academic Press Inc., 2018, pp. 138-153.
[http://dx.doi.org/10.1016/j.jbi.2018.09.002]

[47]   M. Javaid, A. Haleem, S. Rab, R. Pratap Singh, and R. Suman, "Sensors for daily life: A review", In: *Sensors International* vol. 2. KeAi Communications Co., 2021.
[http://dx.doi.org/10.1016/j.sintl.2021.100121]

[48]   R.A. Radouan Ait Mouha, "Internet of Things (IoT)", *J. Data Anal. Inf. Process.*, vol. 9, no. 2, pp. 77-101, 2021.
[http://dx.doi.org/10.4236/jdaip.2021.92006]

[49]   A. Ahad, M. Tahir, M. Aman Sheikh, K.I. Ahmed, A. Mughees, and A. Numani, "Technologies trend towards 5g network for smart health-care using iot: A review", *Sensors (Basel),* vol. 20, no. 14, p. 4047, 2020.
[http://dx.doi.org/10.3390/s20144047] [PMID: 32708139]

[50]   M. Al-rawashdeh, P. Keikhosrokiani, B. Belaton, M. Alawida, and A. Zwiri, "IoT Adoption and Application for Smart Healthcare: A Systematic Review", *Sensors,* vol. 22, MDPI, no. 14, 2022.
[http://dx.doi.org/10.3390/s22145377]

[51]   H. Mrabet, S. Belguith, A. Alhomoud, and A. Jemai, "A survey of IoT security based on a layered architecture of sensing and data analysis", In: *Sensors (Switzerland)* vol. 20. MDPI AG, 2020, no. 13, pp. 1-20.
[http://dx.doi.org/10.3390/s20133625]

[52]   A. D. Boursianis, M. S. Papadopoulou, P. Diamantoulakis, A. Liopa-Tsakalidi, P. Barouchas, G. Salahas, G. Karagiannidis, S. Wan, and S. K. Goudos, "Internet of Things (IoT) and Agricultural Unmanned Aerial Vehicles (UAVs) in smart farming: A comprehensive review," *Inter of Thin*, vol. 18, p. 100187, May 2022.
[http://dx.doi.org/10.1016/j.iot.2020.100187]

[53]   M.A. El Khaddar, and M. Boulmalf, "Smartphone: The Ultimate IoT and IoE Device", In: *in Smartphones from an Applied Research Perspective* InTech, 2017.
[http://dx.doi.org/10.5772/intechopen.69734]

[54]   P. Rajak, A. Ganguly, S. Adhikary, and S. Bhattacharya, "Internet of Things and smart sensors in agriculture: Scopes and challenges", *J. Agric. Food Res.,* vol. 14, p. 100776, 2023.
[http://dx.doi.org/10.1016/j.jafr.2023.100776]

[55]   P. M. Chanal, and M. S. Kakkasageri, "Security and Privacy in IoT: A Survey", *Wireless Personal Communications,* vol. 115, Springer, no. 2, pp. 1667-1693, 2020.
[http://dx.doi.org/10.1007/s11277-020-07649-9]

[56]   G. Manogaran, D. Lopez, C. Thota, K. M. Abbas, S. Pyne, and R. Sundarasekar, "Big Data Analytics in Healthcare Internet of Things," In: H. Qudrat-Ullah and P. Tsasis, Eds, *Innovative Healthcare Systems for the 21st Century*. Cham: Springer, 2017, pp. 263–284.
[http://dx.doi.org/10.1007/978-3-319-55774-8_10]

[57]   A. Morchid, R. El Alami, A.A. Raezah, and Y. Sabbar, "Applications of internet of things (IoT) and sensors technology to increase food security and agricultural Sustainability: Benefits and challenges", *Ain Shams Eng. J.,* vol. 15, no. 3, p. 102509, 2024.
[http://dx.doi.org/10.1016/j.asej.2023.102509]

[58]   A. Carri, A. Valletta, E. Cavalca, R. Savi, and A. Segalini, "Advantages of iot-based geotechnical

monitoring systems integrating automatic procedures for data acquisition and elaboration", *Sensors (Basel)*, vol. 21, no. 6, p. 2249, 2021.
[http://dx.doi.org/10.3390/s21062249] [PMID: 33807083]

[59]   H. Landaluce, L. Arjona, A. Perales, F. Falcone, I. Angulo, and F. Muralter, "A review of IoT sensing applications and challenges using RFID and wireless sensor networks", *Sensors (Switzerland)*, vol. 20, MDPI AG, no. 9, 2020.
[http://dx.doi.org/10.3390/s20092495]

[60]   O. Elijah, T.A. Rahman, I. Orikumhi, C.Y. Leow, and M.H.D.N. Hindia, "An Overview of Internet of Things (IoT) and Data Analytics in Agriculture: Benefits and Challenges", *IEEE Internet Things J.*, vol. 5, no. 5, pp. 3758-3773, 2018.
[http://dx.doi.org/10.1109/JIOT.2018.2844296]

[61]   N.Y. Philip, J.J.P.C. Rodrigues, H. Wang, S.J. Fong, and J. Chen, "Internet of Things for In-Home Health Monitoring Systems: Current Advances, Challenges and Future Directions", *IEEE J. Sel. Areas Comm.*, vol. 39, no. 2, pp. 300-310, 2021.
[http://dx.doi.org/10.1109/JSAC.2020.3042421]

[62]   S. Abdulmalek, "IoT-Based Healthcare-Monitoring System towards Improving Quality of Life: A Review", *Healthcare (Switzerland)*, vol. 10, no. 10, 2022.
[http://dx.doi.org/10.3390/healthcare10101993]

[63]   S. Chakrabarti, and H.N. Saha, "Institute of Electrical and Electronics Engineers. Las Vegas Section, and Institute of Electrical and Electronics Engineers,", *IEEE CCWC-2017 : 2017 IEEE 7th Annual Computing and Communication Workshop and Conference,* 2017.Las Vegas, USA.

[64]   P. Jangra and M. Gupta, "A Design of Real-Time Multilayered Smart Healthcare Monitoring Framework Using IoT," In: *2018 International Conference on Intelligent and Advanced System (ICIAS)*, Kuala Lumpur, Malaysia, 2018, pp. 1-5.
[http://dx.doi.org/10.1109/ICIAS.2018.8540606]

[65]   X. Wu, C. Liu, L. Wang, and M. Bilal, "Internet of things-enabled real-time health monitoring system using deep learning", *Neural Comput. Appl.*, vol. 35, no. 20, pp. 14565-14576, 2023.
[http://dx.doi.org/10.1007/s00521-021-06440-6] [PMID: 34539091]

[66]   J.S. Raj, "A Novel Information Processing in IoT Based Real Time Health Care Monitoring System", *Journal of Electronics and Informatics*, vol. 2, no. 3, pp. 188-196, 2020.
[http://dx.doi.org/10.36548/jei.2020.3.006]

[67]   A.M. Rahmani, "Smart e-Health Gateway: Bringing intelligence to Internet-of-Things based ubiquitous healthcare systems", *In: 2015 12th Annual IEEE Consumer Communications and Networking Conference, CCNC 2015,* Institute of Electrical and Electronics Engineers Inc., pp. 826-834, 2015.
[http://dx.doi.org/10.1109/CCNC.2015.7158084]

[68]   A. Abugabah, N. Nizamuddin, and A.A. Alzubi, "Decentralized telemedicine framework for a smart healthcare ecosystem", *IEEE Access,* vol. 8, pp. 166575-166588, 2020.
[http://dx.doi.org/10.1109/ACCESS.2020.3021823]

[69]   M. Ferre, E. Batista, A. Solanas, and A. Martínez-Ballesté, "Smart health-enhanced early mobilization in intensive care units", *Sensors (Basel),* vol. 21, no. 16, p. 5408, 2021.
[http://dx.doi.org/10.3390/s21165408] [PMID: 34450850]

[70]   M. Ijaz, G. Li, L. Lin, O. Cheikhrouhou, H. Hamam, and A. Noor, "Integration and applications of fog computing and cloud computing based on the internet of things for provision of healthcare services at home", *Electronics (Basel),* vol. 10, no. 9, p. 1077, 2021.
[http://dx.doi.org/10.3390/electronics10091077]

[71]   Y. Xie, L. Lu, F. Gao, S. He, H. Zhao, Y. Fang, J. Yang, Y. An, Z. Ye, and Z. Dong, "Integration of Artificial Intelligence, Blockchain, and Wearable Technology for Chronic Disease Management: A New Paradigm in Smart Healthcare", *Curr. Med. Sci.*, vol. 41, no. 6, pp. 1123-1133, 2021.

[http://dx.doi.org/10.1007/s11596-021-2485-0] [PMID: 34950987]

[72]   R. Pulimamidi, "Govind, and P. Buddha, "The Future Of Healthcare: Artificial Intelligence 's Role In Smart Hospitals And Wearable", *Health Devices,* 2023.

[73]   M.P. Stiegler, and A. Tung, "Is it quality improvement or is it research?: Ethical and regulatory considerations", *Anesth. Analg.,* vol. 125, no. 1, pp. 342-344, 2017.
[http://dx.doi.org/10.1213/ANE.0000000000001815] [PMID: 28207587]

[74]   R.S. Dokholyan, L.H. Muhlbaier, J.M. Falletta, J.P. Jacobs, D. Shahian, C.K. Haan, and E.D. Peterson, "Regulatory and ethical considerations for linking clinical and administrative databases", *Am. Heart J.,* vol. 157, no. 6, pp. 971-982, 2009.
[http://dx.doi.org/10.1016/j.ahj.2009.03.023] [PMID: 19464406]

[75]   A. Wexler, "The practices of do-it-yourself brain stimulation: implications for ethical considerations and regulatory proposals", *J. Med. Ethics,* vol. 42, no. 4, pp. 211-215, 2016.
[http://dx.doi.org/10.1136/medethics-2015-102704] [PMID: 26324456]

[76]   M.J. Brown, and K.L. Smiler, "Ethical Considerations and Regulatory Issues", In: *The Laboratory Rabbit, Guinea Pig, Hamster, and Other Rodents.* Elsevier, 2012, pp. 3-31.
[http://dx.doi.org/10.1016/B978-0-12-380920-9.00001-8]

[77]   S. D. Mamdiwar, Z. Shakruwala, U. Chadha, K. Srinivasan, and C.-Y. Chang, "Recent advances on IoT-assisted wearable sensor systems for healthcare monitoring", *Biosensors,* vol. 11, no. 10, p. 372, 2021.
[http://dx.doi.org/10.3390/bios11100372]

[78]   O.S. Albahri, A.S. Albahri, K.I. Mohammed, A.A. Zaidan, B.B. Zaidan, M. Hashim, and O.H. Salman, "Systematic Review of Real-time Remote Health Monitoring System in Triage and Priority-Based Sensor Technology: Taxonomy, Open Challenges, Motivation and Recommendations", *J. Med. Syst.,* vol. 42, no. 5, p. 80, 2018.
[http://dx.doi.org/10.1007/s10916-018-0943-4] [PMID: 29564649]

[79]   S. Krishnamoorthy, A. Dua, and S. Gupta, "Role of emerging technologies in future IoT-driven Healthcare 4.0 technologies: a survey, current challenges and future directions", *J. Ambient Intell. Humaniz. Comput.,* vol. 14, no. 1, pp. 361-407, 2023.
[http://dx.doi.org/10.1007/s12652-021-03302-w]

[80]   M. Kumar, "Healthcare Internet of Things (H-IoT): Current Trends, Future Prospects, Applications, Challenges, and Security Issues", *Electronics (Switzerland),* vol. 12, no. 9, 2023.
[http://dx.doi.org/10.3390/electronics12092050]

[81]   A. Gautam, R. Mahajan, and S. Zafar, "Quality of service optimization in Internet of medical things for sustainable management", In: *Studies in Systems, Decision, and Control* vol. 311. Springer, 2021, pp. 163-179.
[http://dx.doi.org/10.1007/978-3-030-55833-8_10]

[82]   K. Shafique, B. A. Khawaja, F. Sabir, S. Qazi, and M. Mustaqim, "Internet of things (IoT) for next-generation smart systems: A review of current challenges, future trends and prospects for emerging 5G-IoT scenarios", In: *IEEE Access* vol. 8. , 2020, pp. 23022-23040.
[http://dx.doi.org/10.1109/ACCESS.2020.2970118]

[83]   F. Al-Turjman, M. H. Nawaz, and U. D. Ulusar, "Intelligence in the Internet of Medical Things era: A systematic review of current and future trends", *Computer Communications,* vol. 150, Elsevier B.V., pp. 644-660, 2020.
[http://dx.doi.org/10.1016/j.comcom.2019.12.030]

CHAPTER 9

Ensuring Dosage Adherence in the Digital Era of IoT and AI

Shaweta Sharma[1], Dimple Singh Tomar[2], Sunita[3], K.K. Yashwanth[4] and Akhil Sharma[5,*]

[1] *School of Medical and Allied Sciences, Galgotias University Plot No. 2, Yamuna Expy, Opposite Buddha International Circuit, Sector 17A, Greater Noida, Uttar Pradesh, India*

[2] *Kharvel Subharti College of Pharmacy, Swami Vivekanand Subharti University, Meerut, India*

[3] *Metro College of Health Sciences and Research, Greater Noida, Uttar Pradesh, India*

[4] *Department of Civil Engineering, Aditya University, Surampalem, India*

[5] *R.J. College of Pharmacy, Raipur, Gharbara, Tappal, Khair, Uttar Pradesh, India*

Abstract: A major issue in healthcare is to guarantee that people take their medication regularly. This leads to non-adherence, which in turn results in health problems, high healthcare expenditure, and reduced quality of life among the patients themselves. In this digital world, a combination of the Internet of Things and Artificial Intelligence creates an opportunity that has never been seen before and can be used to tackle these challenges effectively. In this chapter, we will explore the role of IoT and AI in improving medication compliance by outlining some promising benefits, difficulties faced as well as implications for future practice. The use of IoT enables remote monitoring systems that enable medical practitioners to keep track of when drugs are taken instantaneously and remotely. The wearable devices integrated with the internet of Things can check the life signs and how medicine works, thereby offering vital signs on patient health and adherence patterns. Additionally, smooth interconnection with electronic health records enables information sharing and better care integration. Personalized interventions and predictive analytics serve as an ideal complement to IoT from AI. AI-driven systems provide customized alerts and notifications based on the patient's individual profile, preference, and behavioral pattern. Predictive algorithms analyze massive data in order to recognize adherence tendencies as well as potential risk factors, thereby making it possible for proactive interventions designed to avert non-compliance-related complications. Chatbots that are AI-enabled offer continuous assistance in addressing patients' questions regarding medications. However, the current advent of IoT and AI comes with several obstacles. Patient trust and compliance should be considered when it comes to ethical data protection and privacy. Again, to use them effectively, these technologies must be trained by many healthcare

---

** **Corresponding author Akhil Sharma:** R.J. College of Pharmacy, Raipur, Gharbara, Tappal, Khair, Uttar Pradesh, India; E-mail: xs2akhil@gmail.com

Akhil Sharma, Neeraj Kumar Fuloria, Pankaj Kumar Singh & Shaweta Sharma (Eds.)

experts and patients, and they must be educated adequately on this matter. In addition, regulatory frameworks need to change swiftly in order to incorporate digital healthcare advancements while striking a balance between innovation and patient safety/privacy. Finally, utilizing IoT together with AI can greatly help secure medication adherence in the digital era. Healthcare providers can heal patients faster, reduce medical expenditures, and improve overall care quality by using these abilities further. Embracing innovation and collaboration among various stakeholders in healthcare is essential if we are going to maximize the full potentiality of IoT and AI regarding medication adherence.

Keywords: Adherence, Disease, Dosage, Digital, Health, Healthcare, Medicine, Patient.

INTRODUCTION

Dosage adherence means the extent to which a patient follows properly the prescribed dose instructions for medication, such as the dose amount, frequency, timing, and duration of treatment. This is an important aspect of medicine-taking behavior that needs to be addressed if patients are to take their medications optimally in order to achieve therapeutic goals and improve health outcomes. Not following dosage instructions correctly can lead to lowered clinical benefits, increased healthcare expenses, and may even deteriorate a patient's condition. Thus, dosage adherence is a critical factor for the efficacy of treatment regimens and the overall well-being of the patient [1, 2].

The digital age can be seen as a time when advanced technologies are growing at a very fast rate. Also, this technology is becoming part of every aspect of society, business, and daily life. These two technologies are the Internet of Things and Artificial Intelligence, which have been instrumental in changing this era. The expression "Internet of Things" (IoT) refers to the interconnection *via* the internet of computing devices embedded in everyday objects, enabling them to send and receive data. Consequently, this has resulted in the formation of a vast network that interlinks everything from cellphones, watches, and refrigerators to entire cities [3, 4].

Artificial Intelligence (AI) is a term used to describe machines performing tasks that would usually demand human intelligence to do, like learning, problem-solving, pattern recognition, understanding of natural language, and decision-making. In the IoT, AI can analyze consumer behavior and search data through emails, blogs, and social media platforms on how users connect with their products and services [5].

IoT coupled with AI is a powerful combination that can revolutionize our approach to different domains like digital marketing, healthcare, and transportation. In this regard, businesses can gain access to a wealth of data by capitalizing on the vast number of interconnected devices that comprise the IoT. It is up to AI to make such insights actionable by converting them into data sets, which have an uncanny ability to predict the behavior of consumers and guide their personalization. This blending of IoT with AI will lead to real-time customer engagement, predictive analysis, AI-powered chatbots, and a major focus on data safety, creating a giant leap in the field of digital marketing. In the healthcare sector, IoT devices enable businesses to interact with customers in real-time, thereby providing unique personalized experiences that hold the attention of customers. For instance, fitness trackers collect information about physical activities carried out by a person's sleep patterns, among other health aspects, allowing doctors to give individualized advice or treatment options as required [6, 7].

AI and IoT can boost safety, communication, and data collection in the transportation industry. Some examples of this are adaptive cruise control, self-driving cars, and see-through pillars that the automotive industry is deploying to make automobiles more secure and economical. Society and commerce have been revolutionized by the digital age, as well as IoT and AI, thus bringing personalization, efficiency, and innovation, among others. By using these technologies wisely, businesses can obtain useful information that will enable them to make good choices regarding products or services that suit their customers [8, 9].

Adherence to dosage is a significant aspect of healthcare, as it greatly affects the efficiency of medication and the general health of the patient. Adherence refers to how much a patient follows a treatment plan, including taking medication as prescribed with respect to dose, dosing interval, duration of therapy, and other particular instructions given [10]. Failure to follow medical instructions may be associated with negative consequences such as rates of disease progression, decrease in functional capabilities, poor quality of life, increased utilization of medical resources, and eventually even death. In the US alone, non-adherence causes approximately 125000 deaths annually from cardiovascular diseases; up to 23% of nursing home admissions (10% hospitalization), many doctor visits, laboratory tests, and unnecessary treatments would be avoided if patients took their medications as directed [10, 11].

Adherence is influenced by various factors such as patient attitudes and personal traits, disease features, social situations, access to services, poor communication between healthcare providers and patients, lack of knowledge about a drug and its administration, no belief in the necessity of treatment, dread of the side effects of drugs, prolonged use of drugs, complicated prescriptions with numerous medications that have different dosages, expenses coupled with accessibility difficulties. Healthcare practitioners should measure adherence among their clients' populations. They must face all challenges related to drug resistance in order to make it possible for physicians to develop special strategies [12, 13].

Interventions might include recommending that clients write down their drug-taking, advising patients to watch their health situation, simplifying the dosage instructions, employing alternative packaging for drug administration, using a multi-compartment medicines system, tackling beliefs and worries leading to a decrease in adherence, and overcoming practical challenges connected with non-adherence if identified. Dosing adherence is a vital part of healthcare since it is of great importance to how effective medication is as well as an individual's overall health. Medical practitioners need to consider various factors that can impact patients' adherence in order to identify and address difficulties with drug use among them [14, 15].

CHALLENGES IN TRADITIONAL DOSAGE ADHERENCE

Many problems make it difficult for patients to follow their prescriptions as required by traditional medication adherence. These factors include patient education, forgetfulness, complex drug schedules, and limitations on the capacity of health systems [16].

Lack of patient education is one main reason for medication non-adherence. Patients may not appreciate the reason for their medications, the significance of taking them as prescribed, or understand the repercussions caused by non-compliance. Without an adequate understanding of their health problem and treatment, patients may lack the urge to adhere to their drug regimens. Furthermore, misunderstandings in relation to drugs can result in being hesitant or unwilling to observe medication instructions [17].

Another common problem is forgetfulness in traditional dosing compliance. It can be very hard to remember when and how to take drugs, especially for people who have hectic work schedules or mental confusion. Even after making up one's mind, patients may face problems with integrating drug therapy into their lives or sometimes forget about it. This has repeatedly led to missed doses, poor compliance consistency, and, as a result, compromised treatment outcomes [18].

Adherence efforts are made more challenging by complicated medication regimens. Many patients have multiple concurrent prescriptions for different illnesses. Each drug may be accompanied by its applicable dosage plan, administration guidelines, and side effects. It is difficult for patients to manage many medications at once, leading to mistakes or accidental non-compliance.

Missed doses and accidental overdoses can result from confusion among patients about which drugs to take at what time [19].

Also, the healthcare system's constraints create significant obstacles to medication adherence. Patients' ability to adhere to their prescribed regimens may be hindered by inadequate access to healthcare resources, which include limited appointment availability, prescription refills, and medication affordability. Some difficulties experienced include long waits for appointments, delayed filling of prescriptions, or money problems hindering regular purchase of drugs. Moreover, logistics can prevent compliance with drug prescriptions among some groups of patients, like transportation issues and remoteness from medical facilities [20].

Comprehensive approaches that involve patient education, behavioral interventions, and healthcare system improvements are needed to address these challenges. In addition, healthcare providers need to play an important role in educating patients about their medications, ensuring they understand the importance of adherence, and addressing any concerns or misconceptions. The use of plain language explanations or visual aids can be employed as patient-centered communication strategies that increase understanding among patients and enable them to participate actively in the management of their medications [21].

Behavioral interventions such as pill organizers, medication reminders, and adherence counseling can assist in mitigating forgetfulness among patients by initiating strategies to help them blend their daily activities with drug taking. These interventions can come in technological packages like smartphone apps or automated reminder systems that give timely prompts and backup [22].

Furthermore, medication adherence in healthcare is impeded by structural factors. Some of these include improving access to medical services, making prescription refills a less tedious process, and strategies aimed at cutting down on patients' drug budgets. Finally, it enhances seamless change from one healthcare provider to another. It ensures that the patient has all the resources needed to faithfully adhere to their regimen through improved coordination and communication between healthcare providers, pharmacists, and other stakeholders [23].

Traditional medical adherence practices have numerous challenges that necessitate concerted efforts to overcome. Suppose health providers tackle concerns revolving around patient information, memory loss, intricate therapeutic routines, and limitations in healthcare. In that case, patients will be able to comply with their dose prescriptions, thereby resulting in improved treatment results and quality of life [24, 25].

ROLE OF IOT IN MEDICATION ADHERENCE

Medication adherence in the growth of IoT is very important; it provides new ways to deal with the complications involved in making sure patients take their medication as directed. It does this by using interconnected devices and sensors, which ensure real-time monitoring, data collection, and enhancement of patient-provider relationships. The various ways in which IoT contributes to medication adherence are described below.

Remote Monitoring of Medication Intake by IoT

The use of IoT technology in healthcare is essential for monitoring medication intake and combatting problems related to drug adherence. The strategy entails using connected gadgets and detectors to keep track of patients' consumption of drugs, therefore offering health providers and caregivers informative data [26, 27].

Connected Medication Packaging

Technology has discovered a new thing in the form of connected medication packaging. All this is when an indication on such boxes is read or whenever embedding tags of sensors or RFID within them take off a tablet. Through this, data gets to be sent wirelessly, thereby making it possible to monitor medical intake in real-time. Pharmaceutical smart packaging is an emerging trend in the industry, adding sensing or wireless communication capabilities to improve packaging solutions competitiveness [28, 29].

Additionally, this technology can reduce supply chain losses by improving environmental monitoring, supporting enhanced patient adherence through smart adherence packaging, and augmenting security with anti-tamper or unclonable serialization technologies. In clinical trials, smart packaging may facilitate an ecosystem that interweaves measurement and intervention, creating closed-loop feedback that will enable the optimization of medication efficacy. By connecting such cutting-edge hardware to cutting-edge software, researchers are able to study medication behaviors in depth in order to understand habits, identify problems, and suggest appropriate remedies [30].

Medication adherence is another significant problem in the management of chronic illnesses that smart medication packaging can also improve. Studies have proven that smart electronic packaging and device monitoring have a 97% accuracy rate compared to drug levels and markers (70%), pill counts (60%), healthcare professional ratings (50%), and patient self-reporting (27%). NFC-enabled packages for drugs are also an emerging trend as the technology allows for setting reminders, feeding in precise information about the pills, and keeping track of medicines taken through a smartphone application. This technology can help healthcare providers monitor medication use and prevent unnecessary complications among patients with chronic conditions [26].

Wearable Devices

IoT wearables can also be worn to monitor the intake of medication from a remote location. These devices could have attributes such as medicine reminders and the capacity to track them, enabling patients to input when they took their drugs straight from their wearable IoT device. They collected data that may be synchronized with a phone app or cloud-based platform for analysis by healthcare professionals [31, 32]. Various wearable IoT devices are used in remote monitoring of medication intake, which is described below and shown in Fig. (**1**).

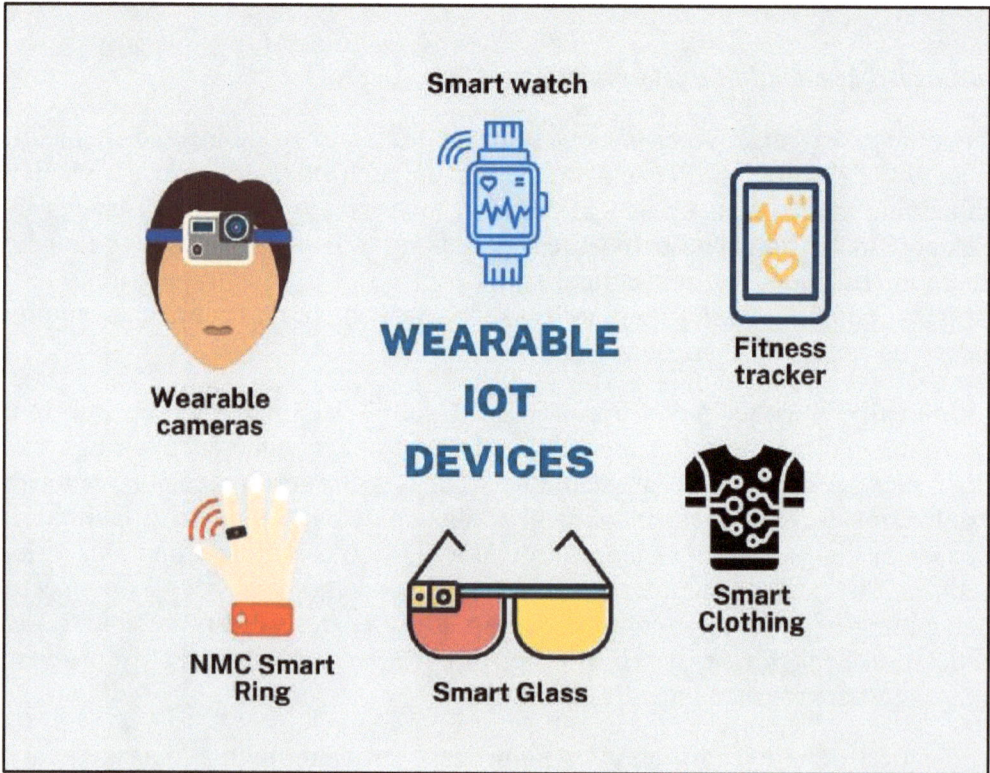

Fig. (1). Wearable IoT devices used in remote monitoring of medication intake.

Smart Watches

Beyond timekeeping, wearable IoT devices are popular, and one of them is smart watches. A digital display is integrated into these devices. They do not only measure physical activities but also keep tabs on heart rates plus sleep rhythms with notifications from smartphones. Likewise, they can operate diverse applications such as fitness tracking, navigation through GPS, communication, and many others. Majorly smart watches track physical activity so that individuals can keep track of their steps taken, distance covered, and calories burnt in a whole day, for instance. Further, smart watches can constantly monitor heart rate, which plays a vital role in determining how good or bad one's cardiovascular fitness is. In addition to that, they can evaluate sleeping patterns, which will eventually help people improve their quality of sleep and obtain more hours of sleep [33].

smart watches are a supplement to smartphones, allowing users to get notifications on calls, text messages, emails, and app alerts directly on their wrists. Notifications from cell phones can, therefore, be received through smart watches, leading to improved user convenience. Some smart watches are fitness trackers; hence, they support apps such as heart rate monitors, which help in tracking the health conditions of individuals who undertake physical exercises. In other words, they are multifunctional gadgets that do the work of the traditional watch plus more advanced features that meet today's lifestyle demands. They have become essential tools for individuals looking to stay connected, track their health and fitness goals, and enhance their overall well-being conveniently and efficiently [34].

Fitness Trackers

Wearable devices, known as activity trackers, fitness bands, or fitness trackers, have been designed specifically to monitor physical activities and exercise. These gadgets are usually fitted with accelerometers that sense movements such as steps taken, distance covered, and calories burnt. In addition to heart rate monitors, some of them come with GPSs as well as other sensors for more detailed information about your activities. In recent years, the popularity of fitness trackers has increased, which means there are now many different types available for purchase. The leading examples of top-rated fitness trackers include the Garmin Venu 3S, Fitbit Charge 6, Apple Watch Series 9, and Fitbit Versa 4 Some features that they offer include GPS tracking, heart rate monitoring, sleep tracking, among others, even blood oxygen level monitoring, *etc* [35, 36].

Fitness trackers help set physical activity milestones and then attain them, helping the user achieve fitness goals such as walking a specific number of times per day or exercising for some time weekly. On the other hand, various fitness trackers contain reminders that alert one to stand up or move around after a long period of being stagnant and socializing tools to motivate and encourage friends and family to stay fit. Amongst other factors, price, features, and compatibility with various devices should be considered when selecting a fitness tracker. Some brands have more expensive gadgets than others; however, they offer more progressive options and better tracking precision. Compatibility of this device with your smartphone or other gadgets is also important, as is the quality of its accompanying software/app [37, 38].

Smart Clothing

The technology of the Internet of Things (IoT) has been incorporated into smart clothing. These can detect and provide information on how users perform different activities, the way they sit or stand, and their biological characteristics. Underneath the fabric or in certain parts of a garment, one may find integrated sensors. In general, smart clothes are employed in monitoring sports performance, postural alignment, and care for chronic illness patients [39].

Smart clothing is becoming more popular due to its potential to change our lifestyles regarding health and fitness tracking. For instance, according to Butler Technologies's report, smart clothing represents a new wave in wearable technology that tracks users' movements while sleeping, health parameters (*e.g.*, heart rate, temperature), sleep patterns, activity levels, *etc.* It can also control devices like smartphones with augmented reality features as well as navigate through new environments. Additionally, it can send messages *via* voice or text, just like ordinary phones [40].

Smart clothing refers to wearable technology that encompasses IoT technology in clothing, enabling them to gather wearer's movement data attitudes, and one such smart clothing is the Levi's Commuter x Jacquard Jacket, which is the first-ever jacquard fabric with conductive fibers. Thus, when you put it on and your phone is inside, it automatically knows and begins connecting as well. You can control your music, pick up calls, and interact with Google Assistant without having to remove the phone from your pocket. Sensoria Fitness Socks are another example of smart wearables that monitor physical activities and track heart rate as well as sleep patterns. The socks have an embedded sensor for measuring pulse rate, which is then wirelessly transmitted over Bluetooth to a smartphone. Users can thus keep track of how much they sweat during each exercise and how their body responds to different training loads [41].

Smart clothes can be used in healthcare monitoring for patients suffering from chronic diseases, too. This includes Neviano Swimwear for women, such as a GPS tracker that can be used to locate the child. This is inclusive of a panic button that sends messages to the parents once they feel threatened. The hat also comes with an emergency SOS call feature; this will alert anyone when something goes wrong with their kid. It is printed electronics that make smart clothing possible by allowing for electronic components like biometric sensors and flexible heaters to be printed onto wafer-thin substrates that flex and stretch along with the garment itself. These electronic components add almost nothing to the weight of the clothing so users find it extremely comfortable and convenient [42, 43].

Smartglasses

IoT wearable glasses are a sort of smart device that can give information about different aspects of the user's activities, such as burnt calories, heart rate, navigation, and exercise duration. Some models also have camera lenses for taking photos or recording videos and can have augmented reality features. They are like ordinary glasses as they are put on but have additional facilities that make them applicable to different situations [44].

Smart glasses are basically a type of computer with the ability to help people perform certain tasks. In most cases, they contain displays that augment information along with what the wearers see Direct View Optics (DVO), which may be implemented in an Optical Head-Mounted Display (OHMD) or embedded into the glass lens of the eye-wear. Other categories of smart glasses have the property of changing their optical specifications, such as programmed sunglasses made to tint by using electricity [45].

Smart glasses are versatile and can be utilized for different reasons, such as sports performance monitoring, posture correction, and healthcare management of patients with chronic ailments. They also serve as navigators by providing maps and current coordinates to the persons concerned. Some smart glasses models also have full lifelogging or activity tracker capabilities that make them suitable for fitness and health tracking [46].

Moreover, some smart glasses models include built-in camera lenses used for taking photos or shooting videos. These cameras can be used in different ways, such as storing memories, recording events, or even broadcasting live on the internet. Additionally, certain smart glasses models have augmented reality features that overlay digital information on users' fields of view [47].

Even though they are relatively new gadgets in the market, these smart glasses offer great potential to transform our interactions with the real world. This is because they possess a unique blend of being functional while being convenient, thus making them beneficial devices for a variety of uses. The technology will advance further, thereby creating more innovative and practical applications for the use of smart glass in the future [48].

NFC Smart Ring

The NFC Smart Ring is a wearable gadget that replaces credit cards, metro cards, and house and car keys using Near Field Communication (NFC) technology. This technology enables users to pay bills, use metro ticketing, unlock doors, and make phone calls. A unique fingerprint scanner is built into the ring, making it safer and more personalised. The NFC Smart Ring is an easy and convenient payment method that lets users pay quickly and securely without any requirement of carrying a plastic card or cash around. In addition to this, it has been designed in such a way that it can withstand water scratches as well as being hypoallergenic, therefore ensuring durability and comfort while being worn [49].

The NFC Smart Ring can function with many different gadgets like smartphones, door locks, and payment terminals. In addition to that, it can share Wi-Fi information, links to websites, and contact information, amongst others. This ring does not need recharging and is therefore convenient for those who want to have a simple life. Besides, the ring can be set to launch apps with particular settings, increasing its performance in different ways. The NFC Smart Ring may transform payment methods and how we interact with our devices as a whole [50].

Wearable Cameras

Devices like wearable cameras allow individuals to take pictures and record videos from their point of view while these are being worn on them. These items are mostly used in such areas as sports and outdoor activities for unmanned documentation of adventures or actions. Additionally, wearable cameras can be utilized within industries like healthcare law enforcement where first-person video is of importance. In a healthcare setting, wearable cameras have been used to gather rich contextual data and provide insights into everyday activities that assist with recall and reminiscence. In one pilot study, the feasibility of using a wearable camera to assess self-care among individuals with heart failure was investigated; these were found feasible and appropriate. Research showed that wearable cameras could capture dieting habits, exercise choices, and occupational sitting time, among other health-related behavioral risk factors. Information obtained from wearable cameras can be employed in addition to other methods of collecting traditional data, such as survey questionnaires [51].

The use of wearable cameras in this field has been documented to provide insights into self-management among people with chronic diseases. Literature review showed that wearable cameras have mainly been employed to record diet, physical activities, daily routines, and stationary behavior. Most studies addressed technical problems or ethical dilemmas arising from the use of wearable cameras, which were taken care of. Additionally, wearable cameras have found application in other sectors, such as police, where they have recorded events and obtained crucial evidence. Furthermore, they can be used either for personal security or to alert the security personnel when necessary. These can serve as an accurate and objective log through the wide range of incidents met by the wearer, ensuring that there is enough information for investigations, thereby safeguarding the patients. This also helps prevent false claims burdening individuals with accused allegations leading to legal suits on hospitals [52].

In healthcare procedures, wearable camera footage can also be useful for training and education, while the practice of real-life scenarios improves staff skills and knowledge leads to better performance, increased efficiency, and improved patient care. In fields such as healthcare, law enforcement, and sports, this offers a new purpose as wearable cameras. For everyday activities, they provide rich contextual data and insights that help in memory recall: health-related behaviors are captured by wearable cameras, importantly through which risk factors may be documented. The self-management of chronic disease can be better understood from the perspective of wearable cameras. Their investigation will protect both patients against false allegations against wearers or organizations making unwarranted claims due to liability [53].

Mobile Apps

Mobile applications enabled by the internet of Things could be used as a handy tool to monitor the remote medication consumption for patients. They come with capabilities such as a pill clock, a book that shows skipped and confirmed doses, a system that can be adjusted to suit different schedules of medicine intake, tracking tablets, dose measurements, activities, and mood, personalized treatment tips, and extensive tests for all cases. Additionally, several programs will enable drug interaction alerts, a health diary, and the sharing of records with physicians [54, 55].

Diabetes, multiple sclerosis, psoriasis, rheumatoid arthritis, anxiety, depression, hypertension, plus many others are some of the conditions these apps are designed to manage. Equally important is their ability to send reminders for refill times as well as scheduled clinic visits and offer email reporting facilities to doctors. Other features that may be present in such applications include but are not limited to mood tracker, weight tracker, blood pressure log, and health diary, which help patients and doctors see how successful treatment has been [56, 57].

Integration with Electronic Health Records (EHR)

IoT technology can be used to optimize health care through integration with EHR with a specific focus on medication management and adherence. Through the integration of EHR, there is enhanced communication and data sharing among IoT devices, health care providers, as well as electronic health record systems, which in turn promotes holistic patient care and therapy coordination [58, 59]. The role of EHR in the enhancement of medication management is described below and summarized in Fig. (2).

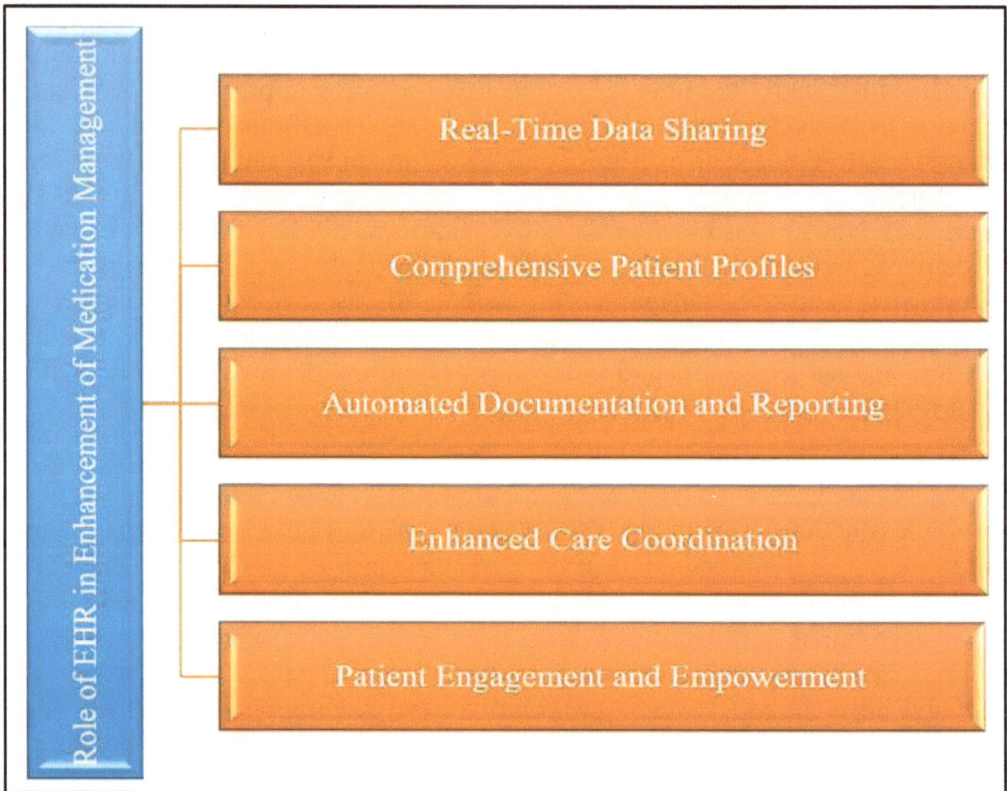

Fig. (2). Role of EHR in enhancement of medication management.

Real-Time Data Sharing

Valuable information about the consumption of drugs, vital statistics, and behavioral characteristics of patients can be collected using IoT gadgets such as smart pill dispensers and wearable health monitors. This happens through integration with EHR, where such data can be sent in real-time to the electronic health record maintained for a patient. It allows medical care providers to access updated data concerning the intake of medicines or development during consultations with patients or even from a distance at any given time [60].

Comprehensive Patient Profiles

Having electronic health records informed by IoT data enables healthcare givers to have a better understanding of the patient's medication past, adherence patterns as well as well-being. With this in mind, the providers can make well-informed decisions when it comes to drug adjustment and treatment plans as well as interventions that cater to a person's personalized requirements [61].

Automated Documentation and Reporting

When it comes to integrating with EHR, the process of streamlining documentation activities becomes automatic, and that will be through a process where the medication adherence information is directly fed into a patient's electronic health record. It reduces the pressure on healthcare givers and eliminates the need for manual data keying, thereby resulting in precise and complete medication records. Furthermore, IoT-generated data can be used to create quality improvement programs as well as reports and analytics for research purposes [62, 63].

Enhanced Care Coordination

The use of EHR systems in healthcare can enhance communication and collaboration between the patient's care providers, including doctors in primary care settings, specialists, druggists, and people caring for him. This coordination is essential in preventing non-adherence or addressing medication non-adherence issues at the right time [64].

Patient Engagement and Empowerment

Medication adherence data can also be accessed by patients *via* patient portals or mobile apps integrated with electronic health records, which enhance patient empowerment and engagement by letting individuals become active participators in their treatment plans, monitor their progress, and communicate more effectively with their healthcare team [65].

Seamless communication, comprehensive data sharing, and collaborative care coordination across the entire healthcare ecosystem are done through integration with EHR. Healthcare providers can leverage IoT technology along with EHR systems to optimize medication therapy, improve patient outcomes, and therefore enhance care delivery quality [66].

ROLE OF AI IN MEDICATION ADHERENCE

The role of AI in medication adherence is a revolutionary one. It brings with it innovative approaches to tackling the myriad challenges involved in ensuring that patients take their medication as recommended. In order to enhance drug compliance and patient outcomes, AI systems employ data analysis algorithms plus machine learning techniques for behavior forecasting and personalized interventions [67].

Personalized Reminders and Notifications

In modern healthcare technology, personalized reminders and notifications are the mainstay of everyday operations as they supply bespoke help to individuals who need assistance in keeping to prescribed medication regimens. Such frameworks can use advanced algorithms and AI to analyze individual patient data, including medication schedules, preferences, and adherence history, so as to send reminders and alerts that meet each patient's unique requirements. Personalized reminders know the subtleties of patient behavior and medication management patterns; thus, patients get notifications in line with their daily habits and inclinations [68].

The reminders may be customized by preferred timing, frequency, and mode of communication, like text messages, emails, mobile app notifications, and automated phone calls, among others. Moreover, adaptive scheduling features ensure that reminders can adapt dynamically to changes in a patient's medication regimen or routine so as to ensure continuity of support. Another approach is a contextual reminder, which considers factors including; patient location, activity level, and current health situation, thereby delivering notifications at the best time possible to ensure adherence. These interactive feedback mechanisms also provide a platform through which patients can confirm that they have taken their drugs on time or give any other responses directly *via* the reminder interface, leading to more engagement and accountability [69].

Predictive Analytics for Identifying Adherence Patterns

In healthcare, predictive analytics is an important tool, especially in medication adherence, by predicting patient behavior through data insights. It can accurately forecast the future behavior of patients and detect their pattern of adherence using its knowledge from past data containing medical history. This big data system provides historical information about previous cases related to drug-taking compliance, patient's demographics, as well as the background of certain diseases all, are used to identify conformity indicators that could explain the variations in drug-taking patterns. These analyses reveal what makes some patients adhere to their medications and others not, leading to a proactive response from healthcare givers toward potential non-compliance issues [70].

Predictive analytics's primary contribution is its ability to trace trends in adherence over time. Predictive models can identify patterns of fluctuation in adherence, the varying rates of medication intake seen among different patient populations, and the reasons why some patients adhere while others do not through examining historical records on adherence. This information helps find a better understanding of the complexities of medication administration and supports the development of focused interventions geared toward individual patient needs [71].

Predictive analytics also enables risk stratification by sorting patients into different groups depending on their probability of non-adherence. Risk scores for each patient help prioritize between healthcare provider interventions and resource allocation for better targeting of those at higher risk of non-adherence. In so doing, health systems focus their intervention efforts optimally and maximize the impact of adherence strategies on patients' outcomes [72].

Additionally, predictive analytics acts as an early warning system to identify patients with at-risk behaviors before problems become serious. Thus, predictive models help healthcare providers quickly detect when people begin deviating from their usual ways and what might happen if they continue along such paths. The idea here is that when non-adherence is identified early enough, it is possible to intervene through personalized reminders, educational interventions, or support programs that target underlying obstacles to adherence and promote behavior change [68].

Behavior Analysis and Intervention

Medication adherence management revolves around behavior analysis and intervention, which are founded on data insights and personalized strategies. In this regard, behavior analysis entails the systematic study of patient behaviors, preferences, and patterns of adherence to determine factors that hinder compliance with medication schedules among others, as well as develop relevant interventions.

Healthcare providers comprehend the complex interactions between medication adherence through the examination of factors such as drug-taking habits, lifestyle variables, socio-economic status, and health beliefs. With the employment of advanced algorithms and machine learning techniques, behavior analysis identifies trends and connections in patients' data, thereby allowing healthcare professionals to develop customized interventions targeting specific barriers to adherence or any other challenge that could affect a positive outcome for their patients [73].

Behavior analysis is fundamental to designing personalized intervention strategies that encourage drug intake. Healthcare providers can develop specific intercessions customized to the needs and wants of each patient once they understand what factors cause non-adherence. These could be personalized reminders and notifications, teaching materials, encouragement from health personnel, or even others, which are tailored to address particular barriers against taking medication as prescribed and consequently empower patients on how to handle their medications. Behavior analysis also assists in guiding the choice of methods for intervention as well as when and how often it should be done to ensure that interventions made suit the patient's goals, aspirations, and change readiness [74].

Behavior analysis has made the most significant contributions to medicine adherence by showing factors that can be changed and thus being able to give interventions that focus on behavior changes. Additionally, behavior analysis allows healthcare workers to conduct interventions aimed at reducing or eliminating barriers to medication adherence, such as a lack of understanding about the importance of medication adherence, forgetfulness, and medication side effects. For instance, educational interventions for patients who are experiencing side effects from their medications or switching them to alternative drugs with fewer adverse effects may be helpful in such situations [75].

Additionally, behavior analysis helps in coming up with flexible remedies that adapt to the changing behaviors of patients. By monitoring how patients respond and adhere to treatment plans over time, healthcare providers can modify their intervention strategies such as therapy intensities medications or introduce new forms of interventions depending on what would work better for the client. Hence, this iterative process of refining the intervention treatments makes sure that these interventions are always pertinent, efficient, and responsive to the changing patient requirements and challenges [76].

Additionally, the use of behavior analysis in health care helps identify patients who are more likely to be non-adherents and, hence intervene earlier to avert adherence-related complications. Consequently, by categorizing patients into different risk groups based on their probability of non-adherence, providers can make better use of limited resources by focusing interventions on those with the greatest need. Such an approach will ensure effective intervention because it concentrates efforts upon those who would most benefit from it, thereby enhancing the impact of adherence interventions on patient outcomes [77].

Medication adherence management requires behavior analysis and intervention, which are crucial in identifying what patients do, addressing barriers to adherence, and developing targeted interventions to enhance medication compliance. With data-driven insights, healthcare providers can individualize interventions based on the needs and preferences of each patient, thus equipping them with the necessary tools to manage their medications efficiently, resulting in enhanced rates of adherence and better patient outcomes. In order to promote medication adherence and improve patient well-being using personalized approaches to medication adherence management by healthcare institutions, behavior analysis and intervention will always be needed [73].

Chatbots for Answering Medication-Related Queries

AI-powered virtual assistant chatbots are known for providing patients with prompt and personalized medication-related information *via* round-the-clock interactive platforms. They enable patients to seek advice, inquire about their medication, or find support on drug-taking procedures. Unlike healthcare providers who may not be available all the time and still offer a solution within 24-hour access to pharmaceutical information or help whenever a patient urgently needs it. By using complex algorithms and having natural language processing skills at their disposal, these chatbots can grasp queries asked by patients in real time and provide relevant answers that suit users' preferences based on accurate data provided [78].

The principal advantage of chatbots is that they can give customized responses to drug-associated questions using personal patient data. By examining patients' age, sex, medication history, adherence patterns, and preferences, chatbots help guide and support them through their medication routines. Whether it is about dosage, side effects, or how to take it, medicine chat-bots offer customer-centralized answers that enable the patients to make choices about their therapy and medication management in an informed manner [79].

Moreover, chatbots work as educational resources, enabling even patients to obtain a comprehensive understanding of their medications. Chatbots educate patients *via* interactive dialogue and multimedia content on the purpose of the medication, how to use it properly, possible side effects, and why they should be taken. Patients can get appropriate information from chatbots that are reliable and easy to get through they understand well about their healthcare needs for drug therapy [80].

Furthermore, medication reminder functions of chatbots can be helpful for notifying and reminding patient when to take their medication at the right time. The reminder feature in the chatbot helps to keep patients on track with their doses of medicine and reduces the chances of missing drugs. Reminders can be sent through SMS, electronic mail, mobile applications, or automated phone calls, thus allowing patients to choose a medium that best suits them based on their preferences [81].

In addition to this, chatbots provide help with medication management by advising patients on their medication organization, storage, and refilling. Patients can receive messages about how to store drugs correctly, what should be done in case they forget to take a dose, how prescriptions can be re-ordered, and how medical appointments might be managed. By giving patients practical advice and support, chatbots enable them to handle the challenge of drug administration more effectively, thus allowing them to adhere to the prescribed doses as strictly as possible [82].

Moreover, chatbots facilitate interactive engagement, allowing patients to ask questions, seek clarification, and express concerns about their medications. Through conversational interactions, chatbots foster patient engagement and encourage active participation in their treatment plans, ultimately promoting medication adherence and patient empowerment [83].

There are several ways through which a chatbot can support a patient with regard to their drugs. This is with the help of AI technology employed in the bots for purposes of enhancing medication management that involves client education on the same as well as adherence mechanisms. For this reason, among others discussed above, it can be stated that chatbots will continue to be an essential tool in facilitating proper drug administration by patients, thereby helping them achieve better health outcomes [84].

Adverse Event Detection and Prevention

Healthcare requires constant monitoring and intervention in order to avoid any untoward incident, and AI is a great tool for achieving this. Hospitals are able to detect earlier when patients get at risk of getting problems that are related to the medication they take by the use of artificial intelligence algorithms together with advanced analytics that can scrutinize massive datasets incorporating things like medication adherence records, health device data, and reports on adverse events. What makes AI useful is the ability to go through substantial amounts of raw information fast enough while at the same time determining connections, which essentially signifies an adverse incident [85].

A proactive surveillance mechanism, artificial intelligence detects deviations from expected norms, as well as identifies patterns that could be associated with an adverse reaction or complication; it keeps monitoring patient health metrics along with medication adherence data and looks for minute changes that might signify drug-induced complications or early warning signs of a drug reaction. Healthcare providers can intervene early enough to prevent adverse outcomes through early detection. Moreover, AI predictive analytics models powered by AI predict the probability of occurrence of these adverse events based on individual risk profiles made up of patient characteristics and medication profiles, among many other factors [86].

The use of predictive models to stratify patients into risk categories and score them allows healthcare providers to prioritize interventions and allocate resources more efficiently, as they concentrate on high-risk patients likely to have adverse events. AI's role in adverse event detection and prevention is reinforced by its real-time monitoring and surveillance functionalities, which help healthcare givers monitor drug-related adverse events across patient populations in real-time. Through data aggregation from multiple sources and the application of machine learning algorithms, AI systems can identify emerging trends or patterns suggestive of adverse events necessitating immediate responses or focused interventions [87].

The potential of AI is maximized by integration with clinical decision support systems, which provide real-time guidance and recommendations to healthcare providers during patient care encounters. By incorporating evidence-based guidelines, best practices, and alerts for potential medication-related risks, AI-driven decision support systems help healthcare providers make informed decisions and prevent adverse events during medication prescribing, administration, and monitoring. Also, these programs can identify potential medication errors or drug interactions that may lead to serious complications [88].

These systems generate alerts and warnings by analyzing medication orders, patient profiles, and clinical data to make healthcare providers aware of potential risks and improve safer medication management practices. Furthermore, artificial intelligence automates adverse event reporting and surveillance processes to enable the identification, documentation, and reporting of medication-related adverse events. AI systems analyze adverse event reports, among other data sources, such as electronic health records, to note patterns in the occurrence of such incidents that help in instituting focused interventions and quality improvement initiatives within healthcare organizations [89].

AI uses data-driven insights, predictive analytics, real-time monitoring, and decision-support capabilities to improve the detection of adverse events and their prevention. AI also contributes to medication safety, healthcare quality, and patient outcomes by providing timely information and actionable insights to empower healthcare providers. As AI technology keeps improving, its significance in detecting and preventing adverse events will be more important for ensuring patient safety as well as optimizing medication management practices [90].

Drawbacks of IoT and AI in Medication Adherence

While AI and IoT offer promising solutions for improving medication adherence, several drawbacks and challenges must be addressed to maximize their effectiveness and ensure patient safety, as summarized in Table **1**.

Table 1. Drawbacks of IoT and AI in medication adherence.

Drawback	Description
Privacy and Security Concerns	The gathering and transmission of IoT devices and AI systems have also been linked to privacy issues and vulnerabilities, including the possibility of data breaches [91].
Reliability and Accuracy	Algorithms of AI and IoT devices can be responsible for mistakes or inaccuracies that may lead to wrong medicine reminders, false adherence monitoring, or mistaken interventions [92].
Digital Divide and Accessibility	Healthcare disparities may worsen if AI and IoT solutions are not utilized by individuals who do not possess smartphones, digital literacy skills, or reliable internet connection [93].
Integration Challenges	Integrating AI and IoT solutions can be difficult in existing health facilities because they may not be compatible with one another, have data integration problems, or interoperability issues [94].
Ethical Considerations	Patient autonomy, consent, algorithmic bias, and equitable healthcare access – are the ethical questions raised by AI and IoT that need transparent and ethical deployment strategies [95].
Cost and Resource Constraints	The requisite investment in technology infrastructure, staff training, and ongoing maintenance is enormous when it comes to deploying IoT and AI solutions for medication adherence [96].
Patient Acceptance and Engagement	The success of AI and IoT adoption is dependent on patient acceptance and engagement, which can be affected by resistance to technology-driven interventions or desire for human interaction [97].

The limitations of these platforms emphasize the need to handle privacy issues, guaranteeing reliability and correctness, diminishing the digital divide, eradicating biases in integration, legal ramifications and ethical concerns, and cost management while encouraging patients' acceptance and involvement, enabling the realization of maximum benefits through AI and IoT aiding adherence to medication [98].

BENEFITS OF IOT AND AI IN IMPROVING MEDICATION ADHERENCE

IoT and AI technologies offer a multitude of benefits in improving medication adherence, which are discussed below and summarized in Fig. (**3**).

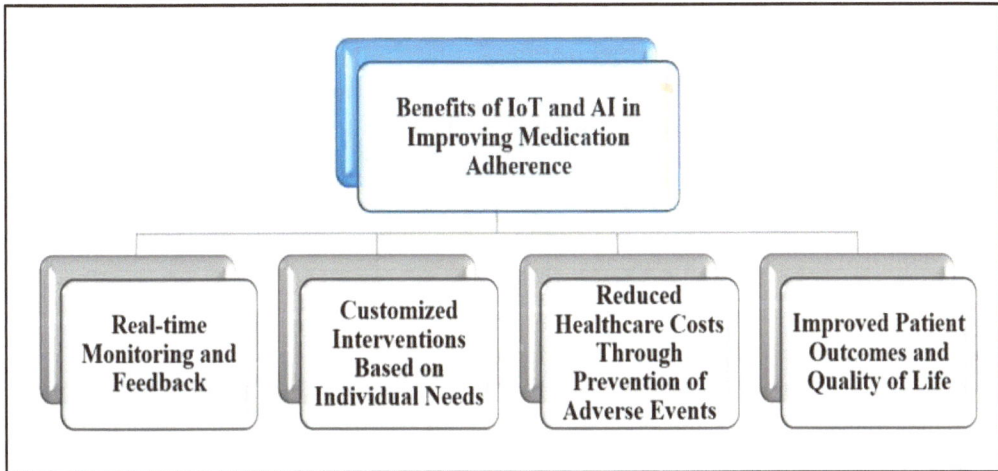

Fig. (3). Benefits of IoT and AI in improving medication adherence.

FUTURE DIRECTIONS AND INNOVATIONS

The future of medication adherence management is set to change healthcare delivery and improve patient outcomes. With more accurate projections about the adherence patterns in AI, and even data analytics, it will be possible for health care providers to intervene proactively and personalise interventions according to individual needs of patients. Personalized medicine approaches which involve genomics as well as pharmacogenomics will tailor medications to fit the respective genetic profiles of a patient thereby optimizing their effectiveness while at the same time minimizing their side effects [99].

Such developments are vital because they allow virtual support and interventions from any place globally, which makes telemedicine and remote monitoring technologies relevant to real-time communication between patients and healthcare providers. In this case, other digital therapeutics alongside behavioral interventions such as mobile health apps together with gamification strategies nurture patients through their treatment plans by reinforcing compliant behaviors throughout, as well as addressing psychological barriers that would deter them from adhering to medication accordingly. Additionally, blockchain technology will be vital in enhancing data security as well as integrity, thus ensuring the provision of tamper-proof records concerning medicinal adherence data while still facilitating the safe sharing of data over healthcare networks across all levels [100].

AR (Augmented Reality) and VR (Virtual Reality) technology will revolutionize patient education regarding drug administration techniques, making them more interactive so that patients can understand how to adhere better. Various smart packaging solutions, including innovative drug delivery systems, adopt IoT sensors together with RFID technologies that help monitor patients' usage of drugs so that reminders improve compliance while improving therapeutic results. By doing so, these innovations play a critical role in driving prospects related to medication adherence management, especially when we take into consideration that collaborative efforts amongst researchers, policymakers, innovators, and technology developers, among others, are enhanced, ultimately resulting in improved patient health status [101].

CONCLUSION

In conclusion, the era of the Internet of Things and Artificial intelligence is an unprecedented opportunity for enhancing medication adherence and improving patient outcomes. Through the utilization of modern technologies, which include IoT devices, AI algorithms, and big data analytics, healthcare practitioners can now monitor drug intake in real-time, predict adherence trends, and tailor interventions to meet individual needs. These developments allow proactive management of drug adherence, thereby leading to improved control of diseases, reduced costs related to medical care, and better life quality among patients with chronic illnesses. However, addressing ethical issues like patient confidentiality, protection of data, and fairness in AI algorithms is necessary for the appropriate and justifiable deployment of these technologies. Furthermore, this includes stakeholders such as providers/payers/ regulators/ tech developers all coming together to move innovation forward so that we can realize IoT & AI's huge potential in relation to medication adherence management. Therefore, embracing opportunities offered by the digital era can change health service delivery at all levels, empowering patients and thus improving well-being globally.

ACKNOWLEDGEMENTS

Authors are highly thankful to their Universities/Colleges for providing library facilities for the literature survey.

REFERENCES

[1]   J. Koerner and M. Bates, "Improving Medication Adherence and Clinical Outcomes Through Connected Drug Delivery Devices," *ONdrugDelivery*, Issue 155, pp. 16–20, Dec. 2023. [Online]. Available: https://www.ondrugdelivery.com/improving-medication-adherence-and-clinical-out-omes-through-connected-drug-delivery-devices/

[2]   B. Jimmy and J. Jose, "Patient medication adherence: Measures in daily practice," *Oman Med. J.*, vol. 26, no. 3, pp. 155–159, May 2011.
[http://dx.doi.org/10.5001/omj.2011.38]

[3]   J. Cleland-Huang, O. C. Z. Gotel, J. H. Hayes, P. Mäder, and A. Zisman, "Software traceability: Trends and future directions," *ACM Comput. Surv.*, vol. 47, no. 2, pp. 1-28, Apr. 2015.
[http://dx.doi.org/10.1145/2593882.2593891]

[4]   M. T. Brown and J. K. Bussell, "Medication adherence: WHO cares?," *Mayo Clin. Proc.*, vol. 86, no. 4, pp. 304–314, Apr. 2011.
[http://dx.doi.org/10.4065/mcp.2010.0575]

[5]   J. Bourbeau and S. J. Bartlett, "Patient adherence in COPD," *Thorax*, vol. 63, no. 9, pp. 831–838, Sep. 2008.
[http://dx.doi.org/10.1136/thx.2007.086041]

[6]   Y. Xu, "Artificial intelligence: A powerful paradigm for scientific research," *Xiv International*, vol. 6, no. 4, pp. 100179, 2021.
[http://dx.doi.org/10.1016/j.xinn.2021.100179]

[7]   I. Ullah, D. Adhikari, X. Su, F. Palmieri, C. Wu, and C. Choi, "Integration of data science with the intelligent IoT (IIoT): current challenges and future perspectives", *Digit. Commun. Netw.,* no. Mar, 2024.
[http://dx.doi.org/10.1016/j.dcan.2024.02.007]

[8]   A. Ullah, S.M. Anwar, J. Li, L. Nadeem, T. Mahmood, A. Rehman, and T. Saba, "Smart cities: the role of Internet of Things and machine learning in realizing a data-centric smart environment", *Complex Intell. Syst.,* vol. 10, no. 1, pp. 1607-1637, 2024.
[http://dx.doi.org/10.1007/s40747-023-01175-4]

[9]   H. Allioui and Y. Mourdi, "Exploring the full potentials of IoT for better financial growth and stability: A comprehensive survey," *Sensors*, vol. 23, no. 19, p. 8015, Sep. 2023.
[http://dx.doi.org/10.3390/s23198015]

[10]   B. Chander, S. Pal, D. De, and R. Buyya, "Artificial intelligence-based Internet of Things for Industry 5.0," in *Recent Advances in Artificial Intelligence and Communication Technologies*, Springer, 2021, pp. 1-16.
[http://dx.doi.org/10.1007/978-3-030-87059-1_1]

[11]   S. Pandya, "A study of the recent trends of immunology: Key challenges, domains, applications, datasets, and future directions," *Sensors*, vol. 21, no. 23, p. 7786, Dec. 2021.
[http://dx.doi.org/10.3390/s21237786]

[12]   D. Jacobs and M. Brewer. APA Practice Guideline Provides Recommendations for Assessing and Treating Patients With Suicidal Behaviors. *Psychiatric Annals.* vol. 34, no. 5, pp. 373-380, 2004.
[http://dx.doi.org/10.3928/0048-5713-20040501-18]

[13]   E. Fenta, B. Ayal, A. Kidie, T. Anagaw, T. Mekonnen, E. Ketema Bogale, S. Berihun, T.D. Tsega, C. Mengistie Munie, T. Talie Fenta, N. Kassie Worku, S. Shiferaw Gelaw, and M.G. Tiruneh, "Barriers to Medication Adherence Among Patients with Non-Communicable Disease in North Wollo Zone Public Hospitals: Socio-Ecologic Perspective, 2023", *Patient Prefer. Adherence,* vol. 18, pp. 733-744, 2024.
[http://dx.doi.org/10.2147/PPA.S452196] [PMID: 38533490]

[14]   P. Kardas, P. Lewek, and M. Matyjaszczyk, "Determinants of patient adherence: a review of systematic reviews", *Front. Pharmacol.,* vol. 4, no. JUL, p. 91, 2013.
[http://dx.doi.org/10.3389/fphar.2013.00091] [PMID: 23898295]

[15]   K. Kvarnström, A. Westerholm, M. Airaksinen, and H. Liira, "Factors contributing to medication adherence in patients with a chronic condition: A scoping review of qualitative research," *Pharmaceutics*, vol. 13, no. 7, p. 1100, Jul. 2021.

[http://dx.doi.org/10.3390/pharmaceutics13071100]

[16] T.F. Blaschke, L. Osterberg, B. Vrijens, and J. Urquhart, "Adherence to medications: insights arising from studies on the unreliable link between prescribed and actual drug dosing histories", *Annu. Rev. Pharmacol. Toxicol.,* vol. 52, no. 1, pp. 275-301, 2012.
[http://dx.doi.org/10.1146/annurev-pharmtox-011711-113247] [PMID: 21942628]

[17] C.M. Fairman, T.S. Nilsen, R.U. Newton, D.R. Taaffe, N. Spry, D. Joseph, S.K. Chambers, Z.P. Robinson, N.H. Hart, M.C. Zourdos, B.C. Focht, C.J. Peddle-McIntyre, and D.A. Galvão, "Reporting of Resistance Training Dose, Adherence, and Tolerance in Exercise Oncology", *Med. Sci. Sports Exerc.,* vol. 52, no. 2, pp. 315-322, 2020.
[http://dx.doi.org/10.1249/MSS.0000000000002127] [PMID: 31436734]

[18] F. Chappell, "Medication adherence in children remains a challenge," *Prescriber,* vol. 26, no. 12, pp. 31–34, Jun. 2015.

[19] S. A. Iacob, D. G. Iacob, and G. Jugulete, "Improving the adherence to antiretroviral therapy, a difficult but essential task for a successful HIV treatment—clinical points of view and practical considerations," *Front. Pharmacol.,* vol. 8, p. 831, Oct. 2017.
[http://dx.doi.org/10.3389/fphar.2017.00831]

[20] C. I. Coleman, "Dosing frequency and medication adherence in chronic disease," *J. Manag. Care Pharm.,* vol. 18, no. 7, pp. 527-539, Jul. 2012.
[http://dx.doi.org/10.18553/jmcp.2012.18.7.527]

[21] Al-Worafi YM, Ming LC, Alseragi WM. Patient Care-Related Issues in the Developing Countries: Patient Education and Counseling. InHandbook of Medical and Health Sciences in Developing Countries: Education, Practice, and Research 2024 Mar 5 (pp. 1-19). Cham: Springer International Publishing.

[22] O. L. Okafor-Muo, H. Hassanin, R. Kayyali, and A. ElShaer, "3D printing of solid oral dosage forms: Numerous challenges with unique opportunities," *J. Pharm. Sci.,* vol. 109, no. 12, pp. 3676-3686, Dec. 2020.
[http://dx.doi.org/10.1016/j.xphs.2020.08.029]

[23] A. Mannan, "Challenges and advances in pediatric pharmaceutical dosage forms," *Int. J. Pharm. Biol. Sci.,* vol. 8, no. 3, pp. 1-10, 2018. [Online]. Available: www.ijpbsonline.com

[24] F. J. Pinto, "Single-pill combination in the management of chronic coronary syndromes: A strategy to improve treatment adherence and patient outcomes?", *Int. J. Cardiol.,* vol. 384, pp. 10–17, Aug. 2023.
[http://dx.doi.org/10.1016/j.ijcard.2023.04.046]

[25] S. Tanna, J. Ogwu, and G. Lawson, "Hyphenated mass spectrometry techniques for assessing medication adherence: Advantages, challenges, clinical applications and future perspectives," *Clin. Chem. Lab. Med.,* vol. 58, no. 5, pp. 643–663, May 2020.
[http://dx.doi.org/10.1515/cclm-2019-0820]

[26] F. Sharmila, M. Nasir, O. A. Hassan, M. Rusydi, and M. Razif, "Smart medication adherence system using IoT for elderly patients," *Prog. Eng. Appl. Technol.,* vol. 3, no. 1, pp. 559–570, 2022.
[http://dx.doi.org/10.30880/peat.2022.03.01.056]

[27] A. Omotosho and P. Ayegba, "Medication adherence: A review and lessons for developing countries," *Int. J. Online Eng. (iJOE),* vol. 15, no. 11, pp. 104–123, 2019.
[http://dx.doi.org/10.3991/ijoe.v15i11.10647]

[28] M. Aldeer, M. Javanmard, and R. P. Martin, "A review of medication adherence monitoring technologies," *Appl. Syst. Innov.,* vol. 1, no. 2, p. 14, Jun. 2018.
[http://dx.doi.org/10.3390/asi1020014]

[29] M. Aldeer and R. P. Martin, "Medication adherence monitoring using modern technology," in *Proc. IEEE 8th Annu. Ubiquitous Comput., Electron. Mobile Commun. Conf. (UEMCON),* New York, NY, USA, 2017, pp. 491–497.

[http://dx.doi.org/10.1109/UEMCON.2017.8249101]

[30]   T. Islam, R. Hassan, S.R. Romy, D. Dellal, and T.R.A. Bin, "Enhancing Medication Adherence with IoT Technology", *Eur. J. Electr. Eng. Comput. Sci.,* vol. 7, no. 5, pp. 7-13, 2023.
[http://dx.doi.org/10.24018/ejece.2023.7.5.557]

[31]   D. Verma, K.R.B. Singh, A.K. Yadav, V. Nayak, J. Singh, P.R. Solanki, and R.P. Singh, "Internet of things (IoT) in nano-integrated wearable biosensor devices for healthcare applications", *Biosens. Bioelectron. X,* vol. 11, p. 100153, 2022.
[http://dx.doi.org/10.1016/j.biosx.2022.100153]

[32]   S. M. A. Iqbal, I. Mahgoub, E. Du, M. A. Leavitt, and W. Asghar, "Advances in healthcare wearable devices," *npj Flexible Electronics*, vol. 5, no. 1, p. 9, Apr. 2021.
[http://dx.doi.org/10.1038/s41528-021-00107-x]

[33]   A. Shrivastava and J. Sjöström, *"Exploring the smartwatch as a tool for medical adherence,"* M.Sc. thesis, Dept. Informatics and Media, Uppsala Univ., Uppsala, Sweden, Jun. 2015. [Online]. Available: https://www.diva-portal.org/smash/get/diva2%3A824289/FULLTEXT01.pdf

[34]   D. Fozoonmayeh, H.V. Le, E. Wittfoth, C. Geng, N. Ha, J. Wang, M. Vasilenko, Y. Ahn, and D.M. Woodbridge, "A Scalable Smartwatch-Based Medication Intake Detection System Using Distributed Machine Learning", *J. Med. Syst.,* vol. 44, no. 4, p. 76, 2020.
[http://dx.doi.org/10.1007/s10916-019-1518-8] [PMID: 32112271]

[35]   R. Lederman, O. Ben-Assuli, and T. H. Vo, "The role of the Internet of Things in Healthcare in supporting clinicians and patients: A narrative review," *Health Policy and Technology*, vol. 10, no. 3, p. 100552, Sep. 2021.
[http://dx.doi.org/10.1016/j.hlpt.2021.100552]

[36]   S. Khan and M. Alam, "Wearable Internet of Things for Personalized Healthcare: Study of Trends and Latent Research," in *Health Informatics: A Computational Perspective in Healthcare*, R. Patgiri, A. Biswas, and P. Roy, Eds. Singapore: Springer, 2021, pp. 43–60.
[http://dx.doi.org/10.1007/978-981-15-9735-0_3]

[37]   E. Chiauzzi, C. Rodarte, and P. DasMahapatra, "Patient-centered activity monitoring in the self-management of chronic health conditions", *BMC Med.,* vol. 13, no. 1, p. 77, 2015.
[http://dx.doi.org/10.1186/s12916-015-0319-2] [PMID: 25889598]

[38]   X. Toh, H.X. Tan, H. Liang, and H.P. Tan, "Elderly medication adherence monitoring with the Internet of Things", *2016 IEEE International Conference on Pervasive Computing and Communication Workshops, PerCom Workshops 2016,* 2016
[http://dx.doi.org/10.1109/PERCOMW.2016.7457133]

[39]   M. Ahsan, S.H. Teay, A.S.M. Sayem, and A. Albarbar, "Smart Clothing Framework for Health Monitoring Applications", *Signals (Basel),* vol. 3, no. 1, pp. 113-145, 2022.
[http://dx.doi.org/10.3390/signals3010009]

[40]   P.K.D. Pramanik, B.K. Upadhyaya, S. Pal, and T. Pal, "Internet of things, smart sensors, and pervasive systems: Enabling connected and pervasive healthcare", In: *Healthcare Data Analytics and Management.* Elsevier, 2019, pp. 1-58.
[http://dx.doi.org/10.1016/B978-0-12-815368-0.00001-4]

[41]   A. K. Yetisen, J. L. Martinez-Hurtado, B. Ünal, A. Khademhosseini, and H. Butt, "Wearables in medicine," *Adv. Mater.*, vol. 30, no. 33, p. 1706910, Jun. 2018.
[http://dx.doi.org/10.1002/adma.201706910]

[42]   S. Nazir, Y. Ali, N. Ullah, and I. García-Magariño, *"Internet of Things for Healthcare Using Effects of Mobile Computing: A Systematic Literature Review,"* Wireless Communications and Mobile Computing, vol. Hindawi Limited, 2019.
[http://dx.doi.org/10.1155/2019/5931315]

[43]   A. Sheth, U. Jaimini, K. Thirunarayan and T. Banerjee, "Augmented personalized health: How smart

data with IoTs and AI is about to change healthcare," In: *IEEE 3rd International Forum on Research and Technologies for Society and Industry (RTSI)*, Modena, Italy, 2017, pp. 1-6.
[http://dx.doi.org/10.1109/RTSI.2017.8065963]

[44]   W. Salehi, G. Gupta, S. Bhatia, D. Koundal, A. Mashat, and A. Belay, *"IoT-Based Wearable Devices for Patients who have Alzheimer Disease,"* Contrast Media and Molecular Imaging, vol. Hindawi Limited, 2022.
[http://dx.doi.org/10.1155/2022/3224939]

[45]   V.V. Meshram, K.R. Patil, V.A. Meshram, and S. Bhatlawande, "SmartMedBox: A Smart Medicine Box for Visually Impaired People Using IoT and Computer Vision Techniques", *Revue d'Intelligence Artificielle*, vol. 36, no. 5, pp. 681-688, 2022.
[http://dx.doi.org/10.18280/ria.360504]

[46]   B. Charyyev, M. Mansouri, and M. H. Gunes, "Modeling the adoption of Internet of Things in healthcare: A systems approach," in *Proc. IEEE Int. Symp. Systems Eng. (ISSE)*, Vienna, Austria, 2021, pp. 1–8.
[http://dx.doi.org/10.1109/ISSE51541.2021.9582493]

[47]   A. Ahad, M. Tahir, M. Aman Sheikh, K.I. Ahmed, A. Mughees, and A. Numani, "Technologies trend towards 5g network for smart health-care using iot: A review", *Sensors (Basel),* vol. 20, no. 14, p. 4047, 2020.
[http://dx.doi.org/10.3390/s20144047] [PMID: 32708139]

[48]   S. Imbesi, M. Corzani, F. Petrocchi, G. Lopane, L. Chiari, and G. Mincolelli, "User-Centered Design of Cues with Smart Glasses for Gait Rehabilitation in People with Parkinson's Disease: A Methodology for the Analysis of Human Requirements and Cues Effectiveness," in *Advances in Simulation and Digital Human Modeling*, vol. 264, S. K. S. Gupta, Ed. Cham, Switzerland: Springer, 2021, pp. 348–358. [Online]. Available: https://doi.org/10.1007/978-3-030-79763-8_42
[http://dx.doi.org/10.1007/978-3-030-79763-8_42]

[49]   M. Aledhari, R. Razzak, B. Qolomany, A. Al-Fuqaha, and F. Saeed, "Biomedical IoT: Enabling Technologies, Architectural Elements, Challenges, and Future Directions", *IEEE Access,* vol. 10, pp. 31306-31339, 2022.
[http://dx.doi.org/10.1109/ACCESS.2022.3159235] [PMID: 35441062]

[50]   U. Hariharan, K. Rajkumar, T. Akilan, and J. Jeyavel, "Smart wearable devices for remote patient monitoring in healthcare 4.0," in Internet of Medical Things: *Remote Healthcare Systems and Applications*, H. D. J. Hemanth and J. Anitha, Eds. Cham, Switzerland: Springer, 2021, pp. 117–135.
[http://dx.doi.org/10.1007/978-3-030-63937-2_7]

[51]   R. Indrakumari, T. Poongodi, P. Suresh, and B. Balamurugan, "The growing role of Internet of things in healthcare wearables", In: *Emergence of Pharmaceutical Industry Growth with Industrial IoT Approach.* Elsevier, 2019, pp. 163-194.
[http://dx.doi.org/10.1016/B978-0-12-819593-2.00006-6]

[52]   M. Alder, M. Alaziz, J. Ortiz, R. E. Howard, and R. P. Martin, "A sensing-based framework for medication compliance monitoring," in *Proc. 1st ACM Int. Workshop Device-Free Human Sensing (DFHS)*, New York, NY, USA, 2019, pp. 52–56.
[http://dx.doi.org/10.1145/3360773.3360886]

[53]   K. Wac and S. Wulfovich, Eds., *Quantifying Quality of Life: Incorporating Daily Life into Medicine*, 1st ed. Cham, Switzerland: Springer, 2022. [Online]. Available: https://link.springer.com/book/10.1007/978-3-030-94212-0. [Accessed: 8 May 2025].

[54]   Shrivastava, T. P., Goswami, S., Gupta, R., & Goyal, R. K. (2023). Mobile app interventions to improve medication adherence among type 2 diabetes mellitus patients: A systematic review of clinical trials. *Journal of Diabetes Science and Technology*, 17(2), 458–466.
[http://dx.doi.org/10.1177/19322968211060060]

[55]   S.A. Ishak, H.Z. Abidin, and M. Muhamad, "Improving medical adherence using smart medicine

cabinet monitoring system", *Indones. J. Electr. Eng. Comput. Sci.,* vol. 9, no. 1, pp. 164-169, 2018.
[http://dx.doi.org/10.11591/ijeecs.v9.i1.pp164-169]

[56]   R.O. Adetunji, M.A. Strydom, M.E. Herselman, and A. Botha, "Augmented Reality Technology: A Systematic Review on Gaming Strategy for Medication Adherence," in *Advances in Human Factors and Ergonomics,* vol. 1, pp. 25–35, 2022. [Online]
[http://dx.doi.org/10.1007/978-3-031-14748-7_3]

[57]   J.E. Pedi Reddy, and A. Chavan, "AI-IoT based Smart Pill Expert System", *Proceedings of the 4th International Conference on Trends in Electronics and Informatics, ICOEI 2020,* Institute of Electrical and Electronics Engineers Inc., pp. 407-414, 2020.
[http://dx.doi.org/10.1109/ICOEI48184.2020.9142946]

[58]   M.P. Gagnon, E.K. Ghandour, P.K. Talla, D. Simonyan, G. Godin, M. Labrecque, M. Ouimet, and M. Rousseau, "Electronic health record acceptance by physicians: Testing an integrated theoretical model", *J. Biomed. Inform.,* vol. 48, pp. 17-27, 2014.
[http://dx.doi.org/10.1016/j.jbi.2013.10.010] [PMID: 24184678]

[59]   T. Heart, O. Ben-Assuli, and I. Shabtai, "A review of PHR, EMR and EHR integration: A more personalized healthcare and public health policy", *Health Policy Technol.,* vol. 6, no. 1, pp. 20-25, 2017.
[http://dx.doi.org/10.1016/j.hlpt.2016.08.002]

[60]   D. Deutscher, D.L. Hart, R. Dickstein, S.D. Horn, and M. Gutvirtz, *Implementing an Integrated Electronic Outcomes and Electronic Health Record Process to Create a Foundation for Clinical Practice Improvement Background and Purpose,* 2008.www.ptjournal.org

[61]   K.K. Jetelina, T.T. Woodson, R. Gunn, B. Muller, K.D. Clark, J.E. DeVoe, B.A. Balasubramanian, and D.J. Cohen, "Evaluation of an electronic health record (EHR) tool for integrated behavioral health in primary care", *J. Am. Board Fam. Med.,* vol. 31, no. 5, pp. 712-723, 2018.
[http://dx.doi.org/10.3122/jabfm.2018.05.180041] [PMID: 30201667]

[62]   R. Pivovarov, and N. Elhadad, "Automated methods for the summarization of electronic health records", *J. Am. Med. Inform. Assoc.,* vol. 22, no. 5, pp. 938-947, 2015.
[http://dx.doi.org/10.1093/jamia/ocv032] [PMID: 25882031]

[63]   M. Cifuentes, M. Davis, D. Fernald, R. Gunn, P. Dickinson, and D.J. Cohen, "Electronic Health Record Challenges, Workarounds, and Solutions Observed in Practices Integrating Behavioral Health and Primary Care", *J. Am. Board Fam. Med.,* vol. 28, no. Suppl 1, suppl. Suppl. 1, pp. S63-S72, 2015.
[http://dx.doi.org/10.3122/jabfm.2015.S1.150133] [PMID: 26359473]

[64]   S.J.C. Lee, K.K. Jetelina, E. Marks, E. Shaw, K. Oeffinger, D. Cohen, N.O. Santini, J.V. Cox, and B.A. Balasubramanian, "Care coordination for complex cancer survivors in an integrated safety-net system: a study protocol", *BMC Cancer,* vol. 18, no. 1, p. 1204, 2018.
[http://dx.doi.org/10.1186/s12885-018-5118-7] [PMID: 30514267]

[65]   M.J. Rantz, M. Skubic, G. Alexander, M. Popescu, M.A. Aud, B.J. Wakefield, R.J. Koopman, and S.J. Miller, "Developing a comprehensive electronic health record to enhance nursing care coordination, use of technology, and research", *J. Gerontol. Nurs.,* vol. 36, no. 1, pp. 13-17, 2010.
[http://dx.doi.org/10.3928/00989134-20091204-02] [PMID: 20047248]

[66]   L. Samal, P.C. Dykes, J.O. Greenberg, O. Hasan, A.K. Venkatesh, L.A. Volk, and D.W. Bates, "Care coordination gaps due to lack of interoperability in the United States: a qualitative study and literature review", *BMC Health Serv. Res.,* vol. 16, no. 1, p. 143, 2016.
[http://dx.doi.org/10.1186/s12913-016-1373-y] [PMID: 27106509]

[67]   Y. Gu, A. Zalkikar, M. Liu, L. Kelly, A. Hall, K. Daly, and T. Ward, "Predicting medication adherence using ensemble learning and deep learning models with large scale healthcare data", *Sci. Rep.,* vol. 11, no. 1, p. 18961, 2021.
[http://dx.doi.org/10.1038/s41598-021-98387-w] [PMID: 34556746]

[68]   El-Mallakh, P., & Findlay, J. (2015). Strategies to improve medication adherence in patients with

schizophrenia: The role of support services. Neuropsychiatric Disease and Treatment, 11, 1077–1090.
[http://dx.doi.org/10.2147/NDT.S56107]

[69]   J. Sumner, A. Bundele, H.W. Lim, P. Phan, M. Motani, and A. Mukhopadhyay, "Developing an Artificial Intelligence-Driven Nudge Intervention to Improve Medication Adherence: A Human-Centred Design Approach", *J. Med. Syst.*, vol. 48, no. 1, p. 3, 2023.
[http://dx.doi.org/10.1007/s10916-023-02024-0] [PMID: 38063940]

[70]   S. Alves Pinho, M. Cruz, F. Ferreira, A. Ramalho, and R. Sampaio, "Improving medication adherence in hypertensive patients: A scoping review," Preventive Medicine, vol. 146, Article 106467, 2021.
[Online]. Available:
[http://dx.doi.org/10.1016/j.ypmed.2021.106467]

[71]   C. Arbuckle, D. Tomaszewski, L. Brown, J. Schommer, D. Morisky, C. Parlett-Pelleriti, and E. Linstead, "Exploring the relationship of digital information sources and medication adherence", *Comput. Biol. Med.*, vol. 109, pp. 303-310, 2019.
[http://dx.doi.org/10.1016/j.compbiomed.2019.04.023] [PMID: 31100583]

[72]   S.I. Mirzadeh, A. Arefeen, J. Ardo, R. Fallahzadeh, B. Minor, J.A. Lee, J.A. Hildebrand, D. Cook, H. Ghasemzadeh, and L.S. Evangelista, "Use of machine learning to predict medication adherence in individuals at risk for atherosclerotic cardiovascular disease", *Smart Health (Amst.)*, vol. 26, p. 100328, 2022.
[http://dx.doi.org/10.1016/j.smhl.2022.100328] [PMID: 37169026]

[73]   L. Robinson, M.A. Arden, S. Dawson, S.J. Walters, M.J. Wildman, and M. Stevenson, "A machine-learning assisted review of the use of habit formation in medication adherence interventions for long-term conditions", *Health Psychol. Rev.*, vol. 18, no. 1, pp. 1-23, 2024.
[http://dx.doi.org/10.1080/17437199.2022.2034516] [PMID: 35086431]

[74]   I. Ahmed, N. S. Ahmad, S. Ali, S. Ali, A. George, H. S. Danish, E. Uppal, J. Soo, M. H. Mobasheri, D. King, B. Cox, and A. Darzi, "Medication adherence apps: Review and content analysis," *JMIR mHealth and uHealth*, vol. 6, no. 3, article e62, Mar. 2018. [Online]
[http://dx.doi.org/10.2196/mhealth.6432]

[75]   I. Ahmed, N. S. Ahmad, S. Ali, S. Ali, A. George, H. S. Danish, E. Uppal, J. Soo, M. H. Mobasheri, D. King, B. Cox, and A. Darzi, "Medication adherence apps: Review and content analysis," *JMIR mHealth uHealth*, vol. 6, no. 3, article e62, Mar. 2018. [Online]. Available: https://doi.org/10.2196/mhealth.6432 . [Accessed: 8 May 2025].

[76]   T. Eckes, U. Buhlmann, H.D. Holling, and A. Möllmann, "Comprehensive ABA-based interventions in the treatment of children with autism spectrum disorder – a meta-analysis", *BMC Psychiatry*, vol. 23, no. 1, p. 133, 2023.
[http://dx.doi.org/10.1186/s12888-022-04412-1] [PMID: 36864429]

[77]   J. B. Leaf, J. H. Cihon, R. Leaf, J. McEachin, N. Liu, N. Russell, L. Unumb, S. Shapiro, and D. Khosrowshahi, "Concerns About ABA-Based Intervention: An Evaluation and Recommendations," *Journal of Autism and Developmental Disorders*, vol. 52, no. 6, pp. 2838–2849, Jun. 2021.
[http://dx.doi.org/10.1007/s10803-021-05137-y]

[78]   M. Mittal, G. Battineni, D. Singh, T. Nagarwal, and P. Yadav, "Web-based chatbot for Frequently Asked Queries (FAQ) in Hospitals", *J. Taibah Univ. Med. Sci.*, vol. 16, no. 5, pp. 740-746, 2021.
[http://dx.doi.org/10.1016/j.jtumed.2021.06.002] [PMID: 34690656]

[79]   C. Ramadhani, "Chatbots in Pharmacy: A Boon or a Bane for Patient Care and Pharmacy Practice?", *Sci. Pharm.*, vol. 2, no. 3, p. 95, 2023.
[http://dx.doi.org/10.58920/sciphar02030001]

[80]   C.N. Ramadhani, "Chatbots in pharmacy: A boon or a bane for patient care and pharmacy practice?", *Sciences of Pharmacy*, vol. 3;2, no. 3, pp. 117-33.001, 2023.
[http://dx.doi.org/10.58920/sciphar02030001]

[81]   A.M. Preininger, B.L. Rosario, A.M. Buchold, J. Heiland, N. Kutub, B.S. Bohanan, B. South, and G.P.

Jackson, "Differences in information accessed in a pharmacologic knowledge base using a conversational agent vs traditional search methods", *Int. J. Med. Inform.*, vol. 153, p. 104530, 2021.
[http://dx.doi.org/10.1016/j.ijmedinf.2021.104530] [PMID: 34332466]

[82] C. Sweeney, C. Potts, E. Ennis, R. Bond, M.D. Mulvenna, S. O'neill, M. Malcolm, L. Kuosmanen, C. Kostenius, A. Vakaloudis, G. Mcconvey, R. Turkington, D. Hanna, H. Nieminen, A-K. Vartiainen, A. Robertson, and M.F. Mctear, "Can Chatbots Help Support a Person's Mental Health? Perceptions and Views from Mental Healthcare Professionals and Experts", *ACM Trans. Comput. Healthc.*, vol. 2, no. 3, pp. 1-15, 2021.
[http://dx.doi.org/10.1145/3453175]

[83] S. Ajmal, A. Abdullah, I. Ahmed, & C. Jalota, "Natural Language Processing in Improving Information Retrieval and Knowledge Discovery in Healthcare Conversational Agents", *J. Artif. Intell. Mach. Learn. Manag.*, vol. 7, no. 1, pp. 34-47, 2023.
[http://dx.doi.org/10.2196/73]

[84] N. Minian, K. Mehra, M. Earle, S. Hafuth, R. Ting-A-Kee, J. Rose, S. Veldhuizen, L. Zawertailo, M. Ratto, O.C. Melamed, and P. Selby, "AI Conversational Agent to Improve Varenicline Adherence: Protocol for a Mixed Methods Feasibility Study", *JMIR Res. Protoc.*, vol. 12, no. 1, p. e53556, 2023.
[http://dx.doi.org/10.2196/53556] [PMID: 38079201]

[85] P. McNair, V. Kilintzis, K. Skovhus Andersen, J. Niès, J-C. Sarfati, E. Ammenwerth, E. Chazard, S. Jensen, R. Beuscart, N. Maglaveras, and V.G. Koutkias, "From adverse drug event detection to prevention. A novel clinical decision support framework for medication safety", *Methods Inf. Med.*, vol. 53, no. 6, pp. 482-492, 2014.
[http://dx.doi.org/10.3414/ME14-01-0027] [PMID: 25377477]

[86] D.O. Klein, R.J.M.W. Rennenberg, R.P. Koopmans, and M.H. Prins, "Adverse event detection by medical record review is reproducible, but the assessment of their preventability is not", *PLoS One*, vol. 13, no. 11, p. e0208087, 2018.
[http://dx.doi.org/10.1371/journal.pone.0208087] [PMID: 30496243]

[87] J.A. Berlin, S.C. Glasser, and S.S. Ellenberg, "Adverse event detection in drug development: recommendations and obligations beyond phase 3", *Am. J. Public Health*, vol. 98, no. 8, pp. 1366-1371, 2008.
[http://dx.doi.org/10.2105/AJPH.2007.124537] [PMID: 18556607]

[88] D.W. Bates, R.S. Evans, H. Murff, P.D. Stetson, L. Pizziferri, and G. Hripcsak, "Policy and the future of adverse event detection using information technology", *J. Am. Med. Inform. Assoc.*, vol. 10, no. 2, pp. 226-228, 2003.
[http://dx.doi.org/10.1197/jamia.M1268] [PMID: 12595412]

[89] D.W. Bates, R.S. Evans, H. Murff, P.D. Stetson, L. Pizziferri, and G. Hripcsak, "Detecting adverse events using information technology", *J. Am. Med. Inform. Assoc.*, vol. 10, no. 2, pp. 115-128, 2003.
[http://dx.doi.org/10.1197/jamia.M1074] [PMID: 12595401]

[90] S. Verman, and A. Anjankar, "A Narrative Review of Adverse Event Detection, Monitoring, and Prevention in Indian Hospitals", *Cureus*, vol. 14, no. 9, p. e29162, 2022.
[http://dx.doi.org/10.7759/cureus.29162] [PMID: 36258971]

[91] G. Latif, A. Shankar, J.M. Alghazo, V. Kalyanasundaram, C.S. Boopathi, and M. Arfan Jaffar, "I-CARES: advancing health diagnosis and medication through IoT", *Wirel. Netw.*, vol. 26, no. 4, pp. 2375-2389, 2020.
[http://dx.doi.org/10.1007/s11276-019-02165-6]

[92] M. Jha and A.K. Bhandari, "Provoking Medication Adherence with Automated IoT System," *IEEE Transactions on Instrumentation and Measurement*, vol. 70, Article 9500893, 2021
[http://dx.doi.org/10.1109/TENSYMP52854.2021.9550893]

[93] F. Firouzi, B. Farahani, M. Ibrahim, and K. Chakrabarty, "Keynote paper: From EDA to IoT eHealth: Promises, challenges, and solutions", *IEEE Trans. Comput. Aided Des. Integrated Circ. Syst.*, vol. 37,

no. 12, pp. 2965-2978, 2018.
[http://dx.doi.org/10.1109/TCAD.2018.2801227]

[94]   T. M. Ghazal, M. K. Hasan, M. T. Alshurideh, H. M. Alzoubi, M. Ahmad, S. S. Akbar, B. Al Kurdi, and I. A. Akour, "IoT for smart cities: Machine learning approaches in smart healthcare—A review," *Future Internet*, vol. 13, no. 8, p. 218, 2021.
[http://dx.doi.org/10.3390/fi13080218]

[95]   P.   Singh,   and   R.   Chaturvedi, *Challenges,   and   Ethical   Considerations,* 2024.www.ijirts.orgwww.ijirts.org

[96]   M.M. Amri, V. Kumar, W.A. Khattak, D. Pandey, and A. Kundu, *Personalized Healthcare in the Age of AI: A Comprehensive Overview of its Applications and Limitations International Journal of Intelligent Automation and Computing,* 2021.https://orcid.org/0000-0001-5501-8484

[97]   S. Marzban, M. Najafi, A. Agolli, and E. Ashrafi, "Impact of Patient Engagement on Healthcare Quality: A Scoping Review", *J. Patient Exp.,* vol. 9, p. 23743735221125439, 2022.
[http://dx.doi.org/10.1177/23743735221125439] [PMID: 36134145]

[98]   A. R. Ahlan and B. I. Ahmad, "An overview of patient acceptance of Health Information Technology in developing countries: A review and conceptual model," *Int. J. Inf. Syst. Proj. Manag.,* vol. 3, no. 1, pp. 29–48, 2015.
[http://dx.doi.org/10.12821/ijispm030102]

[99]   J.L. Bender, A.B. Cyr, L. Arbuckle, and L.E. Ferris, "Ethics and privacy implications of using the internet and social media to recruit participants for health research: A privacy-by-design framework for online recruitment", *J. Med. Internet Res.,* vol. 19, no. 4, p. e104, 2017.
[http://dx.doi.org/10.2196/jmir.7029] [PMID: 28385682]

[100] N. Allahrakha, "Вопросы права в цифровую эпоху. 2023. Том 4. № 2. Ethical Considerations in the Digital Age", *Legal Issues in the Digital Age,* vol. 4, no. 2, pp. 78-121, 2018.
[http://dx.doi.org/10.17323/10.17323/2713-2749.2023.2.78.121]

[101] S. R. Mohd Arifin, "Ethical considerations in qualitative study," *International Journal of Care Scholars*, vol. 1, no. 2, pp. 82–85, Aug. 2018.

CHAPTER 10

Seamless Integration of Technology in Pharmaceuticals

B. Rama Sagar[1], Akanksha Sharma[4], Shaweta Sharma[2], Shekhar Singh[3] and **Akhil Sharma[4,*]**

[1] *Department of Civil Engineering, Aditya University, Surampalem, India*

[2] *School of Medical and Allied Sciences, Galgotias University Plot No. 2, Yamuna Expy, Opposite Buddha International Circuit, Sector 17A, Greater Noida, Uttar Pradesh, India*

[3] *Faculty of Pharmacy, Babu Banarasi Das Northern India Institute of Technology, Lucknow, Uttar Pradesh, India*

[4] *R.J. College of Pharmacy, Raipur, Gharbara, Tappal, Khair, Uttar Pradesh, India*

Abstract: The pharmaceutical industry is the most innovative of all industries due to the integration of technology into its main operations. This chapter examines the impact of technology on pharmaceuticals and highlights some significant achievements as well as their consequences. Revolutionizing the development, discovery, and delivery of drugs by pharmaceutical companies is taking place through the convergence of advanced technologies like Artificial Intelligence (AI), big data analytics, automation, and the Internet of Medical Things (IoMT). The streamlining of manufacturing processes through automation and robotics has enhanced their efficiency and guaranteed accuracy in drug formulation and packaging processes. Meanwhile, big data usage has unveiled very essential information from large datasets, which accelerated the discovery of drugs, identifying new targets, predicting drug interactions, and optimizing clinical trials. AI and Machine Learning (ML) algorithms are giving researchers the ability to develop models that can predict drugs quickly and more accurately. IoMT has made it possible to monitor patients' real-time health metrics from connected devices and sensors, enabling personalized medicine as well as remote patient care. Nevertheless, there are regulatory issues around data privacy, security, and interoperability. To exploit the full potential of technology in pharmaceuticals while maintaining patient safety and privacy, a balance must be struck between innovative ideas and compliance needs. It also highlights the ethical issues that are associated with technology integration, focusing on the significance of ethical frameworks that guide responsible innovations. Further developments in pharmaceutical research, development, and healthcare delivery depend on the industry's capacity to adapt to new technologies and surmount difficulties related to these technologies. The pharmaceutical landscape is bound to change significantly with

---

* **Corresponding author Akhil Sharma:** R.J. College of Pharmacy, Raipur, Gharbara, Tappal, Khair, Uttar Pradesh, India; E-mail: xs2akhil@gmail.com

Akhil Sharma, Neeraj Kumar Fuloria, Pankaj Kumar Singh & Shaweta Sharma (Eds.)

the help of technology integration, which promises a new era of precision medicine-improved patient outcomes through collaboration, innovation, and ethical stewardship.

Keywords: Analytics, Artificial intelligence, Automation, Big data, Drug, Health, Internet of medical things, Internet of things, Medication, Machine learning, Medicine, Patient, Personalized medicine, Robotics, Treatment.

INTRODUCTION

The seamless assimilation of pharmaceuticals involves the harmonious blending of various technological advancements and processes within the pharmaceutical industry to create a cohesive and efficient ecosystem. It consists of the smooth and efficient integration of technologies like automation, data analytics, artificial intelligence, and interconnected devices, among others, in all the stages of drug development, manufacturing, distribution, and patient care [1, 2].

This integration is intended to scrap silos and optimize workflows so as to realize more collaborations and synergies between different departments and stakeholders involved in pharmaceutical operations. By ensuring that technology is merged with this sector, efficiency can be achieved, drug discovery timelines will take a shorter period, product quality can improve, and ultimately, patient healthcare outcomes will be enhanced [3, 4].

Seamless integration also ensures that different technology platforms and systems can work together, making it possible for data to be exchanged across the pharmaceutical value chain without any break. Through this network of interconnections, instantaneous decision-making is enabled in addition to personalized medicine approaches and continuous process improvements [5, 6].

The importance of technology in modern pharmaceutical practices cannot be overstated. Several key reasons why technology plays a vital role in the pharmaceutical industry are discussed below and shown in Fig. (**1**).

The advancement of technology has allowed drug discovery to adopt advanced computational approaches, such as virtual screening, molecular modeling, and simulation. Researchers are able to evaluate vast datasets and more accurately predict drug-target interactions using high-performance computing for faster discovery. Massive amounts of data are generated by the pharmaceutical industry from clinical trials, research studies, patient records, and genomic information. Technology has made it possible to collect, store, and analyze this data, thus revealing information that can be used in decision-making, optimizing the design of clinical trials, and indicating new therapeutic targets [7].

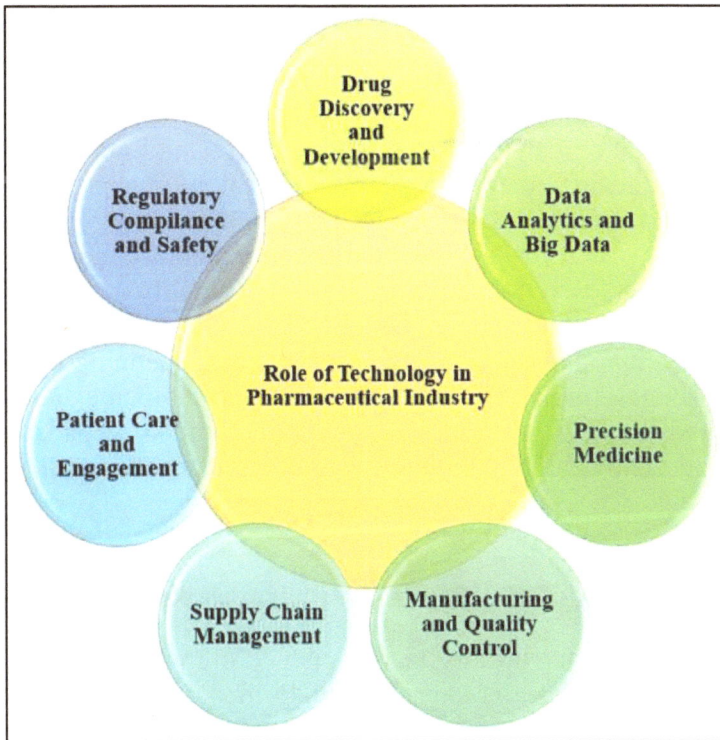

Fig. (1). Role of technology in pharmaceutical industry.

Progressions in technology have given rise to personalized medicine, for example, the ability to read genes and identify biomarkers. Diagnosis and treatment of diseases can be made by analyzing an individual's genetic profile, among other patient-specific details, so that the correct care is provided for every patient, thus minimizing side effects while enhancing efficiency [8]. Robotics and automation have turned around the pharmaceutical manufacturing processes by enhancing effectiveness, lowering mistakes, and ensuring product uniformity. Examples of technically driven advances include continuous processing and real-time monitoring systems that help to scale up production, reduce wastage, and improve compliance with regulations [9].

Supply chain optimization technology plays a vital role in sourcing raw materials, distribution, and logistics. Advanced software systems, such as those that allow inventory tracking in real-time, demand forecasting, temperature-controlled product management, *etc.*, are important to ensure the safe and efficient delivery of pharmaceutical products to patients worldwide. Mobile apps, wearable devices, and telemedicine platforms are some of the digital health technologies that enable patients to take charge of their healthcare processes. These gadgets allow remote monitoring of health indicators, tracking of medication adherence, personal health information, and the ability to have a virtual chat with medical experts, which boosts participation by patients and even improves their overall fitness [10, 11].

Regulatory compliance can be ensured through technologies that support the security, safety, and efficiency of pharmaceutical products. Compliance with regulations is made more efficient by technological solutions such as electronic data capture systems, risk management tools, and regulatory intelligence software, which monitor adverse events and maintain robust quality management systems. Modern pharmaceutical practices benefit from technology in many ways, including driving innovation, improving efficiency, enhancing patient care, and ultimately advancing public health. Pharmaceutical companies have to embrace technological advancements if they are to remain competitive, adapt to changing healthcare trends, and deal with the industry's complex challenges [12, 13].

HISTORICAL PERSPECTIVE

Evolution of Technology Adoption in the Pharmaceutical Industry

A lot of technological innovations have happened in the pharmaceutical industry over the years, which have radically transformed various elements of drug discovery, development, manufacturing, and distribution [14, 15]. Technological evolution in terms of adoption in pharmaceuticals is briefly described below.

Computational Biology and Bioinformatics

In the last decades of the 20th century, computational biology and bioinformatics have been important tools for drug discovery. Computational biology and bioinformatics employ computer algorithms and databases in analyzing biological data, projecting drug-target interactions, and simulating biological processes that facilitate faster identification of potential drug candidates [16 - 18].

Genomics and Personalized Medicine

The development of personalized medicine has been enabled by human genome mapping and advances in genomics. This way, researchers can analyze a person's genetic composition and hence make out genetic differences that affect drug response, thus leading to targeted therapies designed for particular patients [19 - 21].

Biopharmaceuticals and Biotechnology

The use of biopharmaceuticals, like monoclonal antibodies, recombinant proteins, and gene therapies, has been increasingly critical in managing different illnesses.

Some of the intricate biological molecules used as therapy agents are obtained through genetic engineering and protein engineering *via* biotechnology innovations [22].

Big Data and Artificial Intelligence (AI)

The pharmaceutical industry is using big data analytics and AI to extract insights pertaining to disease mechanisms, drug efficacy, and safety from a huge amount of data. Machine learning algorithms have been applied to discover new drug targets, optimize drug candidates, and predict clinical outcomes, thus improving decision-making during the process of developing a medicine [23, 24].

3D Printing and Advanced Manufacturing

3D printing technologies are transforming pharmaceutical manufacturing as they allow for personalized dosage forms, complex drug delivery systems, and individual patient medical devices. Moreover, continuous manufacturing and microfluidics, which are advanced manufacturing technologies, are also being adopted in order to enhance efficiency, flexibility, and quality control in the production of drugs [25 - 28].

Blockchain and Supply Chain Management

Explorations are ongoing in the use of blockchain technology to enhance transparency, traceability, and security in the pharmaceutical supply chain. Blockchain can be used to prevent fake medicine, minimize drug scarcity, and make it easier to comply with regulations by creating a non-changeable record of drug transactions and maintaining information accuracy [29].

Technological advancements in the pharmaceutical industry have been used to improve patient outcomes, increase efficiency, and meet medical needs that were not met. The emergence of fresh technologies and their maturation can lead to further changes within the sector, thus shaping the future of healthcare [30].

Key Milestones in the Integration Process

The combination of two or more companies, divisions, or systems in the pharmaceutical industry is known as an integration process. This is done to achieve synergies, enhance competitiveness, and optimize operations. Key milestones in the integration process are summarized in Table **1**.

Table 1. Key milestones in the integration process.

Milestone	Description
Pre-merger Planning	Strategic planning, careful investigation, compatibility checking, synergy and risk identification, integration roadmap development [31].
Announcement and Regulatory Approval	An official announcement about a merger, specifically the request for regulatory approvals, dealing with antitrust issues, answering regulatory concerns [32].
Integration Planning	Developing strategies for integration, establishing teams, setting timelines, and planning on organizational structure, processes, systems, culture, and communication [33].
Day One Readiness	Preparing for operations post-merger, ensuring systems, processes, and employees are ready, and maintaining customer and supplier relationships [34].
Functional Integration	Aligning operations, systems, and processes, consolidating facilities, harmonizing IT systems, standardizing procedures, and integrating supply chains [35].
Cultural Integration	Aligning values, norms, and behaviors, fostering collaboration and trust, and addressing cultural differences and conflicts [36].
Customer Integration	Integrating sales, marketing, and customer service functions, rationalizing product portfolios, harmonizing pricing and promotion strategies, and ensuring a seamless customer experience [37].
Post-Merger Optimization	Realizing synergies, improving efficiency, driving growth, identifying and implementing cost-saving initiatives, leveraging combined resources and capabilities, and pursuing strategic initiatives [38].
Monitoring and Adjustment	Tracking performance, soliciting feedback, and making adjustments to optimize outcomes [39].
Cultural Evolution	Evolving organizational culture over time through collaboration, adaptation, and fostering a culture of continuous improvement and innovation [40].

CURRENT TECHNOLOGICAL LANDSCAPE

Overview of Current Technologies Used in Pharmaceuticals

The pharmaceutical industry is a dynamic field that employs various advanced technology platforms to guide its course from the drug discovery and development stage to manufacturing and distribution. It is important to note that AI machine learning plays an important role in revolutionizing how processes are done through predictive analysis. The algorithms filter through huge datasets to predict drug-target interactions, hasten lead identification, and optimize molecular structures, thereby speeding up the typically slow drug development pipeline. High-throughput screening (HTS) technologies have similarly evolved side-by-side with automation and data analysis, making it possible for scientists to rapidly screen large compound libraries in search of potential therapeutic agents [41, 42].

The advent of genomics and personalized medicine, which is an approach to tailored treatment based on the mapping of individual genomes, heralds a new era. This leads to the exact identification of biomarkers for disease susceptibility, drug response, and adverse reactions, which could enable the development of personalized therapies depending on someone's genetic constitution. Monoclonal antibodies, recombinant proteins, and gene therapies are some of the major innovations in the field of biopharmaceuticals and biotechnology. These technologies have resulted in a range of disease-specific therapeutic approaches. Using genetic engineering tools and protein engineering kits, which are components of biotechnology, novel, productive, and safe biologics can be produced [43, 44].

The field of digital health and telemedicine has changed significantly, and this way it deals with patients. In drug manufacturing, they are used during clinical trials to gather information, enhance patient enrollment, follow-up study participants, and post-marketing surveillance. Drug production is entering a new era with 3D printing and advanced manufacturing. Personalized dosage forms and intricate drug delivery systems can now be produced using these technologies. Increased efficiency, flexibility, and quality control are some of the benefits that these technologies bring to streamline manufacturing processes [45].

When blockchain and supply chain management combine, they produce new channels of visibility coupled with safety that protect drug supply chains from counterfeiters, inadequacy in provision, and regulatory interventions. Omics Technologies is a group of technologies such as genomics, proteomics, metabolomics, and transcriptomics that provide massive amounts of biological information about disease mechanisms and potential targets for drugs. Virtual Clinical Trials use technological breakthroughs like remote monitoring and telemedicine to simplify trial procedures by speeding up drug development timelines while increasing patient participation [46].

Regenerative Medicine has revolutionized medical treatment landscapes for diseases with high unmet clinical needs through the restoration or replacement of damaged tissues and organs. There is hope in combating diseases through stem cell therapy, tissue engineering, and gene editing, whereas normal treatments have become unsuccessful. Consequently, this brings together technologies from these fields that will lead to more efficient drug discovery, personalized medicines, and improved patient outcomes, thereby creating a new era in pharmaceuticals [47, 48].

Technologies Used in Different Stages of Drug Development

Drug Discovery

Drug discovery is a complex and multidimensional process that involves the use of advanced technologies to explore molecular space. High-throughput screening (HTS) automates the labor-intensive testing of large compound libraries, which expedites the identification of potential drugs. Computational chemistry utilizes computer simulation and modeling techniques to predict how molecules will behave and design new compounds accordingly. Bioinformatics examines biological data and looks at genomics and proteomics to identify possible drug targets and untangle the complicated mechanisms of diseases. Virtual screening uses complex algorithms to search through large chemical databases, thus predicting which chemicals might be good drugs, making it easier for researchers to find suitable candidates [49, 50].

Preclinical Development

During the stage of preclinical development, there is a confluence of different analytical methods aimed at critically assessing the safety, effectiveness, and potential of drug candidates before commencing human studies. The foundation for such studies relies on *in vitro* assays, which involve the examination of compounds within controlled laboratory conditions with cell cultures or biochemical assays. These experiments offer valuable information concerning the biological activities and toxicity of the agent under consideration, thereby providing a basis for future testing. Furthermore, *in vivo* examinations are conducted in animals to study the candidate drug's pharmacokinetics, toxicity, and efficacy parameters. Thus, these investigations may provide a comprehensive understanding of how the candidate interacts with living organisms, which is necessary for its evaluation for human purposes [51].

Pharmacogenomics delves into the complex domain of genetic differences, demonstrating how individual genetic constitutions influence drug response. By exposing these intricacies, pharmacogenomics helps improve strategies for drug development, and it also seems to provide an opportunity for the identification of possible biomarkers that could be used in patient stratification, thus ushering in a new era of personalized medicine that would strictly consider individual genetic make-up when making treatment choices. These approaches, therefore, work together to guide through the labyrinthine preclinical stage, where only the most hopeful prospects move forward into the next levels of clinical evaluation [52].

Clinical Development

The field of clinical development involves a range of advanced technologies that work together to manage clinical trials, which are crucial in the testing of drug effectiveness and safety on human subjects. Clinical Trial Management Systems (CTMS) provide the framework that flawlessly brings about trial planning execution and supervision, thus resulting in better data collection and analysis as well as regulatory compliance. Electronic Data Capture (EDC) systems digitize the clinical trial landscape by improving the quality, accuracy, and efficacy of data management [53].

In addition, these platforms allow for real-time data collection that ensures trial results are quickly available and carefully noted down. Biomarker technologies provide noteworthy insights into patient response and disease progression, the prominence of which is increasing in the industry. By measuring biomarkers in patient samples, these technologies enable precise patient stratification, thereby leading to individualized treatment approaches and making it easier to identify potential subjects for clinical trials. Furthermore, imaging technologies like MRI, PET, and CT scans hold immense power in revealing disease progression and treatment response with unprecedented detail [54, 55].

Clinicians find such imaging modalities extremely useful in evaluating the effectiveness of treatments. This allows doctors to make necessary adjustments promptly and ensure that decisions that have been taken are correct during the journey of the clinical trial. These technologies work together harmoniously towards advancing clinical development, ensuring that new therapies are rigorously assessed within a controlled and closely supervised setting for the eventual delivery of safer and more efficient medical solutions to suffering patients [51, 56].

Regulatory Approval

To ensure compliance and protect public health, pivotal technologies streamline processes in the field of regulatory approval. Regulatory Information Management (RIM) Systems, covering all aspects of regulatory submissions, approvals, and compliance obligations throughout the drug development lifecycle, are central to this process [57, 58]. These systems offer a single point of access for regulatory data and documents and also ensure that all the prospective participants maintain communication and work together according to the existing regulations. In addition, ECTD standardizes the format in which regulatory documents are submitted to health authorities, thereby speeding up the review process and increasing efficiency. Pharmacovigilance Systems stand as vigilant guardians, monitoring the safety of drugs post-market and swiftly detecting adverse events

[59, 60]. Pharmacovigilance systems report such incidents promptly to regulatory agencies, which is valuable for timely response and maintaining optimum levels of safety and efficacy in drugs while ensuring that the most secure and effective treatments reach patients alone. As such, these technologies provide an essential framework for the convoluted pathway to clearance by regulators, thereby protecting public health while facilitating access to life-saving medicines on time [61, 62].

Manufacturing

Pharmaceutical manufacturing is an area in which three revolutionary technologies have changed the way things are done and made sure that they comply with strict quality conditions while at the same time ensuring that efficiency and flexibility are boosted. In this regard, Process Analytical Technology (PAT) has emerged as a steadfast technology for monitoring and controlling manufacturing processes on a real-time basis. PAT ensures manufacturers are able to continuously have insights and information on process critical parameters, which makes product quality and consistency possible since they enable manufacturers to adjust their products in time. In addition, continuous manufacturing is a pace-setter in innovation, hence replacing traditional batch manufacturing with a seamless supply chain and unbroken operations [63].

The change of paradigm does not only increase efficiency by eliminating downtime but also makes it possible for companies to be more flexible and better control their quality, helping them respond faster to changes in the market. Besides, Quality by Design (QbD) is adhered to as a core principle that shapes manufacturing processes with a focus on product quality. QbD, which combines scientific principles and risk-based approaches, makes sure that quality is established in the manufacturing process from the beginning, thus reducing risks and improving outcomes. As such, they are the bedrock of contemporary pharmaceutical manufacturing that fosters innovation, efficiency, and quality excellence in developing drugs that save lives [64].

Post-Market Surveillance

In the arena of post-marketing surveillance, three novel techniques ensure public safety by watching drug safety and efficacy in real-world circumstances. Pharmacovigilance Systems are watchful sentinels that collect vast amounts of data on adverse events and medication errors for analysis so that timely detection and reporting to regulatory authorities is ensured. Underneath this, Real-World Evidence (RWE) draws useful information from various sources, such as electronic health records and insurance claims, to establish a link between drug safety and effectiveness in ordinary clinical practice [65, 66].

RWE is valuable because it uses real-world data to demonstrate how drugs function beyond study settings, thus giving insight for clinical decision-making and regulatory assessments. Moreover, social media monitoring is a quick partner that can evaluate different platforms, such as social media sites and online health forums, in order to identify any potential safety concerns or emerging trends in drug use [67].

Social Media Monitoring keeps track of patients and healthcare professionals to ensure that the pharmaceutical industry always remains watchful in its surveillance of the constantly changing drug safety environment. Thus, it is possible to conclude that these strategies or methods create a very strong foundation for post-market surveillance, which is an important tool that enables regulators, healthcare providers, and pharmaceutical companies to safeguard public health and maintain drugs continuing safety and efficacy [68].

AUTOMATION AND ROBOTICS

Utilization of Automation and Robotics in Manufacturing Processes

Manufacturing processes are increasingly using automation and robotics for increased productivity, quality, safety, and innovation. Workflow optimization, downtime reduction, accuracy assurance, and conformity to requirements, as well as providing new capabilities, products, and services, can be achieved through the use of these technologies. For manufacturing processes, automation and robotics can be employed in different ways, such as fixed automation, programmable automation systems, flexible automation, or intelligent automation [69].

Fixed automation encompasses machines or devices that carry out a specific activity or order of activities precisely and quickly, such as production lines or conveyors. Programmable automation involves machines or devices that can be coded to undertake different tasks or sequences of tasks, for example, CNC machines or robots. Flexible automation comprises devices that reprogramme themselves to run varying tasks or sequences of actions, such as industrial robots or AGVs. Intelligent automation refers to the utilization of machines that are capable of learning from data and changing conditions like AI, machine learning, and vision systems [70].

Automation and robotics are applied across multiple sectors and applications of manufacturing like automotive, food & beverage, electronics, and medical. For example, in the automotive industry, they are used for car assembly, welding, painting, inspection, and testing, as well as material handling and logistics. Use in the food and beverage industry involves processing, packaging, labeling, and distributing products while ensuring their quality and safety. For the electronics industry, automation and robotics are used in making, assembling, soldering, testing, or inspecting components or devices such as PCBs, chips, or smartphones. Lastly, in the medical sector, they are adopted in order to produce, sterilize, and deliver medical devices or supplies like syringes or masks [71].

However, there are also several challenges posed by automation and robotics, including making an initial investment in the cost of equipment and software, integrating systems with existing processes, infrastructure, and workforce, managing change and transition for employees, customers, and suppliers as well as ensuring security, reliability, and sustainability of such systems and data [72].

To ensure the successful use of automation and robotics in manufacturing operations, it is necessary to evaluate requirements and objectives and create a multidisciplinary team comprising engineering, production, quality assurance, safety, and human resource personnel at the stage of planning the implementation of these systems; and also to train and reskill workers so that they can operate using these systems, follow up on the outcomes and implications derived from that while making any appropriate change [73, 74].

Advantages of Automated Systems in Improving Efficiency and Reducing Errors

Automated systems offer numerous advantages in improving efficiency and reducing errors across various industries, including pharmaceuticals, which are described below and summarized in Fig. (**2**).

Automated systems are able to perform tasks at a much faster pace than what could be achieved using manual methods. Hence, productivity and throughput are doubled. For example, pharmaceutical manufacturing processes can take less time when automated systems are used, which can result in quicker delivery of medicines to patients. Automated systems are designed to perform tasks with a lot of exactness and correctness, thus reducing the chances of human mistakes. This is essential, especially in industries where slight errors can lead to severe consequences, for instance, in pharmaceuticals where patients may be harmed due to an incorrect dose or wrong formulation [75].

Automated processes guarantee that performance is constant and conformity to pre-established norms reduces variability in procedures and results. Such uniformity is vital for maintaining the quality of commodities and ensuring adherence to regulatory obligations in areas like pharmaceuticals, where strict quality control is very important. Automated systems can reduce the need for manual labor by automating repetitive or labor-intensive tasks within an organization. For example, pharmaceutical manufacturing can use automated systems to replace all the filling and packaging processes that are manual, thereby reducing labor costs and enhancing efficiency [76].

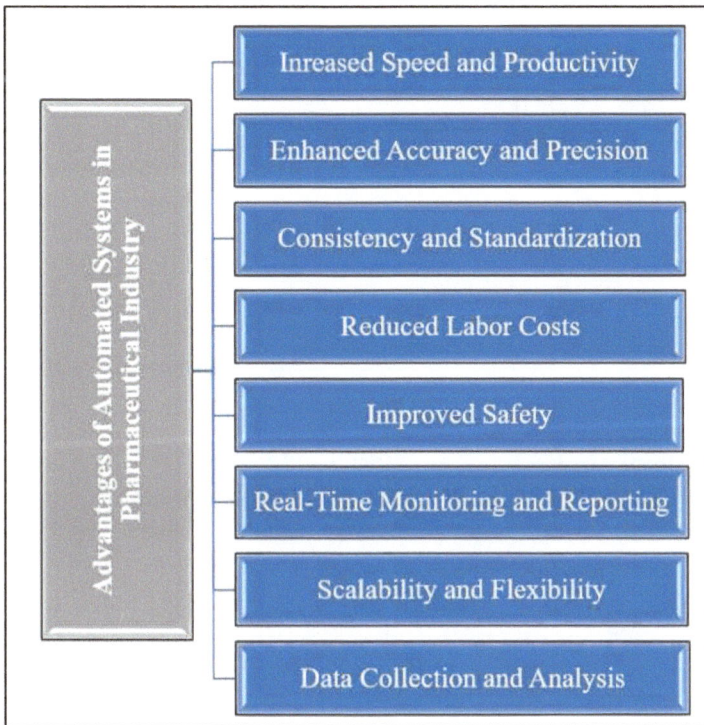

Fig. (2). Advantages of automation systems in pharmaceutical industry.

Automated systems can be used in the workplace to make it safer, reducing hazards and physically demanding tasks for employees. Automation in pharmaceutical production replaces harmful chemicals or pollutants that are dangerous to workers' health. Most of these automated systems usually come with built-in monitoring and reporting provisions that enable the tracking of processes and performance metrics on a real-time basis. This makes it possible to take corrective action before errors can escalate into major mistakes when deviations occur or if there are abnormalities [77].

Scalability and adaptability to changing production needs are often considered when designing automated systems. This can help firms respond quickly to variations in demand or changes in product requirements, resulting in agility and responsiveness in dynamic environments. Automated systems can collect and analyze extensive amounts of data, providing information on the efficiency of processes, quality of products, and performance measurements. This approach, driven by the use of data, empowers businesses to point out where improvement is needed and streamline processes for maximum efficiency and effectiveness. The benefits of using automatic systems to enhance efficiency and reduce mistakes make them indispensable for businesses that want to optimize their operation, enhance productivity, and maintain high standards of quality and safety [78].

BIG DATA AND ANALYTICS

Importance of Big Data in Drug Discovery and Development

Revolutionary in drug discovery and development, big data and analytics are of great importance because they give unique insights into disease mechanisms, treatment outcomes, and targets for drugs. The importance of big data in drug discovery and development is summarized below.

Data-driven Insights

Through big data analytics, researchers can explore vast datasets from different sources, such as genomic data, electronic health records, clinical trial data, and scientific literature. By studying these datasets, researchers may discover relationships, patterns, or even connections that could not easily be observed by conventional means, thus providing them with critical knowledge of disease biology and the potency of drugs [79 - 81].

Clinical Trial Optimization

Clinical trial design and execution are improved by big data analytics, which reveals the patient groups most likely to respond to a given treatment and estimates of probable response based on patient attributes, genetic profiles, and biomarkers. Researchers can enhance trial outcomes, minimize expenses, and boost efficiency by adapting clinical trials to particular subsets of people [82, 83].

Real-world Evidence Generation

Big data analytics exploit real-world information such as electronic health records, insurance claims, wearable devices, and social media to provide real-world evidence of the safety, efficacy, and outcomes of treatment in everyday clinical practice. This kind of evidence complements traditional trial data by providing a better understanding of how drugs perform with different patients and within various settings [84, 85].

Precision Medicine and Personalized Treatment

Precision medicine approaches in big data analytics have been made possible by combining genomic data, clinical phenotypes, and other patient-specific information to modify treatment to suit particular patients. Researchers can identify genetic biomarkers associated with drug response or adverse reactions, stratify patients based on their genetic profiles, and optimize treatment regimens for maximum efficacy and safety [86, 87].

Drug Safety and Pharmacovigilance

Drug safety monitoring and pharmacovigilance are improved by big data analytics, which analyzes large-scale healthcare data to identify adverse drug reactions, medication errors, and drug interactions as they occur. Early detection of safety signals allows researchers to take steps in advance that can help them manage risks and ensure continued drug safety in clinical practice.

Big data and analytics highly influence drug discovery and development as they assist in speeding up the recognition of new drug targets, improving clinical trial layout, facilitating individualized treatment options, and increasing medication safety surveillance. The growth of technology and expansion in datasets means that big data will continue to play a major role in healthcare innovation [88, 89].

Applications of Analytics in Identifying Patterns and Predicting Outcomes

Analytics plays an important part in finding patterns and predicting outcomes in different domains, such as healthcare, finance, marketing, and logistics. Some of the applications of analytics in these areas are discussed below.

Healthcare

Analytics can analyze patient information, *e.g.*, medical background, genetic data, and lifestyle aspects, in order to determine trends, project the probability of certain illnesses, and provide early interventions and individual treatment plans. By assessing clinical details such as patient attributes, therapeutic measures employed, and effects thereof, analytics can foresee possible consequences in relation to a variety of remedies, making it easier for doctors to select the most appropriate treatments for specific patients. Hospital analytic systems are used to ascertain any imbalances in terms of patient flow, resource utilization, and wait times, thus leading to better scheduling or staffing decisions that would increase efficiency within hospitals while at the same time reducing costs [90 - 92].

Finance

Analysis can detect patterns and anticipate risks in finance, such as market volatility, bad loans, and deception, by examining financial data, market trends, and consumer behavior. These predictions can be made possible through analysis of historical market data and economic indicators; this helps in maximizing returns on investments while at the same time reducing the risk involved in investment portfolios that have been optimized. Customer data analytics can be used to differentiate consumers based on specific characteristics and predict their preferences, behavior, age, purchases, and activities online. This can help in creating personalized customer experiences and focused marketing campaigns [93].

Marketing

Marketing data such as campaign performance, customer engagement, and conversion rates can be analyzed by analytics tools in order to identify trends and forecast the efficiency of upcoming marketing campaigns, allowing marketers to improve their strategies and distribute resources more efficiently. Customer purchase history, interaction frequency, and feedback can be used to estimate the lifetime value of customers as well as to identify high-value customers for targeted marketing efforts and retention strategies.

The segmentation of markets using analysis can be done using common features to predict behaviors and interests of individual consumers, thus making marketing messages and product suggestions tailored to particular segments [94].

Logistics

Analytics can analyze historical sales data, market trends, and external factors like climate changes and economic situations to forecast future demand for products and services so that organizations can maximize stock control, production planning, and supply chain logistics. To optimize route planning and scheduling so as to reduce fuel costs, minimize delivery times, and enhance client satisfaction, analytics can inspect transportation data such as traffic patterns, vehicle performance, and delivery schedules. Analytics may assess supply chain information to ascertain possible risks such as alliance disruption, natural disasters, or political instabilities that affect processes of production and come up with remedies to adopt in case of any eventualities [95].

ARTIFICIAL INTELLIGENCE AND MACHINE LEARNING

Role of AI and Machine Learning (ML) in Drug Design and Virtual Screening

AI and ML have revolutionized the field of drug design and virtual screening methodologies, providing unprecedented opportunities for accelerating drug discovery and development [96]. AI and ML are transforming these domains in various ways, which are described below.

Data Analysis and Pattern Recognition

AI and ML algorithms are good at scrutinizing big and complicated data sets like chemical structures, biological interactions, and drug-target relationships. They can recognize patterns, connections, and underlying ties that may not be seen by traditional means through being trained on huge amounts of data, thereby enabling more drug-designing informed decisions [97].

Predictive Modeling and Optimization

AI and ML algorithms are able to produce predictive models that could predict the actions of molecules, anticipate their connections with biological targets, and build drug candidates for potency, selectivity, and safety. Such algorithms can focus on lead compounds by simulating molecular structures and properties to design new drug candidates while optimizing chemical properties for maximal efficacy and minimal side effects [98].

Virtual Screening and Lead Identification

AI and ML algorithms make it possible to screen large compound libraries virtually in order to identify possible drug candidates having the desired pharmacological properties. By using computational models and predictive algorithms, these methods can quickly estimate the binding affinity and activity of millions of compounds against drug targets, thus accelerating lead identification and minimizing the necessity for expensive and time-consuming experimental screening [99].

Biomarker Discovery

Through the use of AI and ML, individualized medical practice is made possible by analyzing patient-specific data, which includes genetic profiles, clinical phenotypes, and treatment outcomes. Such programs can also determine genetic biomarkers connected to drug efficacy or disease advancement, hence allowing for the stratification of patients and the customization of treatment plans to ensure maximum safety and effectiveness.

AI and ML are leveraging the power of data-driven insights, predictive modeling, and computational algorithms to drive innovation in drug design and virtual screening, accelerate the discovery and development of novel therapies, optimize treatment strategies, and ultimately improve patient outcomes [100 - 103].

Examples of AI Applications in Optimizing Clinical Trials and Patient Recruitment

Clinical trials that need to be optimized and patient recruitment processes that must be streamlined are increasingly tapping into AI applications that bring revolutionary solutions for the long-standing issues of healthcare [104]. Examples of AI applications in these areas are summarized below.

Predictive Analytics for Patient Recruitment

The machine learning models can use AI to analyze various information such as EHRs, patient demographics, and historical trial data to forecast the eligibility of patients for clinical trials. These algorithms can examine patient attributes, including medical record histories, in order to identify trial criteria that match them, thereby enhancing the process of patient recruitment by making it quicker and more efficient [105].

Natural Language Processing (NLP) for Protocol Optimization

Clinical trial protocols can be parsed and analyzed by NLP algorithms, which highlight vital eligibility criteria, endpoints, and study procedures. By extracting structured data from unstructured text, NLP offers automated protocol review and optimization to ensure that researchers detect possible inconsistencies, ambiguities, or inefficiencies in the design and implementation of the trials [106].

Risk Prediction and Mitigation

Clinical trial data analysis by AI algorithms can help anticipate potential risks like protocol deviations, patient dropouts, and adverse events. It allows for early identification of risk factors and warning signs, which enables proactive mitigation strategies, including amendment of protocols, targeted interventions, or stratification of patients to reduce the impact on patient safety and trial outcomes [107, 108].

Site Selection and Resource Allocation

Clinical trials can employ AI-powered predictive models that effectively select the best sites and allocate other resources using historical trial data, performance metrics from different sites, and geographical factors. The models also enable sponsors to optimally allocate their resources, minimize trial delays, and improve the odds of success by identifying high-performing sites, logistical challenges, and patient recruitment hotspots [109].

Adaptive Trial Design and Optimization

AI algorithms can analyze current trial data to inform adaptive trial design and optimization measures in real time. Such algorithmic systems allow for dynamic revisions of trial protocols, like escalation of doses, patient stratification, and treatment arm modifications, based on continuous monitoring of patient responses, treatment outcomes, and safety end-points so as to maximize the efficiency and effectiveness of clinical trials [110].

These illustrations show how AI applications in areas such as patient recruitment, optimization of protocols to real-time monitoring, and risk mitigation are transforming clinical trial operations. It is accelerating the pace of medical innovation, improving the outcomes of patients, and revolutionizing how clinical trials are done through predictive analytics and data-driven insights powered by AI [111].

INTERNET OF MEDICAL THINGS (IOMT)

Integration of Connected Devices and Sensors in Pharmaceuticals

Incorporating sensors and connected devices into pharmaceuticals has many uses, like material tracking, the management of the supply chain, clinical studies, and regulatory compliance. Internet of Things (IoT) gadgets can track supply availability in real-time, thus leading to more efficient inventory control and reduced costs. They may also link to automatic cut-offs, which can be employed to manage emergencies from a distance. Such devices are useful in supply chain management by recording and transmitting information obtained from bar codes and RFID tags in order to validate data consistency as well as signal replenishment needs. This assists in perpetuating optimal inventory levels and minimizes the requirement for extra supplies, hence reducing expenditures [112].

During clinical trials, IoT approaches can monitor the way experimental medicine is reacting in real-time, thereby enhancing the quality of test data and improving the treatment process of hazardous reactions. The IoT gadgets are able to accumulate networked data and subsequently send it to integrated software, which will assist in recognizing patient conditions and raising alerts throughout clinical trials. IoT-connected devices also enhance regulatory compliance by continuously sending data to servers and thus confirming quality standards have been met, thereby reducing the amount of manual paperwork and possible margin for error. Insights into production process health can be gained through data analytics software, which can determine areas prone to issues and potential cost overruns, as well as pinpoint inefficiencies, in order to boost productivity and profitability [113].

It can also improve patient connectivity and adherence using IoT-enabled intelligent packaging. Such capsules, as well as other in-built mechanisms, will control medication intake, monitor its effect on patients, send notifications for adherence purposes, and alert clinicians where necessary. One of the merits of incorporating connected devices and sensors into drugs is that it enhances efficiency, minimizes errors, improves patient compliance, and assures regulatory compliance. The application of IoT in this sector will enable the pharmaceutical industry to simplify systems and reduce expenditure while enhancing outcomes for patients [114].

Benefits of IoMT in Remote Patient Monitoring and Personalized Medicine

Remote patient monitoring and personalized medicine have been transformed by the Internet of Medical Things (IoMT), which allows real-time data collection and analysis. IoMT refers to the integration of devices/sensors into computer networks *via* the internet, resulting in remote monitoring of patients and the ability to interact with them. A major advantage of IoMT in remote patient monitoring is the capacity to identify and track health conditions immediately, thus facilitating early detection and management of potential health risks. This is extremely advantageous for patients with long-term diseases as it leads to better patient outcomes and lowers healthcare expenditure [115, 116].

The IoMT has also allowed the personalization of treatment methods to be customized to fit individual patient needs. By analyzing data from IoT devices, providers can recognize patterns and habits that may help in developing personalized treatments for each person's specific needs. Additionally, healthcare can benefit from enhanced operational efficiency and resource management that comes with the adoption of IoT. Through monitoring equipment utilization, patient movement, and staff allocation, hospitals can utilize resources effectively, leading to improved efficiency [117, 118].

The IoMT can improve patient satisfaction and engagement by facilitating virtual visits and better access to healthcare. IoT platforms enable patients to communicate with doctors, undergo tests as well as be checked from far away locations, a situation that eases accessibility and improves ease of use. Furthermore, IoMT can provide data-driven insights and predictive analytics, enabling healthcare professionals to foresee health trends, disease outbreaks, and patient needs. This may promote proactive decision-making through informed choices that finally lead to the creation of new treatments or therapies [119, 120].

IoMT can finally empower patients to take an engaged part in their health management. Wearable devices and health apps provide real-time data on activity levels, heart rate, and sleep patterns, among others, leading individuals to healthier lifestyles as well as preventive measures. IoMT does not come without its share of challenges. Implementing and maintaining IoMT infrastructure in healthcare facilities can be expensive. At the same time, the usability and ease of use of IoT devices may affect how readily they are adopted and used effectively [121, 122].

Data security and privacy are also major concerns with IoMT as private information gets transmitted over the internet. Nonetheless, IoMT has great potential in healthcare. By adopting IoT technology and tackling the challenges that come with it, health institutions can take full advantage of IoMT to make their medical system safer, more personalized, and more effective [123, 124].

CHALLENGES AND CONSIDERATIONS

Technology in pharmaceuticals should be used with data privacy and security as the most crucial factors. Maintaining patient trust and confidentiality requires that they are protected against unauthorized access, breaches, or misuse of their health information for a secure future. As such, a number of data protection measures, like encryption, access controls, and data anonymization, need to be put in place by pharmaceutical companies and healthcare providers in order to ensure patient privacy and security [125, 126].

Another challenge in technology systems is interoperability and integration. The healthcare industry is grappling with how to ensure seamless integration and interoperability of various technologies as it adopts a range of such technologies. The absence of intercom links, fragmentation from patient data sharing, and inefficiencies in care delivery will be the results. Interoperability standards should be accorded top priority by pharmaceutical firms and providers so that they can invest in technology solutions that are easily integrated into other systems [127, 128].

The problem of ethics also encounters other obstacles in the area of the technological utilization of drugs. To achieve equity and fairness in health delivery, eliminate algorithmic biases, and have clear information on responsibility transparency, among others, ethical considerations must guide technology development and implementation at all stages. Ethical values such as beneficence, patient privacy, and autonomy should be held high by healthcare providers and pharmaceutical companies that want to make decisions that are consistent with an ethical perspective. They should infuse their decision-making process with moral injunctions guided by a framework that balances out technology benefits in a way that is fair and responsible [129].

FUTURE DIRECTIONS AND IMPLICATIONS

Integrating technology into pharmaceuticals will shape the future of healthcare and treatment outcomes. Customized therapy and individualized medicine are seen to be on the rise, with reliance on patient-specific facts for medication customization and intervention tailored to personal traits and preferences. Digital therapeutics and remote monitoring of patients are expected to continue gaining popularity as more people become proactive in managing their own health and healthcare providers offer personalized services from remote areas [130].

AI and machine learning will accelerate drug discovery and development, treatment regimen optimization, and clinical decision-making. However, ethical considerations around AI, such as algorithmic biases and the lack of transparency, must be addressed to ensure responsible and equitable use. Developments will influence the future of technology in the pharmaceutical industry in data analytics, interoperability, and data sharing, enabling healthcare providers to gain insights from various sources of data and enhance care coordination. To ensure that the confidentiality and rights of patients are observed as information is shared among different stakeholders, it is important to address issues related to regulation, privacy, and security [131].

The prospect of the integration of technology in pharmaceuticals is good because it can enhance the provision of healthcare, improve patient outcomes, and influence population health. However, all those involved in this area should take into account several factors resulting from these advancements, such as ethics, regulatory problems, and equal access to technology-supported healthcare services. By ensuring that they give priority to patients' interests and taking into consideration ethical standards apart from getting together all those involved, integrating technology into pharmaceuticals would bring a better future for healthcare [132].

CONCLUSION

In conclusion, incorporating technology in pharmaceuticals represents a major change in the way healthcare delivery is conducted and presents unique possibilities for patient care improvement, better treatment outcomes, and scientific discovery. With precision medicine, digital therapeutics, and AI, the future of technology in pharmaceuticals is highly promising because it can transform the way healthcare is provided and experienced. Nevertheless, this future has its own challenges and considerations. Among the factors that must be taken into account include ethical implications, regulatory compliance, data privacy, and accessibility in order to ensure that the advantages of technology are equitably and responsibly realized. The use of technology in pharmaceuticals can create a brighter and more sustainable future for healthcare through the prioritization of patient-centric approaches, ethical principles, and collaboration across stakeholders. By being thoughtful and taking proactive measures, the stakeholders can utilize technology to effect positive changes that could enhance patient outcomes and, hence, ultimately, remodel the healthcare system.

REFERENCE

[1]   A. Johri, A. Sayal, C. N, J. Jha, N. Aggarwal, D. Pawar, V. Gupta, and A. Gupta, "Crafting the techno-functional blocks for Metaverse - A review and research agenda", *Int. J. Inf. Manag. Data Insights,* vol. 4, no. 1, p. 100213, 2024.
[http://dx.doi.org/10.1016/j.jjimei.2024.100213]

[2]   H. Allioui, and Y. Mourdi, "Exploring the Full Potentials of IoT for Better Financial Growth and Stability: A Comprehensive Survey", *Sensors (Basel),* vol. 23, no. 19, p. 8015, 2023.
[http://dx.doi.org/10.3390/s23198015] [PMID: 37836845]

[3]   M. Elahi, S.O. Afolaranmi, J.L. Martinez Lastra, and J.A. Perez Garcia, "A comprehensive literature review of the applications of AI techniques through the lifecycle of industrial equipment", *Discov. Artif. Intell.,* vol. 3, no. 1, p. 43, 2023.
[http://dx.doi.org/10.1007/s44163-023-00089-x]

[4]   J.L. Bender, A.B. Cyr, L. Arbuckle, and L.E. Ferris, "Ethics and privacy implications of using the internet and social media to recruit participants for health research: A privacy-by-design framework for online recruitment", *J. Med. Internet Res.,* vol. 19, no. 4, p. e104, 2017.
[http://dx.doi.org/10.2196/jmir.7029] [PMID: 28385682]

[5]   A. Aldoseri, K.N. Al-Khalifa, and A.M. Hamouda, "Re-Thinking Data Strategy and Integration for Artificial Intelligence: Concepts, Opportunities, and Challenges", *Appl. Sci. (Basel),* vol. 13, no. 12, p. 7082, 2023.
[http://dx.doi.org/10.3390/app13127082]

[6]   M. Soori, B. Arezoo, and R. Dastres, "Digital twin for smart manufacturing, A review", *Sustainable Manufacturing and Service Economics,* vol. 2, p. 100017, 2023.
[http://dx.doi.org/10.1016/j.smse.2023.100017]

[7]   A. Abernethy, L. Adams, M. Barrett, C. Bechtel, P. Brennan, A. Butte, J. Faulkner, E. Fontaine, S. Friedhoff, J. Halamka, M. Howell, K. Johnson, P. Long, D. McGraw, R. Miller, P. Lee, J. Perlin, D. Rucker, L. Sandy, L. Savage, L. Stump, P. Tang, E. Topol, R. Tuckson, and K. Valdes, "The Promise of Digital Health: Then, Now, and the Future," NAM Perspectives, vol. 2022, Jun. 27, 2022.

[8]   P. Dutta, T.M. Choi, S. Somani, and R. Butala, "Blockchain technology in supply chain operations: Applications, challenges and research opportunities", *Transp. Res., Part E Logist. Trans. Rev.,* vol. 142, p. 102067, 2020.
[http://dx.doi.org/10.1016/j.tre.2020.102067] [PMID: 33013183]

[9]   R. Hurry, "Precision Medicine: Tailoring Treatment to the Individual's Genomic Profile," ResearchGate, Nov. 2023.
[http://dx.doi.org/10.13140/RG.2.2.32452.19848]

[10]   S. Nikolicic, M. Kilibarda, M. Maslaric, D. Mircetic, and S. Bojic, "Reducing food waste in the retail supply chains by improving efficiency of logistics operations", *Sustainability (Basel),* vol. 13, no. 12, p. 6511, 2021.
[http://dx.doi.org/10.3390/su13126511]

[11]   Y. Mashayekhy, A. Babaei, X.M. Yuan, and A. Xue, "Impact of Internet of Things (IoT) on Inventory Management: A Literature Survey", *Logistics,* vol. 6, no. 2, p. 33, 2022.
[http://dx.doi.org/10.3390/logistics6020033]

[12]   M. Haji, L. Kerbache, M. Muhammad, and T. Al-Ansari, "Roles of Technology in Improving Perishable Food Supply Chains", *Logistics,* vol. 4, no. 4, p. 33, 2020.
[http://dx.doi.org/10.3390/logistics4040033]

[13]   M. Soori, B. Arezoo, and R. Dastres, "Internet of things for smart factories in industry 4.0, a review," *Inter. Thin. Cyb. Phys. Sys*, vol. 3, pp. 192–204, 2023.
[http://dx.doi.org/10.1016/j.iotcps.2023.04.006]

[14]   C. Martin, "Twin Screw Extruders as Continuous Mixers for Thermal Processing: a Technical and Historical Perspective", *AAPS PharmSciTech,* vol. 17, no. 1, pp. 3-19, 2016.
[http://dx.doi.org/10.1208/s12249-016-0485-3] [PMID: 26883259]

[15]   by Luan Paula Linden, L. P. Linden, *"Pharmaceutical industry perspectives on factors that influence the adoption and diffusion of drugs in the UK: Four case studies,"* Ph.D. thesis, The University of Birmingham, United Kingdom, 2012.

[16]   D. Consoli, and A. Mina, "An evolutionary perspective on health innovation systems", *J. Evol. Econ.,* vol. 19, no. 2, pp. 297-319, 2009.
[http://dx.doi.org/10.1007/s00191-008-0127-3]

[17]   J. Weitzel, H. Pappa, G.M. Banik, A.R. Barker, E. Bladen, N. Chirmule, J. DeFeo, J. Devine, S. Emrick, T.K. Hout, M.S. Levy, G.N. Mahlangu, B. Rellahan, J. Venema, and W. Workman, "Understanding Quality Paradigm Shifts in the Evolving Pharmaceutical Landscape: Perspectives from the USP Quality Advisory Group", *AAPS J.,* vol. 23, no. 6, p. 112, 2021.
[http://dx.doi.org/10.1208/s12248-021-00634-5] [PMID: 34654974]

[18]   L.M. Mayr, and P. Fuerst, "The future of high-throughput screening", *SLAS Discov.,* vol. 13, no. 6, pp. 443-448, 2008.
[http://dx.doi.org/10.1177/1087057108319644] [PMID: 18660458]

[19]   D.A. Pereira, and J.A. Williams, "Origin and evolution of high throughput screening", *Br. J. Pharmacol.,* vol. 152, no. 1, pp. 53-61, 2007.
[http://dx.doi.org/10.1038/sj.bjp.0707373] [PMID: 17603542]

[20]   Y.F. Lu, D.B. Goldstein, M. Angrist, and G. Cavalleri, "Personalized medicine and human genetic diversity", *Cold Spring Harb. Perspect. Med.,* vol. 4, no. 9, p. a008581, 2014.
[http://dx.doi.org/10.1101/cshperspect.a008581] [PMID: 25059740]

[21]   R. Tutton, "Personalizing medicine: Futures present and past", *Soc. Sci. Med.,* vol. 75, no. 10, pp. 1721-1728, 2012.
[http://dx.doi.org/10.1016/j.socscimed.2012.07.031] [PMID: 22906526]

[22]   A. Zhang, H. Sun, P. Wang, Y. Han, and X. Wang, "Future perspectives of personalized medicine in traditional Chinese medicine: A systems biology approach", *Complement. Ther. Med.,* vol. 20, no. 1-2, pp. 93-99, 2012.
[http://dx.doi.org/10.1016/j.ctim.2011.10.007] [PMID: 22305254]

[23]   H. Luan, P. Geczy, H. Lai, J. Gobert, S.J.H. Yang, H. Ogata, J. Baltes, R. Guerra, P. Li, and C.C. Tsai, "Challenges and Future Directions of Big Data and Artificial Intelligence in Education", *Front. Psychol.,* vol. 11, p. 580820, 2020.
[http://dx.doi.org/10.3389/fpsyg.2020.580820] [PMID: 33192896]

[24]   B. Chin-Yee, and R. Upshur, "Three problems with big data and artificial intelligence in medicine", *Perspect. Biol. Med.,* vol. 62, no. 2, pp. 237-256, 2019.
[http://dx.doi.org/10.1353/pbm.2019.0012] [PMID: 31281120]

[25]   R.K. Grigsby, ""Telemedicine: Theory and Practice7", *Telemed. J.,* vol. 3, no. 2, pp. 185-187, 1997.
[http://dx.doi.org/10.1089/tmj.1.1997.3.185]

[26]   K. Narayanan and A. Bakshi, "History and Future of Digital Health in the World and India," itihaasa Research and Digital, Nov. 2021. [Online]. Available: https://itihaasa.com/public/pdf/History_and_Future_of_Digital_Health_in_the_World_and_India.pdf. [Accessed: 8 May 2025].

[27] B. Stanberry, "Telemedicine: barriers and opportunities in the 21st century", *J. Intern. Med.,* vol. 247, no. 6, pp. 615-628, 2000.
[http://dx.doi.org/10.1046/j.1365-2796.2000.00699.x] [PMID: 10886483]

[28] C. A. Grant, M. T. Izatt, R. D. Labrom, G. N. Askin, and V. Glatt, "Use of 3D printing in complex spinal surgery: historical perspectives, current usage and future directions," *Tech in Ortho*, vol. 31, no. 3, pp. 172–180, 2016.
[http://dx.doi.org/10.1097/BTO.0000000000000186]

[29] M. Attaran, "The rise of 3-D printing: The advantages of additive manufacturing over traditional manufacturing", *Bus. Horiz.,* vol. 60, no. 5, pp. 677-688, 2017.
[http://dx.doi.org/10.1016/j.bushor.2017.05.011]

[30] B. Wang, "The Future of Manufacturing: A New Perspective", *Engineering (Beijing),* vol. 4, no. 5, pp. 722-728, 2018.
[http://dx.doi.org/10.1016/j.eng.2018.07.020]

[31] O.H. Laguna, P.F. Lietor, F.J.I. Godino, and F.A. Corpas-Iglesias, "A review on additive manufacturing and materials for catalytic applications: Milestones, key concepts, advances and perspectives", *Mater. Des.,* vol. 208, p. 109927, 2021.
[http://dx.doi.org/10.1016/j.matdes.2021.109927]

[32] J. Nihtilä, "R&D–Production integration in the early phases of new product development projects," *J. Eng. Tech. Manag*, vol. 16, no. 1, pp. 55–81, Mar. 1999.
[http://dx.doi.org/10.1016/S0923-4748(98)00028-9]

[33] J. Shaw, J. Gutberg, P. Wankah, M. Kadu, C.S. Gray, A. McKillop, G.R. Baker, M. Breton, and W.P. Wodchis, "Shifting paradigms: Developmental milestones for integrated care", *Soc. Sci. Med.,* vol. 301, p. 114975, 2022.
[http://dx.doi.org/10.1016/j.socscimed.2022.114975] [PMID: 35461081]

[34] C. Grant, L. Nagel-Picioruş, R. Nagel-Picioruş, and R. Sârbu, "Milestones in implementation of an integrated management system in the health sector. Case study radiologische netzwerk rheinland", 2016. Available from: http://creativecommons.org/licenses/by/4.0/

[35] J. Verrollot, A. Tolonen, J. Harkonen, and H. Haapasalo, "Supply capability creation process: Key milestone criteria and activities", *J. Ind. Eng. Manag.,* vol. 10, no. 3, pp. 495-521, 2017.
[http://dx.doi.org/10.3926/jiem.2375]

[36] K. McCormack, J. Willems, J. van den Bergh, D. Deschoolmeester, P. Willaert, M. Indihar Štemberger, R. Škrinjar, P. Trkman, M. Bronzo Ladeira, M. Paulo Valadares de Oliveira, V. Bosilj Vuksic, and N. Vlahovic, "A global investigation of key turning points in business process maturity", *Bus. Process. Manag. J.,* vol. 15, no. 5, pp. 792-815, 2009.
[http://dx.doi.org/10.1108/14637150910987946]

[37] Exner, K., Damerau, T., & Stark, R. (2016). Innovation in Product-Service System Engineering Based on Early Customer Integration and Prototyping. Procedia CIRP, 47, 30–35
[http://dx.doi.org/10.1016/j.procir.2016.03.084]

[38] Lāce, K., & Kirikova, M. (2021). Post-merger Integration Specific Requirements Engineering Model. In Perspectives in Business Informatics Research (Vol. 430, pp. 115–129). Springer.
[http://dx.doi.org/10.1007/978-3-030-87205-2_8]

[39] K. Muruganandan, A. Davies, J. Denicol, and J. Whyte, "The dynamics of systems integration: Balancing stability and change on London's Crossrail project", *Int. J. Proj. Manag.,* vol. 40, no. 6, pp. 608-623, 2022.
[http://dx.doi.org/10.1016/j.ijproman.2022.03.007]

[40] C. Heintz, "Scientific cognition and cultural evolution: theoretical tools for integrating cognitive and social studies of science", 2007.

[41] B.S. Aharonson, and M.A. Schilling, "Mapping the technological landscape: Measuring technology

distance, technological footprints, and technology evolution", *Res. Policy,* vol. 45, no. 1, pp. 81-96, 2016.
[http://dx.doi.org/10.1016/j.respol.2015.08.001]

[42]   S. Kauffman, J. Lobo, and W. G. Macready, "Optimal search on a technology landscape," *J. Econ. Behav. Organ.,* vol. 43, no. 2, pp. 141–166, Oct. 2000.

[43]   N. Singh, "Big data technology: developments in current research and emerging landscape", *Enterprise Inf. Syst.,* vol. 13, no. 6, pp. 801-831, 2019.
[http://dx.doi.org/10.1080/17517575.2019.1612098]

[44]   R. Tierney, W. Hermina, and S. Walsh, "The pharmaceutical technology landscape: A new form of technology roadmapping", *Technol. Forecast. Soc. Change,* vol. 80, no. 2, pp. 194-211, 2013.
[http://dx.doi.org/10.1016/j.techfore.2012.05.002]

[45]   T.M.I. Mahlia, Z.A.H.S. Syazmi, M. Mofijur, A.E.P. Abas, M.R. Bilad, H.C. Ong, and A.S. Silitonga, "Patent landscape review on biodiesel production: Technology updates", *Renew. Sustain. Energy Rev.,* vol. 118, p. 109526, 2020.
[http://dx.doi.org/10.1016/j.rser.2019.109526]

[46]   C. Barrington-Leigh, and M. Ouliaris, "The renewable energy landscape in Canada: A spatial analysis", In: *Renewable and Sustainable Energy Reviews.* vol. Vol. 75. Elsevier Ltd, 2017, pp. 809-819.
[http://dx.doi.org/10.1016/j.rser.2016.11.061]

[47]   Y. Hamada, A. Penn-Nicholson, S. Krishnan, D. M. Cirillo, A. Matteelli, R. Wyss, C. M. Denkinger, M. X. Rangaka, M. Ruhwald, and S. G. Schumacher, "Are mRNA based transcriptomic signatures ready for diagnosing tuberculosis in the clinic? – A review of evidence and the technological landscape," *EBioMedicine*, vol. 82, pp. 104174, Aug. 2022.

[48]   I. Spitsberg, S. Brahmandam, M.J. Verti, and G.W. Coulston, "Technology landscape mapping: At the heart of Open Innovation: Technology landscape maps can help organizations build awareness of strategic technologies and identify opportunities at the intersection of emerging technologies and customer needs", *Res. Technol. Manag.,* vol. 56, no. 4, pp. 27-35, 2013.
[http://dx.doi.org/10.5437/08956308X5604107]

[49]   A.B. Deore, J.R. Dhumane, R. Wagh, and R. Sonawane, "The Stages of Drug Discovery and Development Process", *Asian J. Pharm. Res. Dev.,* vol. 7, no. 6, pp. 62-67, 2019.
[http://dx.doi.org/10.22270/ajprd.v7i6.616]

[50]   S.K.M. Haque, and E.S. Ratemi, "Drug Development and Analysis Review", *Pharm. Chem. J.,* vol. 50, no. 12, pp. 837-850, 2017.
[http://dx.doi.org/10.1007/s11094-017-1543-1]

[51]   A. Ocana, A. Pandiella, L.L. Siu, and I.F. Tannock, "Preclinical development of molecular-targeted agents for cancer", *Nat. Rev. Clin. Oncol.,* vol. 8, no. 4, pp. 200-209, 2011.
[http://dx.doi.org/10.1038/nrclinonc.2010.194] [PMID: 21135887]

[52]   H. S. Newton and M. A. Dobrovolskaia, "Immunophenotyping: Analytical approaches and role in preclinical development of nanomedicines," *Adv. Drug Deliv. Rev.,* vol. 185, p. 114281, Jun. 2022.
[http://dx.doi.org/10.1016/j.addr.2022.114281]

[53]   J. Mateo, C.J. Lord, V. Serra, A. Tutt, J. Balmaña, M. Castroviejo-Bermejo, C. Cruz, A. Oaknin, S.B. Kaye, and J.S. de Bono, "A decade of clinical development of PARP inhibitors in perspective", *Ann. Oncol.,* vol. 30, no. 9, pp. 1437-1447, 2019.
[http://dx.doi.org/10.1093/annonc/mdz192] [PMID: 31218365]

[54]   E. S. Newlands, M. F. G. Stevens, S. R. Wedge, R. T. Wheelhouse, and C. Brock, "Temozolomide: a review of its discovery, chemical properties, pre-clinical development and clinical trials," *Cancer Treat. Rev.,* vol. 23, no. 1, pp. 35–61, Jan. 1997.
[http://dx.doi.org/10.1016/S0305-7372(97)90019-0]

[55]   M-K. Yeh, Hsin-I Chang, and Ming-Yen Cheng, "Clinical development of liposome based drugs: formulation, characterization, and therapeutic efficacy", *Int. J. Nanomedicine,* vol. 7, pp. 49-60, 2011. [http://dx.doi.org/10.2147/IJN.S26766] [PMID: 22275822]

[56]   D. Lebwohl, "Clinical development of platinum complexes in cancer therapy: an historical perspective and an update," *Eur. J. Cancer*, vol. 34, no. 10, pp. 1522–1534, 1998.

[57]   S. Faivre, G. Demetri, W. Sargent, and E. Raymond, "Molecular basis for sunitinib efficacy and future clinical development", *Nat. Rev. Drug Discov.,* vol. 6, no. 9, pp. 734-745, 2007. [http://dx.doi.org/10.1038/nrd2380] [PMID: 17690708]

[58]   U. Kalinke, D.H. Barouch, R. Rizzi, E. Lagkadinou, Ö. Türeci, S. Pather, and P. Neels, "Clinical development and approval of COVID-19 vaccines", *Expert Rev. Vaccines,* vol. 21, no. 5, pp. 609-619, 2022. [http://dx.doi.org/10.1080/14760584.2022.2042257] [PMID: 35157542]

[59]   J. Wang, and S.C. Chow, "On the regulatory approval pathway of biosimilar products", *Pharmaceuticals (Basel),* vol. 5, no. 4, pp. 353-368, 2012. [http://dx.doi.org/10.3390/ph5040353] [PMID: 24281406]

[60]   P. Fernandes, and E. Martens, "Antibiotics in late clinical development", *Biochem. Pharmacol.,* vol. 133, pp. 152-163, 2017. [http://dx.doi.org/10.1016/j.bcp.2016.09.025] [PMID: 27687641]

[61]   I.L. Carolina, A. Antònia, O. Mercè, and V. Antonio, "Regulatory and clinical development to support the approval of advanced therapies medicinal products in Japan", In: *Expert Opin. Biol. Ther.* vol. 22. Taylor and Francis Ltd., 2022, no. 7, pp. 831-842. [http://dx.doi.org/10.1080/14712598.2022.2093637]

[62]   S. Rawat, and A. Gupta, "Regulatory Requirements for Drug Development and Approval in United States: A Review", *Pharm. Res.,* vol. 1, 2011. Available from: www.asianpharmaonline.org

[63]   G. Detela, and A. Lodge, "Manufacturing process development of ATMPs within a regulatory framework for EU clinical trial & marketing authorisation applications", *Cell Gene Ther. Insights,* vol. 2, no. 4, pp. 425-452, 2016. [http://dx.doi.org/10.18609/cgti.2016.056]

[64]   P. Ulrich, G. Blaich, A. Baumann, R. Fagg, A. Hey, A. Kiessling, S. Kronenberg, R.H. Lindecrona, S. Mohl, W.F. Richter, J. Tibbitts, F. Crameri, and L. Weir, "Biotherapeutics in non-clinical development: Strengthening the interface between safety, pharmacokinetics-pharmacodynamics and manufacturing", *Regul. Toxicol. Pharmacol.,* vol. 94, pp. 91-100, 2018. [http://dx.doi.org/10.1016/j.yrtph.2018.01.013] [PMID: 29355662]

[65]   A. Badnjević, L.G. Pokvić, A. Deumić, and L.S. Bećirović, "Post-market surveillance of medical devices: A review", In: *Technology and Health Care* vol. 30. IOS Press BV, 2022, no. 6, pp. 1315-1329. [http://dx.doi.org/10.3233/THC-220284]

[66]   C. Zippel, and S. Bohnet-Joschko, "Post market surveillance in the german medical device sector – current state and future perspectives", *Health Policy,* vol. 121, no. 8, pp. 880-886, 2017. [http://dx.doi.org/10.1016/j.healthpol.2017.06.005] [PMID: 28697849]

[67]   R. Kingston, K. Sioris, J. Gualtieri, A. Brutlag, W. Droege, and T.G. Osimitz, "Post-market surveillance of consumer products: Framework for adverse event management", *Regul. Toxicol. Pharmacol.,* vol. 126, p. 105028, 2021. [http://dx.doi.org/10.1016/j.yrtph.2021.105028] [PMID: 34481892]

[68]   K.D. Hill, B.H. Goldstein, M.J. Angtuaco, P.Y. Chu, and G.A. Fleming, "Post-market surveillance to detect adverse events associated with Melody ® valve implantation", *Cardiol. Young,* vol. 27, no. 6, pp. 1090-1097, 2017. [http://dx.doi.org/10.1017/S1047951116002092] [PMID: 27829472]

[69]   T. Grift, Q. Zhang, N. Kondo, and K. C. Ting, "A review of automation and robotics for the bio-industry," *Journal of Biomechatronics Engineering*, vol. 1, no. 1, pp. 37–54, 2008.

[70]   Soori M, Jough FK, Dastres R, Arezoo B. Robotical automation in CNC machine tools: a review. acta mechanica et automatica. 2024;18(3).

[71]   S.M.S. Elattar, "Automation and robotics in construction: Opportunities and challenges," *Emirates J. Eng. Res.*, vol. 13, no. 2, pp. 21–26, 2008.

[72]   T.R. Kurfess, *Robotics, and automation handbook.* CRC Press, 2005.

[73]   T. Bock, "Construction automation and robotics," In: C. Balaguer and M. Abderrahim, Eds, *Robotics and Automation in Construction,*. Rijeka, Croatia: InTech, 2008, pp. 20–42.
[http://dx.doi.org/10.5772/5861]

[74]   R. Galin and R. Meshcheryakov, "Automation and robotics in the context of Industry 4.0: the shift to collaborative robots," *IOP Conf. Ser. Mater. Sci. Eng.*, vol. 537, p. 032073, 2019.
[http://dx.doi.org/10.1088/1757-899X/537/3/032073]

[75]   S.A. Mohamed, M.A. Mahmoud, M.N. Mahdi, and S.A. Mostafa, "Improving Efficiency and Effectiveness of Robotic Process Automation in Human Resource Management", *Sustainability (Basel)*, vol. 14, no. 7, p. 3920, 2022.
[http://dx.doi.org/10.3390/su14073920]

[76]   M. Tatasciore, V.K. Bowden, T.A.W. Visser, and S. Loft, *Should We Just Let the Machines Do It? The Benefit and Cost of Action Recommendation and Action Implementation Automation*, 2021.

[77]   N. Menachemi, and T.H. Collum, "Benefits and drawbacks of electronic health record systems", *Risk Manag. Healthc. Policy,* vol. 4, pp. 47-55, 2011.
[http://dx.doi.org/10.2147/RMHP.S12985] [PMID: 22312227]

[78]   C.W. Lam, and E. Jacob, "Implementing a laboratory automation system: experience of a large clinical laboratory", *SLAS Technol.,* vol. 17, no. 1, pp. 16-23, 2012.
[http://dx.doi.org/10.1177/2211068211430186] [PMID: 22357604]

[79]   K. Venkatram, and M.A. Geetha, "Review on big data & analytics - Concepts, philosophy, process, and applications", *Cybern. Inf. Technol.,* vol. 17, no. 2, pp. 3-27, 2017.
[http://dx.doi.org/10.1515/cait-2017-0013]

[80]   Vassakis, K., Petrakis, E., & Kopanakis, I. (2018). Big Data Analytics: Applications, Prospects and Challenges. In Mobile Big Data (pp. 3–20). Springer.
[http://dx.doi.org/10.1007/978-3-319-67925-9_1]

[81]   S. Erevelles, N. Fukawa, and L. Swayne, "Big Data consumer analytics and the transformation of marketing", *J. Bus. Res.,* vol. 69, no. 2, pp. 897-904, 2016.
[http://dx.doi.org/10.1016/j.jbusres.2015.07.001]

[82]   I. Hernandez, and Y. Zhang, "Using predictive analytics and big data to optimize pharmaceutical outcomes", *Am. J. Health Syst. Pharm.,* vol. 74, no. 18, pp. 1494-1500, 2017.
[http://dx.doi.org/10.2146/ajhp161011] [PMID: 28887351]

[84]   S. Khozin, G.M. Blumenthal, and R. Pazdur, "Real-world Data for Clinical Evidence Generation in Oncology", *J. Natl. Cancer Inst.,* vol. 109, no. 11, 2017.
[http://dx.doi.org/10.1093/jnci/djx187] [PMID: 29059439]

[85]   T. Geldof, I. Huys, and W. Van Dyck, "Real-World Evidence Gathering in Oncology: The Need for a Biomedical Big Data Insight-Providing Federated Network", *Front. Med. (Lausanne),* vol. 6, p. 43, 2019.
[http://dx.doi.org/10.3389/fmed.2019.00043] [PMID: 30906740]

[86]   D. Cirillo, and A. Valencia, "Big data analytics for personalized medicine", *Curr. Opin. Biotechnol.,* vol. 58, pp. 161-167, 2019.
[http://dx.doi.org/10.1016/j.copbio.2019.03.004] [PMID: 30965188]

[87] T. Hulsen, S. S. Jamuar, A. R. Moody, J. H. Karnes, O. Varga, S. Hedensted, R. Spreafico, D. A. Hafler, and E. F. McKinney, "From big data to precision medicine," *Front. Med.*, vol. 6, Mar. 2019. [http://dx.doi.org/10.3389/fmed.2019.00034]

[88] G. Trifirò, J. Sultana, and A. Bate, "From Big Data to Smart Data for Pharmacovigilance: The Role of Healthcare Databases and Other Emerging Sources", *Drug Saf.*, vol. 41, no. 2, pp. 143-149, 2018. [http://dx.doi.org/10.1007/s40264-017-0592-4] [PMID: 28840504]

[89] A. Bate, R.F. Reynolds, and P. Caubel, "The hope, hype and reality of Big Data for pharmacovigilance", *Ther. Adv. Drug Saf.*, vol. 9, no. 1, pp. 5-11, 2018. [http://dx.doi.org/10.1177/2042098617736422] [PMID: 29318002]

[90] M.S. Islam, M.M. Hasan, X. Wang, H.D. Germack, and M. Noor-E-Alam, "Noor-E, M. -Alam, "A systematic review on healthcare analytics: Application and theoretical perspective of data mining,"", *Healthcare (Basel)*, vol. 6, no. 2, p. 54, 2018. [http://dx.doi.org/10.3390/healthcare6020054] [PMID: 29882866]

[91] A. Belle, R. Thiagarajan, S.M.R. Soroushmehr, F. Navidi, D.A. Beard, and K. Najarian, "Big data analytics in healthcare", *BioMed Res. Int.*, vol. 2015, pp. 1-16, 2015. [http://dx.doi.org/10.1155/2015/370194] [PMID: 26229957]

[92] N. Mishra, D. Silakari, G. Proudyogiki Vishwavidyalaya, C. Sc, and R. Gandhi Proudyogiki Vishwavidyalaya, *Predictive Analytics: A Survey. Trends, Applications, Opportunities & Challenges*, 2012.

[93] D. Broby, "The use of predictive analytics in finance", *J. Finance Data Sci.*, vol. 8, pp. 145-161, 2022. [http://dx.doi.org/10.1016/j.jfds.2022.05.003]

[94] S.L. France, and S. Ghose, *Marketing Analytics: Methods. Practice, Implementation, and Links to Other Fields*, 2018.

[95] E. Ilie-Zudor, A. Ekárt, Z. Kemeny, C. Buckingham, P. Welch, and L. Monostori, "Advanced predictive-analysis-based decision support for collaborative logistics networks", *Supply Chain Manag.*, vol. 20, no. 4, pp. 369-388, 2015. [http://dx.doi.org/10.1108/SCM-10-2014-0323]

[96] R. Gupta, D. Srivastava, M. Sahu, S. Tiwari, R.K. Ambasta, and P. Kumar, "Artificial intelligence to deep learning: machine intelligence approach for drug discovery", *Mol. Divers.*, vol. 25, no. 3, pp. 1315-1360, 2021. [http://dx.doi.org/10.1007/s11030-021-10217-3] [PMID: 33844136]

[97] K. S. (King S. Fu), *Applications of Pattern Recognition* CRC Press, 1982.

[98] Y. Zeng, Z. Zhang, and A. Kusiak, "Predictive modeling and optimization of a multi-zone HVAC system with data mining and firefly algorithms", *Energy*, vol. 86, pp. 393-402, 2015. [http://dx.doi.org/10.1016/j.energy.2015.04.045]

[99] T. Lengauer, Ed., *Bioinformatics: From Genomes to Therapies*, vol. 1, Wiley-VCH, 2008.

[100] V.D. Mouchlis, A. Afantitis, A. Serra, M. Fratello, A.G. Papadiamantis, V. Aidinis, I. Lynch, D. Greco, and G. Melagraki, "Advances in de novo drug design: From conventional to machine learning methods", *Int. J. Mol. Sci.*, vol. 22, no. 4, p. 1676, 2021. [http://dx.doi.org/10.3390/ijms22041676] [PMID: 33562347]

[101] W. Sun, P.E. Sanderson, and W. Zheng, "Drug combination therapy increases successful drug repositioning", *Drug Discov. Today*, vol. 21, no. 7, pp. 1189-1195, 2016. [http://dx.doi.org/10.1016/j.drudis.2016.05.015] [PMID: 27240777]

[102] B. Gülbakan, R.K. Özgül, A. Yüzbaşıoğlu, M. Kohl, H.P. Deigner, and M. Özgüç, "Discovery of biomarkers in rare diseases: innovative approaches by predictive and personalized medicine", *EPMA J.*, vol. 7, no. 1, p. 24, 2016. [http://dx.doi.org/10.1186/s13167-016-0074-2] [PMID: 27980697]

[103] R.D. Beger, M.A. Schmidt, and R. Kaddurah-Daouk, "Current concepts in pharmacometabolomics, biomarker discovery, and precision medicine", *Metabolites,* vol. 10, no. 4, p. 129, 2020.
[http://dx.doi.org/10.3390/metabo10040129] [PMID: 32230776]

[104] S. Askin, D. Burkhalter, G. Calado, and S. El Dakrouni, "Artificial Intelligence Applied to clinical trials: opportunities and challenges", *Health Technol. (Berl.),* vol. 13, no. 2, pp. 203-213, 2023.
[http://dx.doi.org/10.1007/s12553-023-00738-2] [PMID: 36923325]

[105] J.T. Beck, M. Rammage, G.P. Jackson, A.M. Preininger, I. Dankwa-Mullan, M.C. Roebuck, A. Torres, H. Holtzen, S.E. Coverdill, M.P. Williamson, Q. Chau, K. Rhee, and M. Vinegra, "Artificial Intelligence Tool for Optimizing Eligibility Screening for Clinical Trials in a Large Community Cancer Center", *JCO Clin. Cancer Inform.,* vol. 4, no. 4, pp. 50-59, 2020.
[http://dx.doi.org/10.1200/CCI.19.00079] [PMID: 31977254]

[106] Y.R. Chillakuru, S. Munjal, B. Laguna, T.L. Chen, G.R. Chaudhari, T. Vu, Y. Seo, J. Narvid, and J.H. Sohn, "Development and web deployment of an automated neuroradiology MRI protocoling tool with natural language processing", *BMC Med. Inform. Decis. Mak.,* vol. 21, no. 1, p. 213, 2021.
[http://dx.doi.org/10.1186/s12911-021-01574-y] [PMID: 34253196]

[107] S. Faisal, J. Ivo, S. Abu Fadaleh, and T. Patel, "Exploring the Value of Real-Time Medication Adherence Monitoring: A Qualitative Study", *Pharmacy (Basel),* vol. 11, no. 1, p. 18, 2023.
[http://dx.doi.org/10.3390/pharmacy11010018] [PMID: 36827656]

[108] R. Baembitov, M. Kezunovic, K.A. Brewster, and Z. Obradovic, "Incorporating Wind Modeling Into Electric Grid Outage Risk Prediction and Mitigation Solution", *IEEE Access,* vol. 11, pp. 4373-4380, 2023.
[http://dx.doi.org/10.1109/ACCESS.2023.3234984]

[109] T. Soha, L. Papp, C. Csontos, and B. Munkácsy, "The importance of high crop residue demand on biogas plant site selection, scaling and feedstock allocation – A regional scale concept in a Hungarian study area", *Renew. Sustain. Energy Rev.,* vol. 141, p. 110822, 2021.
[http://dx.doi.org/10.1016/j.rser.2021.110822]

[110] R. Lin, P.F. Thall, and Y. Yuan, "An adaptive trial design to optimize dose-schedule regimes with delayed outcomes", *Biometrics,* vol. 76, no. 1, pp. 304-315, 2020.
[http://dx.doi.org/10.1111/biom.13116] [PMID: 31273750]

[111] F.P. Cerqueira, A.M.C. Jesus, and M.D. Cotrim, ""Adaptive design: A review of the technical, statistical, and regulatory aspects of implementation in a clinical trial", In: *Therapeutic Innovation and Regulatory Science.* SAGE Publications Inc., 2019.
[http://dx.doi.org/10.1177/2168479019831240]

[112] P. Manickam, S.A. Mariappan, S.M. Murugesan, S. Hansda, A. Kaushik, R. Shinde, and S.P. Thipperudraswamy, "Artificial Intelligence (AI) and Internet of Medical Things (IoMT) Assisted Biomedical Systems for Intelligent Healthcare", *Biosensors (Basel),* vol. 12, no. 8, p. 562, 2022.
[http://dx.doi.org/10.3390/bios12080562] [PMID: 35892459]

[113] C. Intelligence and Neuroscience, "Retracted: Internet of Medical Things (IoMT)-Based Smart Healthcare System: Trends and Progress", *Comput. Intell. Neurosci.,* vol. 2023, no. 1, p. 9768292, 2023.
[http://dx.doi.org/10.1155/2023/9768292] [PMID: 38074388]

[114] S. Razdan, and S. Sharma, "Internet of Medical Things (IoMT): Overview, Emerging Technologies, and Case Studies", In: *IETE Technical Review (Institution of Electronics and Telecommunication Engineers, India)* vol. 39. Taylor and Francis Ltd., 2022, no. 4, pp. 775-788.
[http://dx.doi.org/10.1080/02564602.2021.1927863]

[115] K.S. Adewole, Cloud-based IoMT framework for cardiovascular disease prediction and diagnosis in personalized E-health care. *Intelligent IoT Systems in Personalized Health Care.* Elsevier, 2020, pp. 105-145.
[http://dx.doi.org/10.1016/B978-0-12-821187-8.00005-8]

[116] A. A, F. Dahan, R. Alroobaea, W.Y. Alghamdi, F. Hajjej, and K. Raahemifar, "A smart IoMT based architecture for E-healthcare patient monitoring system using artificial intelligence algorithms", *Front. Physiol.,* vol. 14, p. 1125952, 2023.
[http://dx.doi.org/10.3389/fphys.2023.1125952] [PMID: 36793418]

[117] O. AlShorman, B. AlShorman, M. Al-khassaweneh, and F. Alkahtani, "A review of internet of medical things (IoMT) - based remote health monitoring through wearable sensors: a case study for diabetic patients", *Indones. J. Electr. Eng. Comput. Sci.,* vol. 20, no. 1, pp. 414-422, 2020.
[http://dx.doi.org/10.11591/ijeecs.v20.i1.pp414-422]

[118] M.A. Khan, I.U. Din, B.S. Kim, and A. Almogren, "Visualization of Remote Patient Monitoring System Based on Internet of Medical Things", *Sustainability (Basel),* vol. 15, no. 10, p. 8120, 2023.
[http://dx.doi.org/10.3390/su15108120]

[119] S. K. Polu, "IoMT Based Smart Health Care Monitoring System," Int. J. Innov. Res. Sci. Technol., vol. 5, no. 11, pp. 58–64, 2019. [Online]. Available: Available from: www.ijirst.org

[120] A. Ciuffi, "The benefits of integration", *Clin. Microbiol. Infect.,* vol. 22, no. 4, pp. 324-332, 2016.
[http://dx.doi.org/10.1016/j.cmi.2016.02.013] [PMID: 27107301]

[121] S. Talapatra and G. Santos, "Circular Economy and Quality Management within the Furniture Sector: An Exploratory Study," in *Proc. 1st Conf. Qual. Innov. Sustain.* (ICQIS 2019), Valença, Portugal, June 2019, pp. 3–20. [Online]. [Accessed: 8 May 2025].
[http://dx.doi.org/10.1007/978-3-319-67925-9_1]

[122] G.K. Kiriiri, P.M. Njogu, and A.N. Mwangi, "Exploring different approaches to improve the success of drug discovery and development projects: a review", *Future J. Pharm. Sci.,* vol. 6, no. 1, p. 27, 2020.
[http://dx.doi.org/10.1186/s43094-020-00047-9]

[123] Y. Tanrikulu, B. Krüger, and E. Proschak, "The holistic integration of virtual screening in drug discovery", *Drug Discov. Today,* vol. 18, no. 7-8, pp. 358-364, 2013.
[http://dx.doi.org/10.1016/j.drudis.2013.01.007] [PMID: 23340112]

[124] S. Mathur, and J. Sutton, "Personalized medicine could transform healthcare (Review)", In: *Biomedical Reports* vol. 7. Spandidos Publications, 2017, no. 1, pp. 3-5.
[http://dx.doi.org/10.3892/br.2017.922]

[125] L.J. Schneiderman, N.S. Jecker, and A.R. Jonsen, "Medicine and public issues medical futility: its meaning and ethical implications", 1990. Available from: http://annals.org/

[126] J.E. Hunter, F.L. Schmidt, and J. Rauschenberger, Methodological, Statistical, and Ethical Issues in the Study of Bias in Psychological Tests. *Perspectives on Bias in Mental Testing.* Springer US, 1984, pp. 41-99.
[http://dx.doi.org/10.1007/978-1-4684-4658-6_2]

[127] M. Sarkis, A. Bernardi, N. Shah, and M.M. Papathanasiou, "Emerging challenges and opportunities in pharmaceutical manufacturing and distribution", *Processes (Basel),* vol. 9, no. 3, p. 457, 2021.
[http://dx.doi.org/10.3390/pr9030457]

[128] S. Byrn, "Achieving continuous manufacturing for final dosage formation: Challenges and how to meet them continuous symposium novartis-mit center for continuous manufacturing", 2014.

[129] E. Jovanov, A. Milenkovic, C. Otto, and P.C. de Groen, "A wireless body area network of intelligent motion sensors for computer assisted physical rehabilitation", *J. Neuroeng. Rehabil.,* vol. 2, no. 1, p. 6, 2005.
[http://dx.doi.org/10.1186/1743-0003-2-6] [PMID: 15740621]

[130] G.D. Logan, *Skill and Automaticity: Relations.* Implications, and Future Directions, 1985.

[131] C. Austin, and F. Kusumoto, "The application of Big Data in medicine: current implications and future directions", *J. Interv. Card. Electrophysiol.,* vol. 47, no. 1, pp. 51-59, 2016.

[http://dx.doi.org/10.1007/s10840-016-0104-y] [PMID: 26814841]

[132] R.T. Liu, "Stress generation: Future directions and clinical implications", *Clin. Psychol. Rev.,* vol. 33, no. 3, pp. 406-416, 2013.
       [http://dx.doi.org/10.1016/j.cpr.2013.01.005] [PMID: 23416877]

CHAPTER 11

Healthcare Outcomes Amplified by Data Insights

N. Bhaskara Rao[1], Shaweta Sharma[2], Sunita[3], Akanksha Sharma[4] and Akhil Sharma[4,*]

[1] *Department of Civil Engineering, Aditya University, Surampalem, India*

[2] *School of Medical and Allied Sciences, Galgotias University Plot No. 2, Yamuna Expy, Opposite Buddha International Circuit, Sector 17A, Greater Noida, Uttar Pradesh, India*

[3] *Metro College of Health Sciences and Research, Greater Noida, Uttar Pradesh, India*

[4] *R.J. College of Pharmacy, Raipur, Gharbara, Tappal, Khair, Uttar Pradesh, India*

Abstract: The level of success in healthcare can be assessed by patient care improvements, treatment efficiency, and overall quality of health provision. The aim of clinical outcomes is challenging and influenced by several factors, such as patient demography, disease profile, treatment methods, and healthcare delivery systems. Over the past years, there has been an increase in healthcare information available and new ways to improve outcomes through data-driven decisions. This chapter is about how data insights can improve healthcare outcomes. It starts by explaining why healthcare outcomes are important in gauging the effectiveness of health interventions. Problems associated with health care delivery, such as different responses to treatment, escalating costs, and gaps in access to services, will be explored throughout this chapter. Healthcare providers can obtain useful information regarding trends in patient health, treatment effectiveness, and disease evolution when they use data from varied sources such as electronic health records, medical imaging, and wearable devices. Consequently, this acquired evidence enhances decision-making, personalized treatment approaches, and proactive interventions to optimize healthcare outcomes. The use of data insights ranging from predictive analytics for early disease detection to personalized medicine based on individual genetic profiles gives an unprecedented opportunity to improve patient outcomes, reducing clinical workflow redundancy and minimizing overall healthcare budgets. However, the chapter also recognizes the ethical, legal, and technical challenges of leveraging healthcare data. Concerns regarding patient privacy, data security, and algorithmic bias must be addressed to realize the full potential of data-driven healthcare. In conclusion, the chapter highlights the transformative impact of data insights into healthcare outcomes and calls for continued investment and innovation in data-driven approaches to improve patient care and population health.

* **Corresponding author Akhil Sharma:** R.J. College of Pharmacy, Raipur, Gharbara, Tappal, Khair, Uttar Pradesh, India; E-mail: xs2akhil@gmail.com

Keywords: Data insights, Digital, Disease, Electronic health records, Health, Healthcare, Machine learning algorithms, Medicine, Patient, Predictive modeling, Real-time monitoring, Wearable devices.

INTRODUCTION

The healthcare system's cornerstone is healthcare outcomes, which are the results and repercussions of medical interventions, treatments, and healthcare services. The efficiency, efficacy, and quality of care delivered can be assessed by these outcomes and their impact on patients' health welfare as well as the overall performance of the health systems [1].

The essence of healthcare outcomes is their ability to ascertain the effectiveness of clinical treatments. They serve as indices by which healthcare practices can measure their goal attainment in terms of patients' health. Healthcare intervention outcomes give important insights into the effectiveness of different treatment and therapeutic approaches for managing chronic conditions, preventing diseases, or treating acute illnesses [2].

Healthcare outcome is still the major determinant in the overall assessment of healthcare service quality. As a result, this allows healthcare professionals and institutions to evaluate their performance on specific clinical guidelines and best practices. Healthcare entities can identify areas that need improvement and adopt evidence-based practices through outcomes, enabling them to improve patient safety [3].

Healthcare outcomes have broader implications for healthcare system performance and public health beyond individual patient encounters. Policymakers and public health officials can evaluate the effectiveness of public health interventions, healthcare policies, and preventive measures through monitoring population-level outcomes. It helps them allocate resources efficiently, make informed decisions, and address health disparities to enhance overall population health outcomes [4].

Moreover, healthcare results are intimately connected to the satisfaction and experiences of patients. Such positive outcomes include enhanced health, relief from symptoms, and a better quality of life, which patients value in healthcare encounters. These positive outcomes lead to long-term loyalty and relationships between patients and healthcare providers or systems [5].

Besides making patients feel better, good results in healthcare can save costs to both patients and health systems. Better health outcomes may reduce the need for medical interventions, drugs, and hospital stays, thus lowering healthcare costs.

Likewise, by focusing on interventions and practices that result in a positive outcome, healthcare facilities can optimize resource utilization and minimize this unnecessary use of health services [6].

On the other hand, negative results in health care may also be disadvantageous for patients, healthcare providers, and systems at large. For instance, outcomes below standard can result in extended sicknesses, disabilities, or complications among individuals, thereby leading to reduced living standards and increased medical expenses. These results potentially reduce patients' trust in healthcare workers and organizations, thus hampering patient-focused service provision [7].

The concept of data-driven insights has become a powerful tool across industries, including healthcare, in today's society. Data insights are meaningful information that can be acted upon, derived from analyzing huge amounts of data. Such perspectives or patterns revealed by this correlation may help organizations make decisions, foster innovation and identify areas for growth [8].

Healthcare data insights are useful in enhancing patient outcomes, transforming care delivery, and optimizing healthcare operations. Healthcare providers and organizations can learn more about the health condition of patients, trends in diseases, effectiveness of treatment, and patterns of healthcare use by utilizing the abundant health data produced within systems like Electronic Health Records (EHRs), medical imaging, genetic information, and patient-generated data [9].

Clinical decision-making is an important area where data insights can make a major difference. Healthcare providers can use data analytics and machine learning algorithms to analyze patient data and formulate personalized treatment plans for the patient's specific needs. For instance, prediction models based on analytics can help identify persons with a high chance of developing certain diseases or experiencing adverse events, thereby facilitating preventive interventions and proactive steps that enhance patient results [10].

Further, data analytics can enable evidence-based medicine by transforming clinical data and research into practical guidelines for medical practice. Medical personnel can access extensive databases and clinical decision support systems that offer real-time recommendations and guidance using current medical information and treatment techniques. This ensures that patient care is consistent with contemporary norms and regulations, enhancing better clinical results as well as the safety of patients [11].

Data insights have extensive implications for population health management and public health surveillance beyond clinical care. Public health agencies and healthcare organizations can use population-level data to discover patterns of diseases, identify and trace outbreaks, and detect disparities in healthcare access and outcomes. Stakeholders may develop focused interventions and allocate resources properly for pressing public health challenges utilizing predictive modeling and data visualization techniques [12].

Additionally, healthcare organizations can use data insights to drive continuous quality improvement and operational efficiency. Healthcare leaders can identify areas for improvement by looking at performance metrics such as how long patients stay in the hospital, hospital readmission rates, and patient satisfaction scores. Moreover, data analytics entails optimizing resource allocation, streamlining workflows, and lowering healthcare costs through improved inventory management, staffing scheduling, and patient flow optimization [13].

In the world of research and innovation, the progressions in medical technology are fueled by data insights. This can be achieved by collecting and analyzing large clinical and genomic datasets to help identify new biomarkers, therapeutic targets, and treatment modalities for various diseases. Furthermore, data-driven approaches result in precision medicine and personal healthcare solutions considering genetic differences among individuals and lifestyle and environmental factors [14].

Data insights, which can help unlock the full potential of healthcare, are faced with several obstacles, such as lack of data interoperability, privacy concerns, quality problems in data, and the need for professionals in data analysis. Healthcare organizations need to invest in strong data infrastructure, cybersecurity measures, and data governance frameworks that can ensure the ethical use and security of patients' information [15].

TYPES OF HEALTHCARE DATA

Healthcare data includes a huge amount of information collected and produced in the healthcare domain. This type of information is used for different purposes, such as clinical decision-making, research, healthcare delivery, and population health management [16]. Types of healthcare data are summarized in Fig. (**1**) and discussed below.

Medical Imaging Data

Modern healthcare relies heavily on medical imaging data, which provides detailed images of the human body to help diagnose, prepare treatment plans, and monitor medical conditions. The main imaging modalities and their uses are explained below [17].

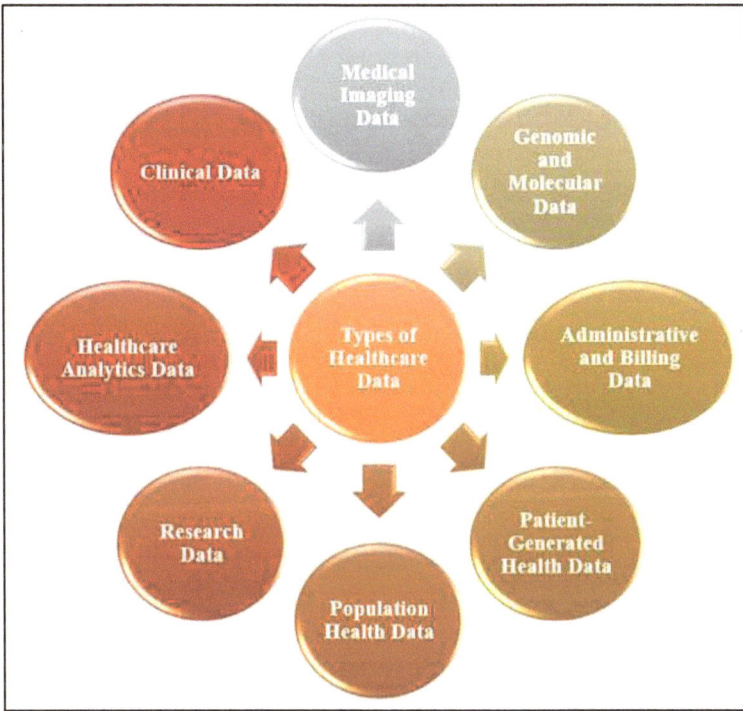

Fig. (1). Types of healthcare data.

X-rays

X-rays are produced through electromagnetic radiation to create two-dimensional images of internal body structures, especially bones and soft tissues. X-rays usually diagnose bone fractures, joint dislocations, dental problems, and diseases like pneumonia that affect the chest [18].

Computed Tomography (CT)

Detailed cross-sectional images of the body can be made by combining multiple X-ray images taken from different angles into CT scans. These scans help determine and assess different ailments such as traumatic injuries, tumors, vascular disorders, and brain, abdominal and chest abnormalities [19].

Magnetic Resonance Imaging (MRI)

MRI uses strong magnets and radio waves to produce clear images of the body's inside, such as its soft tissues, organs, and brain. For diagnosis of neurological abnormalities or disorders, musculoskeletal injuries, spinal cord deformities, or diseases that involve heart and blood vessels, MRI is most useful [20].

Ultrasound

Ultrasound technology employs high-frequency sound waves that create live pictures of the body's internal organs, blood flow, and tissues. It is frequently used in prenatal examinations, watching fetal growths, diagnosing conditions affecting the abdomen and pelvis, checking heart performance and circulatory system, and helping clinicians perform minimally invasive procedures such as biopsies or injections [21].

Positron Emission Tomography (PET)

PET scans use radioactive tracers that emit positrons, which are detected by a PET scanner, to render three-dimensional images of metabolism within the body. PET scans are broadly employed for cancer diagnosis and staging, evaluation of brain activity about neurological disorders, and assessment of heart disease [22].

Medical imaging data helps medical practitioners see the internal body parts, find out about deviations, and make precise treatment decisions. They have become an important tool for diagnosing various medical conditions ranging from fractures and tumors to cardiovascular diseases and nerve disorders. Medicinal imaging data shows a complete understanding of the body's intricate structures and functions, thereby enabling early detection, precise diagnosis, and personalized therapeutic plans that eventually enhance patient outcomes and healthcare quality in general [23].

Genomic and Molecular Data

A transformative frontier in healthcare is represented by genomic and molecular data, providing insights into diseases' genetic and molecular basis and individual variability in treatment responses that have never been seen before. Our comprehension of genetic disease, inherited traits, and complex illnesses has been altered by the advent of genomic data, which encompasses all the genetic information in an organism's DNA. Advances in genomic sequencing technology now make it possible for scientists to read the whole human genome, decode it, and identify specific variations in DNA sequences. This development has paved the way for personalized medicine based on patients' genetic profiles [24].

Transcriptome data collection, which highlights gene expression patterns, enhances our understanding of the mechanism behind gene activation or suppression under different physiological conditions or diseases. Biomarkers molecular signatures can be identified by researchers using these transcriptomic data for specific diseases and treatment responses, which might improve diagnosis accuracy and prognosis and influence therapeutic choice. Proteome information enhances the knowledge of cellular processes and disease mechanisms by capturing the entire set of proteins in any cell type, tissue, or organism.

Biomarker discovery, drug target identification, and drug development are facilitated by proteomic analyses through which protein targets for therapeutic intervention are revealed, and the efficacy, safety, and mechanisms of action of drugs are assessed. In terms of the molecular landscape of health and disease, these provide a complete overview that enables researchers and healthcare providers to unravel the complexities of diseases to design targeted therapies that would eventually improve patient outcomes.

The possibility to revolutionize health provision may arise from using these multidimensional data sets, which can be combined with clinical information and other omics data to reach a new era in healthcare where treatments are developed based on distinctive genetic or molecular make-ups of individual patients. The increasing accessibility and advancement in the technologies used for genomics and molecular studies have raised hopes for more efficient therapeutic approaches, improved patient care, and advanced knowledge about human biology [25].

Administrative and Billing Data

Administrative and billing data are a basic element of the healthcare system since they explain healthcare utilization, financial transactions, and efficiency in operation. They represent a wide range of information about healthcare services, insurance coverage, reimbursement, and expenditures that form the basis for financing, reimbursement, and policy-making processes in healthcare. Administrative data mainly collects most demographic details about patients necessary for identification due to their demographics, insurance information, or contact details, hence aiding in patient registration as well as communication within different healthcare organizations [26].

On the contrary, financial data relating to healthcare interactions are contained in billing data, which gives an account of what went down and the related charges. Revenue cycle management, claims processing, and reimbursement discussions between providers and payers heavily depend on these types of information. Moreover, administrative and billing data permit healthcare analytics that helps stakeholders analyze healthcare utilization patterns, detect service delivery trends, and assess the financial performance of healthcare organizations. Through putting together administrative and billing data, healthcare leaders can now gain insights into the allocation of resources, operational efficiency, and income growth, thus making informed decisions for strategic planning [27].

Moreover, healthcare policy formulation also depends on administrative and billing data. This is important because it helps monitor healthcare spending, evaluate the effectiveness of healthcare policies, and ensure that they are enforced as regulatory bodies require. However, some challenges have prevented maximizing billing and administration in healthcare, such as privacy concerns, data accuracy, and interoperability. Healthcare organizations are increasingly adopting electronic administration processes and billing through interoperable health information systems, making administrative and billing data more useful for evidence-based decision-making, improving care delivery and financial sustainability.

The administrative and billing data in the health sector are fundamental since they give information about patients' demographics, how they use healthcare services, and their financial transactions, which are crucial for effective healthcare management, policy development, and regulation. The administrative and billing data utilized by healthcare players can help them allocate resources efficiently, simplify operations, and enhance healthcare services quality and productivity to be advantageous for all patients, payers, and providers [28].

Patient-Generated Health Data

Patient-generated health data (PGHD) is an emerging source of information in the healthcare industry, providing useful knowledge about patients' daily lives and their well-being levels. PGHD comprises a wide range of patient-derived health-related information from numerous devices or applications like mobile medical apps, e-patient portals, and wearables. These data sources capture a wide range of information, including vital signs, physical activity levels, sleep patterns, dietary habits, symptom reports, medication adherence, and patient-reported outcomes. By empowering patients to actively participate in their care and monitor their health away from traditional clinical settings, PGHD holds promise for enhancing patient engagement, promoting self-management, and improving health outcomes [29].

Additionally, PGHD helps providers see a bigger picture of patient's health and behavior, allowing for personalized care planning, making decisions regarding treatment, and managing diseases. For instance, wearable devices for remote monitoring of vital signs and symptom monitoring enable healthcare providers to locate any signs of deterioration at early stages, thereby intervening before it leads to complications or hospital readmission. Furthermore, traditional clinical assessments and laboratory tests can be supplemented by PGHD, which gives real-time information on patients' treatment responses, medication compliance, and lifestyle changes.

This patient-centered care delivery model promotes coordination of care that is more effective among patients and providers, leading to shared decisions and improved quality of care. Nonetheless, some obstacles, such as data precision, unity of data, compatibility, and privacy concerns, hamper the extensive application and meaningful use of PGHD in healthcare practice. Healthcare organizations are responsible for providing secure data collection, transmission, and storage of PGHD by establishing strong data governance policies, security practices, and interoperability requirements. Additionally, healthcare providers must plan ways to adopt PGHD into clinical workflows that consider patients general health status when interpreting this information and include them in EHRs and clinical decision support systems.

The PGHD continues to evolve as it gains pace in the healthcare sector. Against this background, the stakeholders must join hands and deal with the challenges they face and maximize the use of PGHD to change healthcare delivery, enhance patient capability, and improve general health. Patient-generated health data represents a paradigm shift in healthcare, empowering patients to take an active role in managing their health and enabling healthcare providers to deliver more personalized, proactive, patient-centered care. By leveraging PGHD, healthcare organizations can enhance care quality, promote patient engagement, and drive improvements in health outcomes, ultimately advancing the goal of achieving better health for all [30].

Population Health Data

The public health data constitute a wide-ranging and complete record, which offers an overview of health behaviors, outcomes, and status of entire populations or communities. It includes demographic, clinical, environmental, and social determinants of health; this way, a comprehensive view of health issues at the population level can be obtained. Many sources, such as public health surveillance systems, epidemiological studies and health surveys, vital statistics, administrative records, and socioeconomic indicators, contribute to population health data. Public health officials, policymakers, and healthcare organizations can identify health trends, monitor disease prevalence, and assess risk factors by aggregating and analyzing these diverse data sets while prioritizing interventions that improve population health outcomes [31].

For example, health disparities among different demographic groups, geographic regions, or socioeconomic strata can be identified using population health data, which can help target interventions in social determinants of health like poverty, education, housing, and healthcare access. Additionally, populations health statistics promote active public health endeavors that let stakeholders implement evidence-based approaches to reducing the toll from non-contagious illnesses such as cancer, preventing infectious disease outbreaks, and cultivating healthy community behaviors. Moreover, population health data form a basis for policy-making on health and resource allocation decisions while providing policymakers with evidence to develop effective public health policies, programs, and initiatives [32].

The levering of population health data by healthcare organizations facilitates the implementation of population health management strategies aimed at improving health outcomes, reducing healthcare costs, and enhancing the overall well-being of populations. Nevertheless, there are still significant barriers to maximizing the utility of population health data, such as data interoperability, privacy concerns, data quality, and limited access to comprehensive datasets. Healthcare organizations and public health agencies should work together to overcome these obstacles and create a strong data infrastructure, governance frameworks, and analytical capabilities that will enable the maximum utilization of population health data [33].

While population health is growing, stakeholders should keep up with innovation and fully use such technologies as Artificial Intelligence (AI), Machine Learning (ML), and big data analytics to find actionable insights into population health data and improve health outcomes at the population level. Public health practice, policy development, and healthcare delivery benefit from population health data, which gives a holistic picture of different groups of people's health status and requirements. Population health data can identify disparities in health care, prioritize interventions, and implement evidence-based approaches for promoting equity in health, preventing diseases, and enhancing the general well-being of communities [34].

Research Data

Scientific inquiry relies heavily on research data, which comprises various clinical trial protocols, study participant demographics, clinical assessments, laboratory test results, imaging findings, genetic analyses, and adverse event reports. The information contained herein is collected during different types of research, such as disease mechanisms evaluation trials for treatment effectiveness or even new healthcare interventions. These data are mainly collected from activities such as clinical trials, observational studies, and projects to investigate disease mechanisms, assess treatment efficacy, or develop new healthcare interventions, including a wide range of information [35].

Collecting and analyzing research data systematically helps researchers test hypotheses, generate new information, and validate scientific discoveries that aid clinical decision-making and healthcare policies. For instance, data from research from Randomized Controlled Trials (RCTs) provide strong evidence about the effectiveness and safety of drug interventions, medical devices, and surgical procedures, which are essential in regulatory approval and clinical practice guidelines. Furthermore, observational and cohort studies offer insights into disease risk factors, natural history, and long-term outcomes to inform disease prevention strategies and public health measures. Additionally, research data is crucial in translational research because it helps bridge the gap between basic science discoveries and clinical applications [36].

Developments of new diagnoses, therapeutics, and interventions in clinical practice are facilitated as a result of translating laboratory findings. This leads to the improvement of outcomes for patients with unmet medical needs. Furthermore, research data enhances collaboration and knowledge sharing among scientists, enabling them to repeat studies, verify results, or do more experiments on earlier research, thus moving scientific explanations forward. Nevertheless, challenges such as data sharing, reproducibility, and data management remain significant barriers to maximizing the value of research data.

Addressing these challenges requires research institutions and funding agencies to increasingly adopt policies and guidelines on data sharing, stewardship, and transparency. Moreover, developing data infrastructure, computational tools, and data analytic methodologies has allowed researchers to use big data and machine learning to extract insights from vast research data. Given the increasing volume and sophistication of research datasets, stakeholders must intensify their efforts to promote standardization, interoperability, and governance to safeguard the integrity, privacy, and accessibility of scientific information.

Advancement of scientific knowledge, better healthcare outcomes, and innovation depend on research data. Researchers can produce fresh ideas, develop evidence-based interventions, and enhance patient care quality through organized collection, analysis, and dissemination of research data. Stakeholders must work together to overcome biomedical data difficulties and employ modern technologies for optimal usage in health domains [37].

Healthcare Analytics Data

Healthcare analytics data is a wealth of information from analyzing various healthcare datasets: operational, financial, clinical, and administrative. These data sources are collected from healthcare establishments such as insurance companies, clinics, hospitals, and laboratories. They inform decision-making, improve healthcare delivery, and enhance patient outcomes. Healthcare analytics comprises several analytical techniques and tools, including descriptive, predictive, and prescriptive analytics, designed to draw meaningful insights from complicated healthcare data [38].

Descriptive analytics involves summarizing and pictorially representing data to appreciate historical events, models, and performance indices such as patient age, disease prevalence, utilization rates, or quality measures. The predictive analysis utilizes statistical modeling, machine learning algorithms, and data mining methodologies to estimate future happenings or results like disease outbreaks, hospital readmission, or patient deterioration based on historical data patterns and risk factors. Prescriptive analytics goes beyond that and suggests the right actions or interventions to reach desired outcomes, such as customized treatment plans, resource allocation approaches, and care coordination initiatives founded on predictive modeling and decision support algorithms.

Healthcare analytics data are essential in healthcare organizations' performance measurement, quality improvement, and population health management initiatives. By analyzing healthcare analytics data, the stakeholders can identify prospects for streamlining processes, lowering costs, and improving quality across the care continuum. For example, analytics data enables healthcare providers to monitor Key Performance Indicators (KPIs), track patient outcomes, and benchmark their performance against industry standards to drive continuous improvement efforts. Similarly, analytics data can help healthcare payers evaluate provider performance, manage risk, and optimize network utilization, ensuring efficient care delivery at manageable costs [39].

Moreover, healthcare analytics is essential for population health management strategies implemented to improve people's health outcomes, reduce the cost of healthcare, and address healthcare disparities within communities. When collected together and analyzed at a group level, public health facilities and healthcare establishments can know the populations with a high chance of suffering from diseases; they can then apply prevention efforts and prioritization or allocation of resources toward population health issues. Despite this, challenges like data standards, quality of data, and privacy have not been addressed fully, hindering the maximum value of healthcare analytics datasets. Therefore, there is a need for strong data infrastructure as well as governance frameworks and analytical capabilities that guarantee the reliability, consistency, and safety of healthcare analytics data [40].

Additionally, creating a data-driven culture and developing analytic skills among healthcare players are indispensable for fully exploiting healthcare analytics data to improve healthcare delivery and patient outcomes. Healthcare organizations use this information to enlighten their decision-making through Evidence-Based

Decision Making (EBDM), performance improvement, and population health management efforts. By employing sophisticated analytical methods in conjunction with appropriate tools, significant stakeholders can unleash healthcare analytics to its full potential to optimize care delivery, improve patients' experiences, and reach better health outcomes for individuals and communities [36].

Clinical Data

Clinical data is collected either during patient treatment or clinical trials and comprises information gathered at medical facilities, hospitals, clinics, or practices, such as administrative and demographic details, diagnoses, treatments, prescription drugs, laboratory tests, and physiologic monitoring data- including hospitalization records and patient insurance information. Therefore, clinical data enhances patient care and medical research [41]. The tabular representation of different types of clinical data commonly found in healthcare is shown in Table **1**.

IMPORTANCE OF MEASURING HEALTHCARE OUTCOMES

There are several reasons why measuring healthcare outcomes is important; it helps understand healthcare providers' performance, quality, and efficiency. The significance of the measurement of healthcare outcomes is discussed below.

Assessment of Treatment Effectiveness

The success or failure of medical interventions and treatments in achieving desired health goals for patients is indicated by healthcare outcomes. Different treatment modalities can be assessed based on the effectiveness of symptom relief, disease remission, or functional improvement by measuring such outcomes, enabling healthcare providers to tailor care plans that will optimize patient outcomes [51].

Quality Improvement

Healthcare organizations can use healthcare outcome monitoring to evaluate performance against established benchmarks and standards like best practices and clinical guidelines. By identifying differences in outcomes and analyzing the root causes of suboptimal performances, healthcare providers can implement focused quality improvement efforts that improve the safety, effectiveness, and patient-centeredness of care delivery [52].

Table 1. Different types of clinical data commonly found in healthcare.

Type of Clinical Data	Description	Examples
Demographic	Information about patient demographics such as age, gender, ethnicity, and location.	Age, gender, ethnicity, address [42]
Vital Signs	Measurements indicate the body's basic functions, including temperature, heart rate, blood pressure, and respiratory rate.	Temperature, heart rate, blood pressure, respiratory rate [43]
Laboratory Results	Data from diagnostic tests performed on patient samples, including blood, urine, and tissue samples.	Complete blood count (CBC), blood glucose levels, and cholesterol levels [44].
Medical History	Details about past illnesses, surgeries, medications, allergies, and family medical history.	Previous diagnoses, surgical procedures, medications, and allergies [45].
Medication Records	Information about prescribed medications, including dosage, frequency, and duration of use.	Medication names, dosage, frequency, and start/end dates [46].
Diagnostic Imaging	Results from medical imaging tests such as X-rays, MRI scans, CT scans, and ultrasounds.	X-ray images, MRI scans, and CT scan reports [47].
Clinical Notes	Narrative descriptions of patient encounters, including symptoms, observations, and treatment plans.	Progress notes, consultation notes, and discharge summaries [48].
Procedure Records	Document medical procedures performed on patients, including surgeries, treatments, and interventions.	Surgical procedures, and therapeutic interventions [49]
Immunization Records	Records of vaccinations received by patients, including vaccine types and administration dates.	Vaccine names, and administration dates [50].

Resource Allocation

Measuring healthcare outcomes helps in the efficient allocation of resources by healthcare organizations, besides prioritizing interventions that significantly impact patient outcomes. Healthcare providers can improve resource allocation, cut waste, and improve the worth of their healthcare delivery by identifying high-value interventions while at the same time reducing low-value or unnecessary services [53].

Patient-Centered Care

The impact of medical treatments, as seen by patients, is the main source of useful information about health care outcomes. In this regard, using patient-reported outcomes and preferences in measuring outcomes results in a higher commitment to patients' goals, values, and choices, leading to more satisfied and engaged patients [54].

Informed Decision-Making

Patients, healthcare providers, and policymakers are given the ability to make informed choices regarding healthcare outcomes through healthcare outcomes data. Healthcare interventions like treatment options and resource allocation can be chosen based on synthesizing evidence about different interventions' effectiveness and safety. Outcome measurement combines evidence of effective and safe interventions to support shared decision-making, enabling stakeholders to choose the most appropriate and evidence-based care paths [55].

Continuous Learning and Innovation

Healthcare outcomes measurement categorizes the healthcare organization into a culture characterized by continuous learning and improvement. Analyzing outcomes data enables healthcare providers to learn more about the areas for innovation, trial new care delivery models, and incorporate best practices in their clinical workflows, thereby facilitating the progress of healthcare systems and enhancing patient results over time [56].

Accountability and Transparency

Healthcare outcomes measurement enhances accountability and transparency in healthcare delivery by offering stakeholders impartial measurements to evaluate performance and track development towards established goals. This promotes public reporting of outcome data, signifying the organization's commitment to quality and safety and its responsibility to patients, payers, and regulatory agencies.

Measuring healthcare outcomes is very important as it helps assess the efficacy of treatment, quality improvement, optimal allocation of resources, patient-centered care delivery, decision-making, innovation, and accountability in healthcare delivery. By prioritizing the measurement of outcomes and integrating outcome data into clinical practice, healthcare organizations can achieve better health results for individuals and populations while improving overall value and efficiency in healthcare provision [57].

EXAMPLES OF HEALTHCARE OUTCOMES

Patient Recovery Rates

The proportion of patients who recover from a given condition or disease after medical treatment is being measured. For instance, in a surgical setting, recovery rates could mean the fraction of patients who have successfully recuperated from surgery without complications or adverse events [58].

Mortality Rates

Mortality rates describe the number of deaths in a given population or group of patients during a certain period. Healthcare providers often monitor mortality rates to evaluate the efficacy of operative procedures, drugs, and disease management programs [59].

Hospital Readmission Rates

Hospital readmission rates measure the number of patients returning to the hospital after discharge. High readmission rates may mean poor care coordination, poor medicine management, or lack of follow-up after discharge, necessitating interventions designed to reduce them [60].

Length of Stay

The term 'length of stay' refers to the time patients spend in a healthcare facility such as a hospital or rehabilitation center for a particular episode of care. When stays are short, it might mean that care is efficient and treatment successful, but prolonged stays may indicate complications or difficulties encountered during discharge [61].

Functional Status Improvement

Functional status improvement measures the extent to which patients regain or improve their ability to perform activities of daily living (ADLs) or functional tasks following medical treatment or rehabilitation. This outcome is particularly relevant for patients undergoing physical therapy, occupational therapy, or rehabilitation services [62].

Patient Satisfaction Scores

Patient satisfaction scores assess patients' perceptions of the quality, accessibility, and responsiveness of healthcare services received. These scores may be based on surveys, feedback forms, or patient-reported experience measures (PREMs), and they provide valuable insights into patients' experiences and preferences for care delivery [63].

Quality of Life Improvements

Measuring the quality of life improvement patients gain from healthcare interventions involves evaluating their overall mental, physical, social, and other emotional well-being. To illustrate, treatments for chronic illnesses like cancer, diabetes, or chronic pain can improve patients' quality of life by reducing symptoms, enhancing function, and promoting health and happiness in an individual's life [64].

Complication Rates

The complication rate estimates the number of complications or adverse events that arise from healthcare procedures, treatments, or interventions. By tracking complication rates, healthcare providers can identify opportunities for improvement and implement preventive measures to improve patient safety.

These are some of the healthcare outcomes that are frequently evaluated and tracked in different healthcare settings. Every outcome would give insights into the efficacy, safety, and quality of healthcare services delivered, enabling providers and organizations to gauge their performance, make requisite improvements in quality, and eventually improve patient care or outcomes [65].

CHALLENGES IN HEALTHCARE OUTCOMES

Achieving optimal healthcare outcomes is a complex endeavor often hindered by various challenges, ranging from clinical to systemic issues. The key challenges in healthcare are described below and summarized in Fig. (**2**).

Variability in Treatment Effectiveness

Health outcomes in healthcare can change greatly between patients depending on genetics, concurrent illnesses, class lines, and lifestyle changes. Health providers face a major difficulty because there are wide variations in the efficacy of these treatments in selecting interventions and managing patient's experiences to maximize results [66].

Rising Healthcare Costs

The escalating healthcare costs are a barrier to optimal outcomes because they create financial impediments to access, deviations in care, and inefficiencies in healthcare delivery systems. Higher costs can curtail patients' access to timely and appropriate treatment, leading to delays or non-adherence to treatment guidelines and disparities in health outcomes among the various socioeconomic groups [67].

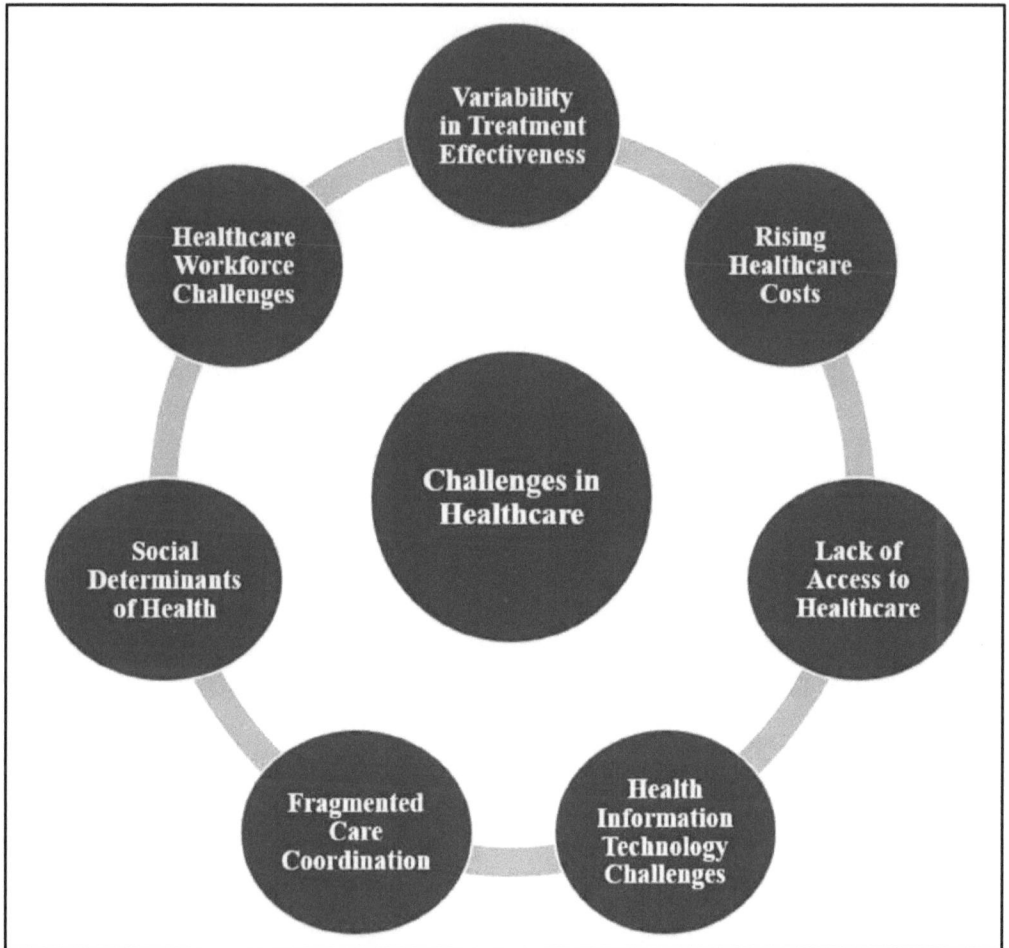

Fig. (2). Challenges in healthcare.

Lack of Access to Healthcare

Health disparities arise from gaps in the availability of healthcare facilities and services that include primary care, specialty care, and preventative services. Access to healthcare depends on several factors, such as geographical location, insurance coverage, social status, and cultural obstacles. These factors can impede timely and appropriate medical care, contributing to uneven health outcomes among different people [68].

Health Information Technology (HIT) Challenges

Although Health Information Technology (HIT) promises to improve healthcare delivery and outcomes, the realization of its prospects is hampered by problems like interoperability, data security, and usability. Moreover, incoherent systems, piecemeal records, and concerns over confidentiality and safety prevent the smooth sharing of patient records and the application of analytical findings from optimizing treatment provision and results [69].

Fragmented Care Coordination

The continuity of treatment, communication, and collaboration between health teams may be disrupted by fragmentation in care delivery across various healthcare settings, providers, and specializations. Because of poor coordination of care, patient outcomes may be compromised by omissions in care, repeated tests or procedures, mistakes in medication administration, and harmful incidents that eventually reduce patient satisfaction levels [70].

Social Determinants of Health

Social determinants of health like socioeconomic status, education, housing, and access to healthy food and transportation significantly influence health outcomes. Addressing social determinants of health requires a multi-sectoral approach involving collaboration between healthcare providers, community organizations, policymakers, and other stakeholders to address underlying social, economic, and environmental factors that impact the health of individuals [71].

Healthcare Workforce Challenges

Delivering high-quality care and achieving optimal outcomes are hindered by healthcare workforce shortages, workforce burnout, and workforce distribution imbalances. As such, patient access to timely and appropriate care can be limited due to insufficient staff levels, lack of specialty providers, or geographical maldistribution of health professionals, causing delays in diagnosis and treatment and poorer health outcomes [72].

Adopting a comprehensive multi-dimensional approach, including policy interventions, health system reforms, investment in health infrastructures, and collaboration among stakeholders along the healthcare continuum, is necessary to address these challenges. By addressing all these challenges together, healthcare systems can achieve closer, optimal outcomes for everyone [69].

ROLE OF DATA INSIGHTS ON HEALTHCARE OUTCOMES

Data insights are facilitated by enhanced care delivery and informed decisions for healthcare providers and other stakeholders, including policymakers, to optimize treatment and improve continuous quality. These are actionable pieces of information that help improve healthcare results. The role of data insights in healthcare outcomes is explained below and in Fig. (**3**).

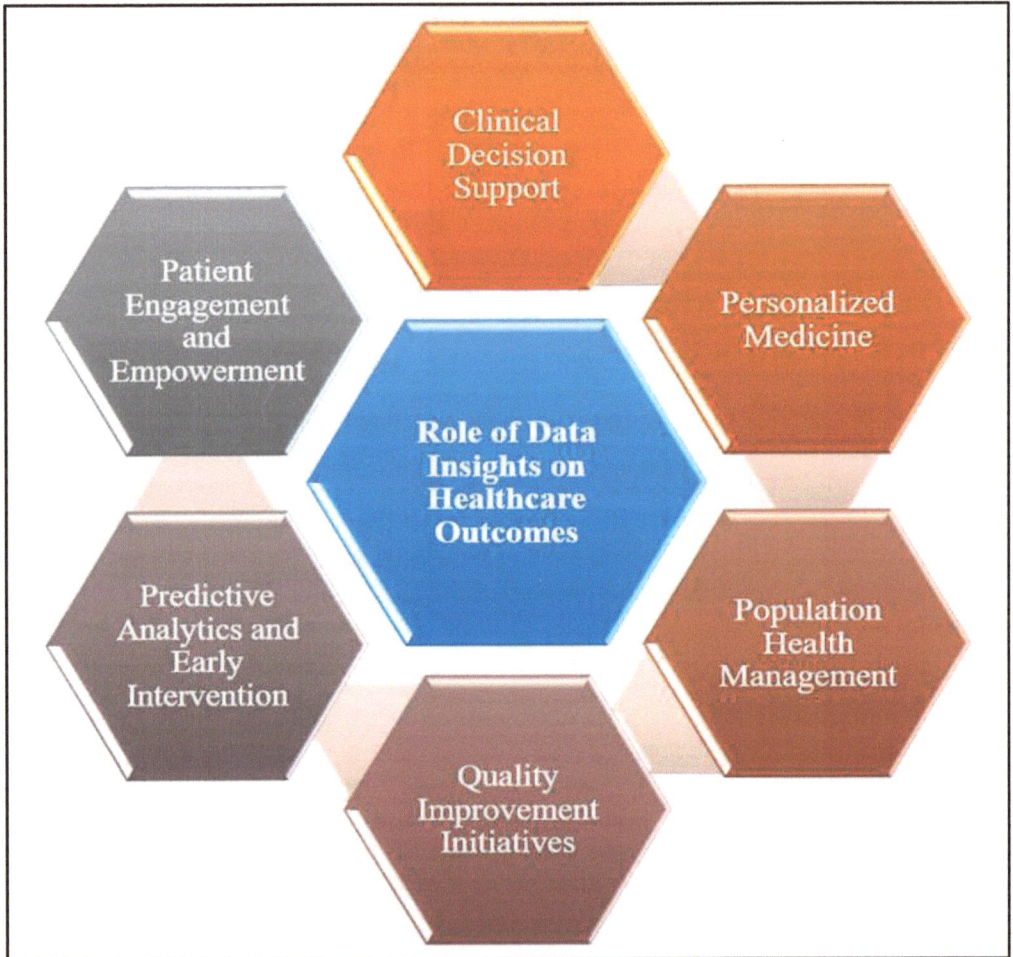

Fig. (3). Role of data insights on healthcare outcomes.

Clinical Decision Support

Data insights from clinical sources like EHRs and medical imaging support clinical decisions. Clinical decision support systems can diagnose diseases, prescribe suitable therapies, and forecast patient outcomes by reviewing patient data, patterns, and risk determinants. Through this process, healthcare providers make better clinical decisions and improve patient outcomes [73].

Personalized Medicine

Genomic, molecular, and patient-generated health data can provide information that enables personalized medicine approaches that consider individual patient traits, preferences, and genetic profiles. The use of predictive analytics and modeling by healthcare providers has the potential to identify the best treatment plans, forecast responsiveness to treatments, and divide patients based on their characteristics to optimize therapies while minimizing adverse effects that may result in better health results [74, 75].

Quality Improvement Initiatives

Improving the health of patients is always a goal that organizations strive to achieve while ensuring data insights are available. This involves measuring the key performance indicators, tracking healthcare outcomes, and comparing them to industry-wide standards, enabling healthcare institutions to ascertain their weaknesses that need improvement so they can devise relevant quality improvement measures and assess how these impact patient outcomes as well as care delivery processes thereby leading to higher levels of care provision and safety of patients [76].

Predictive Analytics and Early Intervention

Predictive analytics and machine learning algorithms generate data insights that identify high-risk patients early, including predicting adverse events such as hospital readmissions, complications, or disease progression. By analyzing patient data and risk factors, healthcare providers can intervene proactively, implement prevention strategies, and optimize care management models to minimize risks, prevent negative outcomes, and enhance patient results [77].

Patient Engagement and Empowerment

Using patient-reported outcomes and data insights from PGHD, patients can participate in their care actively; they can monitor their health and make informed choices on their health behaviors and treatment options. Health providers can engage patients in shared decision-making, offer personalized health coaching, and promote self-management strategies that improve patient satisfaction, adherence to treatment plans, and overall health outcomes through leveraging data analytics and digital healthcare technologies [78].

Evidence-based decision-making, personalized medicine, population health management, quality improvement initiatives, predictive analytics, and patient engagement efforts are among the ways data insights can play a big role in improving healthcare outcomes. Data analytics backed by information-driven insights help healthcare organizations optimize care delivery and improve patient outcomes, thus leading to better health for individuals and populations [79].

CHALLENGES AND CONSIDERATIONS

In healthcare, numerous challenges and limitations must be addressed to make the most of data analytics and improve patient outcomes through such a system. Transparent and accountable decision-making processes in algorithms should be used to address biases. In addition, they should undergo rigorous validation and testing to ascertain fairness, accuracy, and ongoing monitoring with appropriate mitigation of data pre-processing, data collection bias, and development of models. Also, there are quality and integrity issues with data since it may be inaccurate, incomplete, or unreliable, invalidating or compromising the reliability of decisions derived from data. Accurate, complete, and reliable healthcare data require instituting policies for data governance, measures to assure the quality of such information, and protocols for data validation [80 - 82].

Further, complex technical challenges like data integration, scalability, and computational complexity can hinder the application of data-driven approaches in healthcare. To overcome these technical challenges and fully exploit the power of big data analytics in improving healthcare outcomes, it is vital to build a strong back-end infrastructure for data, take advantage of advanced analytics tools and technologies, and invest in expertise in data science. Finally, cultural and organizational challenges such as lack of interoperability, resistance to culture change, or even a siloed approach to database management can become obstacles to embracing any form of a data-driven health system [83].

It is essential to overcome these cultural and organizational barriers and drive meaningful improvements in patients' outcomes through data-driven healthcare initiatives by promoting a data-driven culture, fostering interdisciplinary collaboration, and providing training and support for healthcare professionals. To implement data-driven approaches in healthcare, we need to consider several aspects, such as technical, organizational, cultural, and regulatory ones, while dealing with its challenges and limitations. When these challenges are effectively addressed, the transformative potential of data analytics can be unlocked by healthcare organizations, leading to significant improvements in patient outcomes, quality of care, and healthcare delivery [84 - 86].

FUTURE DIRECTIONS AND INNOVATIONS

The way healthcare is operated will change in the future due to emerging trends and technologies that are revolutionizing its delivery. One of these areas includes using precision medicine for individual care based on the person's genetic composition, biomarkers, and lifestyle. Precision medicine, through the use of clinical data analytics, genomics, data from a patient's own body, and clinical tests, is used to design drugs that target specific diseases, predict the probability of illnesses, as well as enhance treatments, hence leading to more effective personalized care [87].

Furthermore, integrating Artificial Intelligence (AI) and machine Learning (ML) into healthcare can improve diagnostic accuracy, forecast disease development, and maximize clinical decision-making. Machines powered by AI to diagnose predictive analytics models and chatbots allow professionals in the field to handle vast amounts of data, recognize patterns, and provide useful information that can be employed in therapeutic fields. In addition, digital health technologies are making remote monitoring possible through wearable gadgets, telehealth platforms, and mHealth applications, thereby changing healthcare delivery through mobile health apps for telemedicine consultations and patient engagement [88].

The technologies provide a proactive role for patients in their health management, better access to care and communication, and cooperation between patients and providers. In addition, adopting interoperable health information systems and data exchange platforms is improving care coordination, allowing for the sharing of patient data across various healthcare settings without any hitches and enabling population health management efforts. By breaking down silos and fostering collaboration among healthcare stakeholders, interoperability initiatives enhance care continuity, reduce duplicative tests and procedures, and improve patient safety and outcomes. Future directions and innovations in healthcare, including precision medicine, AI-driven analytics, digital health technologies, and interoperable health information systems, hold immense promise for revolutionizing healthcare delivery, advancing patient-centered care, and addressing the evolving needs of patients and populations in the digital age [89, 90].

CONCLUSION

In conclusion, integrating data insights and innovative technologies is poised to transform healthcare delivery, improve patient outcomes, and address longstanding challenges in the healthcare system. Healthcare organizations can unlock new insights by utilizing data analytics, precision medicine, AI, and digital health technologies that will enable them to make better decisions while personalizing care for different patients. However, to realize the data-based health sector's complete potential, one needs to address ethical challenges, guarantee the privacy of patients and the security of data, and comply with legislation such as GDPR and HIPAA. Additionally, it is important to consider other issues like algorithmic bias in healthcare and the readiness of healthcare workers for better results when implementing new data-driven approaches in healthcare. In healthcare, the future directions and innovations to be considered are precision medicine, AI-based analysis, digital health technologies, and interoperable health information systems, which have a lot of promise in revolutionizing healthcare delivery, advancing patient-centered care, and improving individual and population health outcomes. Healthcare organizations can successfully navigate the changing terrain of data-driven healthcare and achieve the same objective by embracing innovation, encouraging collaboration, and putting patient-first. The future of health care is promising when there are unlimited opportunities for innovations, transformation, and better global health outcomes through continued utilization of data insights and technological advancements in the sector.

REFERENCES

[1]   M. Cowing, C. M. Davino-Ramaya, K. Ramaya, and J. Szmerekovsky, "Health care delivery performance: service, outcomes, and resource stewardship," *The Perm. J*, vol. 13, no. 4, pp. 72–78, 2009.

[2]   D. Bhati, M.S. Deogade, and D. Kanyal, "Improving Patient Outcomes Through Effective Hospital Administration: A Comprehensive Review", *Cureus,* vol. 15, no. 10, p. e47731, 2023.
[http://dx.doi.org/10.7759/cureus.47731] [PMID: 38021686]

[3]   S. Dash, S.K. Shakyawar, M. Sharma, and S. Kaushik, "Big data in healthcare: management, analysis and future prospects", *J. Big Data,* vol. 6, no. 1, p. 54, 2019.
[http://dx.doi.org/10.1186/s40537-019-0217-0]

[4]   N. Lloyd, A. Kenny, and N. Hyett, "Evaluating health service outcomes of public involvement in health service design in high-income countries: a systematic review", *BMC Health Serv. Res.,* vol. 21, no. 1, p. 364, 2021.
[http://dx.doi.org/10.1186/s12913-021-06319-1] [PMID: 33879149]

[5]   L. Pantaleon, "Why measuring outcomes is important in health care", *J. Vet. Intern. Med.,* vol. 33, no. 2, pp. 356-362, 2019.
[http://dx.doi.org/10.1111/jvim.15458] [PMID: 30784125]

[6]   S. Marzban, M. Najafi, A. Agolli, and E. Ashrafi, "Impact of Patient Engagement on Healthcare Quality: A Scoping Review", *J. Patient Exp.,* vol. 9, p. 23743735221125439, 2022.
[http://dx.doi.org/10.1177/23743735221125439] [PMID: 36134145]

[7]   B. Prakash, "Patient satisfaction", *J. Cutan. Aesthet. Surg.,* vol. 3, no. 3, pp. 151-155, 2010.
[http://dx.doi.org/10.4103/0974-2077.74491] [PMID: 21430827]

[8]   U. Sivarajah, M.M. Kamal, Z. Irani, and V. Weerakkody, "Critical analysis of Big Data challenges and analytical methods", *J. Bus. Res.,* vol. 70, pp. 263-286, 2017.
[http://dx.doi.org/10.1016/j.jbusres.2016.08.001]

[9]   N. Mehta, A. Pandit, and S. Shukla, "Transforming healthcare with big data analytics and artificial intelligence: A systematic mapping study", *J. Biomed. Inform.,* vol. 100, p. 103311, 2019.

[http://dx.doi.org/10.1016/j.jbi.2019.103311] [PMID: 31629922]

[10] S.A. Alowais, S.S. Alghamdi, N. Alsuhebany, T. Alqahtani, A.I. Alshaya, S.N. Almohareb, A. Aldairem, M. Alrashed, K. Bin Saleh, H.A. Badreldin, M.S. Al Yami, S. Al Harbi, and A.M. Albekairy, "Revolutionizing healthcare: the role of artificial intelligence in clinical practice", *BMC Med. Educ.,* vol. 23, no. 1, p. 689, 2023.
[http://dx.doi.org/10.1186/s12909-023-04698-z] [PMID: 37740191]

[11] K. Batko, and A. Ślęzak, "The use of Big Data Analytics in healthcare", *J. Big Data,* vol. 9, no. 1, p. 3, 2022.
[http://dx.doi.org/10.1186/s40537-021-00553-4] [PMID: 35013701]

[12] J. Budd, B.S. Miller, E.M. Manning, V. Lampos, M. Zhuang, M. Edelstein, G. Rees, V.C. Emery, M.M. Stevens, N. Keegan, M.J. Short, D. Pillay, E. Manley, I.J. Cox, D. Heymann, A.M. Johnson, and R.A. McKendry, "Digital technologies in the public-health response to COVID-19", *Nat. Med.,* vol. 26, no. 8, pp. 1183-1192, 2020.
[http://dx.doi.org/10.1038/s41591-020-1011-4] [PMID: 32770165]

[13] D. Zhang, L.G. Pee, S.L. Pan, and J. Wang, "Information practices in data analytics for supporting public health surveillance", *J. Assoc. Inf. Sci. Technol.,* vol. 75, no. 1, pp. 79-93, 2024.
[http://dx.doi.org/10.1002/asi.24841]

[14] A. Holzinger, K. Keiblinger, P. Holub, K. Zatloukal, and H. Müller, "AI for life: Trends in artificial intelligence for biotechnology", *N. Biotechnol.,* vol. 74, pp. 16-24, 2023.
[http://dx.doi.org/10.1016/j.nbt.2023.02.001] [PMID: 36754147]

[15] N.S. Abul-Husn, and E.E. Kenny, "Personalized Medicine and the Power of Electronic Health Records", *Cell,* vol. 177, no. 1, pp. 58-69, 2019.
[http://dx.doi.org/10.1016/j.cell.2019.02.039] [PMID: 30901549]

[16] P. Nong, J. Adler-Milstein, S. Kardia, and J. Platt, "Public perspectives on the use of different data types for prediction in healthcare", *J. Am. Med. Inform. Assoc.,* vol. 31, no. 4, pp. 893-900, 2024.
[http://dx.doi.org/10.1093/jamia/ocae009] [PMID: 38302616]

[17] T. Lefèvre, C. Rondet, I. Parizot, and P. Chauvin, "Applying multivariate clustering techniques to health data: the 4 types of healthcare utilization in the Paris metropolitan area", *PLoS One,* vol. 9, no. 12, p. e115064, 2014.
[http://dx.doi.org/10.1371/journal.pone.0115064] [PMID: 25506916]

[18] Suryanarayana, C., & Norton, M. G. (1998). X-ray diffraction: A practical approach. Springer. ISBN 978-0-306-45744-9.

[19] W.A. Kalender, "X-ray computed tomography", *Phys. Med. Biol.,* vol. 51, no. 13, pp. R29-R43, 2006.
[http://dx.doi.org/10.1088/0031-9155/51/13/R03] [PMID: 16790909]

[20] S. Arshiya Ara, G. Katti, and A. Shireen, "Magnetic resonance imaging (MRI)-A review", 2011. Available from: https://www.researchgate.net/publication/279471369

[21] W.D. O'Brien Jr, "Ultrasound–biophysics mechanisms", *Prog. Biophys. Mol. Biol.,* vol. 93, no. 1-3, pp. 212-255, 2007.
[http://dx.doi.org/10.1016/j.pbiomolbio.2006.07.010] [PMID: 16934858]

[22] A. Gallamini, C. Zwarthoed, and A. Borra, "Positron emission tomography (PET) in oncology", *Cancers (Basel),* vol. 6, no. 4, pp. 1821-1889, 2014.
[http://dx.doi.org/10.3390/cancers6041821] [PMID: 25268160]

[23] M. Pennant, Y. Takwoingi, L. Pennant, C. Davenport, A. Fry-Smith, A. Eisinga, L. Andronis, T. Arvanitis, J. Deeks, and C. Hyde, "A systematic review of positron emission tomography (PET) and positron emission tomography/computed tomography (PET/CT) for the diagnosis of breast cancer recurrence", *Health Technol. Assess.,* vol. 14, no. 50, pp. 1-103, 2010.
[http://dx.doi.org/10.3310/hta14500] [PMID: 21044553]

[24] M. Kanehisa, S. Goto, Y. Sato, M. Furumichi, and M. Tanabe, "KEGG for integration and

interpretation of large-scale molecular data sets", *Nucleic Acids Res.,* vol. 40, no. D1, pp. D109-D114, 2012.
[http://dx.doi.org/10.1093/nar/gkr988] [PMID: 22080510]

[25]   T.A. Knijnenburg, J.G. Vockley, N. Chambwe, D.L. Gibbs, C. Humphries, K.C. Huddleston, E. Klein, P. Kothiyal, R. Tasseff, V. Dhankani, D.L. Bodian, W.S.W. Wong, G. Glusman, D.E. Mauldin, M. Miller, J. Slagel, S. Elasady, J.C. Roach, R. Kramer, K. Leinonen, J. Linthorst, R. Baveja, R. Baker, B.D. Solomon, G. Eley, R.K. Iyer, G.L. Maxwell, B. Bernard, I. Shmulevich, L. Hood, and J.E. Niederhuber, "Genomic and molecular characterization of preterm birth", *Proc. Natl. Acad. Sci. USA,* vol. 116, no. 12, pp. 5819-5827, 2019.
[http://dx.doi.org/10.1073/pnas.1716314116] [PMID: 30833390]

[26]   S. M. Cadarette and L. Wong, "An introduction to health care administrative data," Can. J. Hosp. Pharm., vol. 68, no. 3, pp. 232–237, May–Jun. 2015,
[http://dx.doi.org/10.4212/cjhp.v68i3.1457]

[27]   L. Eisler, G. Huang, K.E.M. Lee, J.A. Busse, M. Sun, A.Y. Lin, L.S. Sun, and C. Ing, "Identification of perioperative pulmonary aspiration in children using quality assurance and hospital administrative billing data", *Paediatr. Anaesth.,* vol. 28, no. 3, pp. 218-225, 2018.
[http://dx.doi.org/10.1111/pan.13319] [PMID: 29341336]

[28]   B.K. Potter, D. Manuel, K.N. Speechley, I.A. Gutmanis, M.K. Campbell, and J.J. Koval, "Is there value in using physician billing claims along with other administrative health care data to document the burden of adolescent injury? An exploratory investigation with comparison to self-reports in Ontario, Canada", *BMC Health Serv. Res.,* vol. 5, no. 1, p. 15, 2005.
[http://dx.doi.org/10.1186/1472-6963-5-15] [PMID: 15720709]

[29]   M. Shapiro , D. Johnston , J. Wald , D. Mon Patient-generated health data. RTI International, April. 2012 Apr;813:814.

[30]   H.S.L. Jim, A.I. Hoogland, N.C. Brownstein, A. Barata, A.P. Dicker, H. Knoop, B.D. Gonzalez, R. Perkins, D. Rollison, S.M. Gilbert, R. Nanda, A. Berglund, R. Mitchell, and P.A.S. Johnstone, "Innovations in research and clinical care using patient-generated health data", *CA Cancer J. Clin.,* vol. 70, no. 3, pp. 182-199, 2020.
[http://dx.doi.org/10.3322/caac.21608] [PMID: 32311776]

[31]   G.C. Patton, C. Coffey, S.M. Sawyer, R.M. Viner, D.M. Haller, K. Bose, T. Vos, J. Ferguson, and C.D. Mathers, "Global patterns of mortality in young people: a systematic analysis of population health data", *Lancet,* vol. 374, no. 9693, pp. 881-892, 2009.
[http://dx.doi.org/10.1016/S0140-6736(09)60741-8] [PMID: 19748397]

[32]   A.D. Lopez, C.D. Mathers, M. Ezzati, D.T. Jamison, and C.J.L. Murray, "Global and regional burden of disease and risk factors, 2001: systematic analysis of population health data", 2006. Available from: www.thelancet.com
[http://dx.doi.org/10.1016/S0140-6736(06)68770-9]

[33]   C.H.R Greenow. Quality of Data in Perinatal Population Health Databases: a Systematic Review. *Academia.* 2019.

[34]   V. Etches, J. Frank, E.D. Ruggiero, and D. Manuel, "Measuring population health: a review of indicators", *Annu. Rev. Public Health,* vol. 27, no. 1, pp. 29-55, 2006.
[http://dx.doi.org/10.1146/annurev.publhealth.27.021405.102141] [PMID: 16533108]

[35]   H. Nassaji, "Qualitative and descriptive research: Data type versus data analysis", *Lang. Teach. Res.,* vol. 19, no. 2, pp. 129-132, 2015.
[http://dx.doi.org/10.1177/1362168815572747]

[36]   J. N. Morgan and J. A. Sonquist, "Problems in the analysis of survey data, and a proposal," *J. American Stat. Assoc,* vol. 58, no. 302, pp. 415–434, Jun. 1963.

[37]   G. Meyerowitz-Katz, and L. Merone, "A systematic review and meta-analysis of published research data on COVID-19 infection fatality rates", *Int. J. Infect. Dis.,* vol. 101, pp. 138-148, 2020.

[http://dx.doi.org/10.1016/j.ijid.2020.09.1464] [PMID: 33007452]

[38]   M.S. Islam, M.M. Hasan, X. Wang, H.D. Germack, and M. Noor-E-Alam, "-Alam, "A systematic review on healthcare analytics: Application and theoretical perspective of data mining,"", *Healthcare (Basel)*, vol. 6, no. 2, p. 54, 2018.
[http://dx.doi.org/10.3390/healthcare6020054] [PMID: 29882866]

[39]   A. Sharma, R. Malviya, and R. Gupta, "Big data analytics in healthcare", *Cognitive Intelligence and Big Data in Healthcare*, vol. 8, pp. 257-301, 2022.

[40]   A. Belle, R. Thiagarajan, S.M.R. Soroushmehr, F. Navidi, D.A. Beard, and K. Najarian, "Big data analytics in healthcare", *BioMed Res. Int.*, vol. 2015, pp. 1-16, 2015.
[http://dx.doi.org/10.1155/2015/370194] [PMID: 26229957]

[41]   M. Alings and A. Wilde, "'Brugada' syndrome: clinical data and suggested pathophysiological mechanism," *Circulation*, vol. 99, no. 5, pp. 666–673, 1999.

[42]   A. El-Said, R. Patil, B. Leone, A. Gulani, M.P. Abrams, A. Momin, and J. Simms-Cendan, "Assessing the Impact of Demographic Factors on Presenting Conditions or Complaints Among Internal Medicine Patients in an Underserved Population in Central Florida", *Cureus*, vol. 14, no. 8, p. e27811, 2022.
[http://dx.doi.org/10.7759/cureus.27811] [PMID: 36106221]

[43]   M. Kebe, R. Gadhafi, B. Mohammad, M. Sanduleanu, H. Saleh, and M. Al-Qutayri, "Human vital signs detection methods and potential using radars: A review", *Sensors (Basel)*, vol. 20, no. 5, p. 1454, 2020.
[http://dx.doi.org/10.3390/s20051454] [PMID: 32155838]

[44]   R.B. Ford and E. Mazzaferro, *Kirk and Bistner's Handbook of Veterinary Procedures and Emergency Treatment*, 9th ed. Saunders: Philadelphia, 2011.

[45]   S.K. Bell, T. Delbanco, J.G. Elmore, P.S. Fitzgerald, A. Fossa, K. Harcourt, S.G. Leveille, T.H. Payne, R.A. Stametz, J. Walker, and C.M. DesRoches, "Frequency and Types of Patient-Reported Errors in Electronic Health Record Ambulatory Care Notes", *JAMA Netw. Open*, vol. 3, no. 6, p. e205867, 2020.
[http://dx.doi.org/10.1001/jamanetworkopen.2020.5867] [PMID: 32515797]

[46]   T.P. Ryan, R.D. Morrison, J.J. Sutherland, S.B. Milne, K.A. Ryan, J.S. Daniels, A. Misra-Hebert, J.K. Hicks, E. Vogan, K. Teng, and T.M. Daly, "Medication adherence, medical record accuracy, and medication exposure in real-world patients using comprehensive medication monitoring", *PLoS One*, vol. 12, no. 9, p. e0185471, 2017.
[http://dx.doi.org/10.1371/journal.pone.0185471] [PMID: 28957369]

[47]   J.J. Sutherland, R.D. Morrison, C.D. McNaughton, T.M. Daly, S.B. Milne, J.S. Daniels, and T.P. Ryan, "Assessment of Patient Medication Adherence, Medical Record Accuracy, and Medication Blood Concentrations for Prescription and Over-the-Counter Medications", *JAMA Netw. Open*, vol. 1, no. 7, p. e184196, 2018.
[http://dx.doi.org/10.1001/jamanetworkopen.2018.4196] [PMID: 30646345]

[48]   K. Denecke, and D. Reichenpfader, "Sentiment analysis of clinical narratives: A scoping review", *J. Biomed. Inform.*, vol. 140, p. 104336, 2023.
[http://dx.doi.org/10.1016/j.jbi.2023.104336] [PMID: 36958461]

[49]   A. Bali, D. Bali, N. Iyer, and M. Iyer, "Management of medical records: facts and figures for surgeons", *J. Maxillofac. Oral Surg.*, vol. 10, no. 3, pp. 199-202, 2011.
[http://dx.doi.org/10.1007/s12663-011-0219-8] [PMID: 22942587]

[50]   C. Lahariya, "A brief history of vaccines & vaccination in India," *Ind J Med Res*, vol. 139, no. 4, pp. 491–511, 2014.

[51]   C. Jenkinson, "Measuring health and medical outcomes", *Routledge*, vol. 18, 2013.

[52]   N.A. Kampstra, N. Zipfel, P.B. van der Nat, G.P. Westert, P.J. van der Wees, and A.S. Groenewoud, "Health outcomes measurement and organizational readiness support quality improvement: a

systematic review", *BMC Health Serv. Res.,* vol. 18, no. 1, p. 1005, 2018.
[http://dx.doi.org/10.1186/s12913-018-3828-9] [PMID: 30594193]

[53]   D.N. Kleinmuntz, Resource allocation decisions.*Advances in Decision Analysis: From Foundations to Applications.* Cambridge University Press, 2007, pp. 400-418.
[http://dx.doi.org/10.1017/CBO9780511611308.021]

[54]   P. Korhonen, and M. Syrjänen, "Resource allocation based on efficiency analysis", *Manage. Sci.,* vol. 50, no. 8, pp. 1134-1144, 2004.
[http://dx.doi.org/10.1287/mnsc.1040.0244]

[55]   H. Bekker, "Informed decision making: an annotated bibliography and systematic review Review", 1999. Available from: www.hta.ac.uk/htacd.htm
[http://dx.doi.org/10.3310/hta3010]

[56]   B.K. Rimer, P.A. Briss, P.K. Zeller, E.C.Y. Chan, and S.H. Woolf, "Informed decision making: What is its role in cancer screening?", *Cancer,* vol. 101, no. S5, suppl. Suppl., pp. 1214-1228, 2004.
[http://dx.doi.org/10.1002/cncr.20512] [PMID: 15316908]

[57]   M.C. Lodge, "Accountability and transparency in regulation: Critiques, doctrines, and instruments", 1998. Available from: https://www.researchgate.net/publication/30528322

[58]   A.E. Sharma, M. Knox, V.L. Mleczko, and J.N. Olayiwola, "The impact of patient advisors on healthcare outcomes: a systematic review", *BMC Health Serv. Res.,* vol. 17, no. 1, p. 693, 2017.
[http://dx.doi.org/10.1186/s12913-017-2630-4] [PMID: 29058625]

[59]   R.G. Parrish, "Measuring population health outcomes," *Prev. Chro. Dis*, vol. 7, no. 4, p. A71, 2010 [date]

[60]   J. Wong, M. Murray Horwitz, L. Zhou, and S. Toh, "Using machine learning to identify health outcomes from electronic health record data", *Curr. Epidemiol. Rep.,* vol. 5, no. 4, pp. 331-342, 2018.
[http://dx.doi.org/10.1007/s40471-018-0165-9] [PMID: 30555773]

[61]   A.B. Comfort, L.A. Peterson, L.E. Hatt, and A. Comfort, "Effect of health insurance on the use and provision of maternal health services and maternal and neonatal health outcomes: a systematic review", *J. Health Popul. Nutr.,* vol. 31, no. 4, suppl. Suppl. 2, pp. 81-105, 2013.
[PMID: 24992805]

[62]   A.F. Al-Assaf, "Health care quality : an international perspective. World Health Organization, Regional Office for South-", *East Asia (Piscataway),* 2001.

[63]   M.A.K Wood, "Practical considerations in the measurement of outcomes in healthcare," *Ochsner J,* vol. 1, no. 4, pp. 187–194, Oct. 1999.

[64]   M. Zwarenstein, J. Goldman, and S. Reeves, "Interprofessional collaboration: Effects of practice-based interventions on professional practice and healthcare outcomes", In: *Cochrane Database of Systematic Reviews* John Wiley and Sons Ltd, 2009, p. 3.
[http://dx.doi.org/10.1002/14651858.CD000072.pub2]

[65]   I. Wiklund, "Assessment of patient-reported outcomes in clinical trials: the example of health-related quality of life", *Fundam. Clin. Pharmacol.,* vol. 18, no. 3, pp. 351-363, 2004.
[http://dx.doi.org/10.1111/j.1472-8206.2004.00234.x] [PMID: 15147288]

[66]   O.E. Oleribe, J. Momoh, B.S.C. Uzochukwu, F. Mbofana, A. Adebiyi, T. Barbera, R. Williams, and S.D. Taylor Robinson, "Identifying key challenges facing healthcare systems in Africa and potential solutions", *Int. J. Gen. Med.,* vol. 12, pp. 395-403, 2019.
[http://dx.doi.org/10.2147/IJGM.S223882] [PMID: 31819592]

[67]   S. C. Brailsford, "Tutorial: Advances and challenges in healthcare simulation modeling," In: S. G. Henderson, B. Biller, M.-H. Hsieh, J. Shortle, J. D. Tew, and R. R. Barton, Eds. *Proc. 2007 Winter Simulation Conf.*, 2007.

[68]   G.J. Joyia, R.M. Liaqat, A. Farooq, and S. Rehman, "Internet of medical things (IOMT): Applications,

benefits and future challenges in the healthcare domain", *J. Commun.,* vol. 12, no. 4, pp. 240-247, 2017.
[http://dx.doi.org/10.12720/jcm.12.4.240-247]

[69]   S. Anand and S. K. Routray, "Issues and challenges in healthcare narrowband IoT," *Proc. Int. Conf. Inventive Commun. Comput. Technol.* (ICICCT), 2017, pp. 486-489.
[http://dx.doi.org/10.1109/ICICCT.2017.7975247]

[70]   A. Kasthuri, "Challenges to healthcare in India - The five A's", *Indian J. Community Med.,* vol. 43, no. 3, pp. 141-143, 2018.
[http://dx.doi.org/10.4103/ijcm.IJCM_194_18] [PMID: 30294075]

[71]   M. Helfert, "Challenges of business processes management in healthcare", *Bus. Process. Manag. J.,* vol. 15, no. 6, pp. 937-952, 2009.
[http://dx.doi.org/10.1108/14637150911003793]

[72]   J. Emanuele and L. Koetter, "Workflow opportunities and challenges in healthcare," Siemens Medical Solutions USA, Inc., United States, 2007. Available from: https://www.researchgate.net/publication/252065707

[73]   W.F. Shah, "The Future of Healthcare Data Intelligence: Ethical Insights and Evolutionary Pathway", *J. Med. Healthc.,* no. Jun, pp. 1-7, 2022.
[http://dx.doi.org/10.47363/JMHC/2022(4)252]

[74]   Adedolapo Omotosho, Anthony Anyanwu, S.O. Dawodu, A. Omotosho, A. Anyanwu, and C.P. Maduka, "Comparative review of big data analytics and GIS in healthcare decision-making", *World Journal of Advanced Research and Reviews,* vol. 20, no. 3, pp. 1293-1302, 2023.
[http://dx.doi.org/10.30574/wjarr.2023.20.3.2589]

[75]   V. Tresp, J.M. Overhage, M. Bundschus, S. Rabizadeh, P.A. Fasching, and S. Yu, "Going Digital: A Survey on Digitalization and Large Scale Data Analytics in Healthcare", Online Available from: http://arxiv.org/abs/1606.08075

[76]   M.J. Ward, K.A. Marsolo, and C.M. Froehle, "Applications of business analytics in healthcare", *Bus. Horiz.,* vol. 57, no. 5, pp. 571-582, 2014.
[http://dx.doi.org/10.1016/j.bushor.2014.06.003] [PMID: 25429161]

[77]   S. Kumar, and M. Singh, "Big data analytics for healthcare industry: impact, applications, and tools", *Big Data Mining and Analytics,* vol. 2, no. 1, pp. 48-57, 2019.
[http://dx.doi.org/10.26599/BDMA.2018.9020031]

[78]   W. He, S. Nazir, and Z. Hussain, "Big Data Insights and Comprehensions in Industrial Healthcare: An Overview", In: *Mobile Information Systems* Hindawi Limited, 2021.
[http://dx.doi.org/10.1155/2021/6628739]

[79]   Temidayo Olorunsogo, O.A. Elufioye, T. Olorunsogo, O.F. Asuzu, N.L. Nduubuisi, and A.I. Daraojimba, "Data analytics in healthcare: A review of patient-centric approaches and healthcare delivery", *World Journal of Advanced Research and Reviews,* vol. 21, no. 2, pp. 1750-1760, 2024.
[http://dx.doi.org/10.30574/wjarr.2024.21.2.0246]

[80]   G.L. Douglas, S.R. Zwart, and S.M. Smith, "Space food for thought: Challenges and considerations for food and nutrition on exploration missions", *J. Nutr.,* vol. 150, no. 9, pp. 2242-2244, 2020.
[http://dx.doi.org/10.1093/jn/nxaa188] [PMID: 32652037]

[81]   E. Irani, "The Use of Videoconferencing for Qualitative Interviewing: Opportunities, Challenges, and Considerations", *Clin. Nurs. Res.,* vol. 28, no. 1, pp. 3-8, 2019.
[http://dx.doi.org/10.1177/1054773818803170] [PMID: 30470151]

[82]   E.A. Romero-Sandoval, J.E. Fincham, A.L. Kolano, B.N. Sharpe, and P.A. Alvarado-Vázquez, "Cannabis for Chronic Pain: Challenges and Considerations", *Pharmacotherapy,* vol. 38, no. 6, pp. 651-662, 2018.
[http://dx.doi.org/10.1002/phar.2115] [PMID: 29637590]

[83] E. I. Obeagu, C. N. Anyanwu, and G. U. Obeagu, "Challenges and Considerations in Managing Blood Transfusion for Individuals with HIV," *Elite Journal of HIV*, vol. 2, no. 2, pp. 1–17, 2024. Available from: https://www.researchgate.net/publication/378856593

[84] M. Kosinski, S.C. Matz, S.D. Gosling, V. Popov, and D. Stillwell, "Facebook as a research tool for the social sciences: Opportunities, challenges, ethical considerations, and practical guidelines", *Am. Psychol.*, vol. 70, no. 6, pp. 543-556, 2015.
[http://dx.doi.org/10.1037/a0039210] [PMID: 26348336]

[85] C. Lim, K.J. Kim, and P.P. Maglio, "Smart cities with big data: Reference models, challenges, and considerations", *Cities,* vol. 82, pp. 86-99, 2018.
[http://dx.doi.org/10.1016/j.cities.2018.04.011]

[86] R. Spake, and C.P. Doncaster, "Use of meta-analysis in forest biodiversity research: key challenges and considerations", *For. Ecol. Manage.,* vol. 400, pp. 429-437, 2017.
[http://dx.doi.org/10.1016/j.foreco.2017.05.059]

[87] A. Nair, O. Guldiken, S. Fainshmidt, and A. Pezeshkan, "Innovation in India: A review of past research and future directions", *Asia Pac. J. Manage.,* vol. 32, no. 4, pp. 925-958, 2015.
[http://dx.doi.org/10.1007/s10490-015-9442-z]

[88] A. De Massis, F. Frattini, and U. Lichtenthaler, "Research on Technological Innovation in Family Firms", *Fam. Bus. Rev.,* vol. 26, no. 1, pp. 10-31, 2013.
[http://dx.doi.org/10.1177/0894486512466258]

[89] D. W. Rattner, "Future directions in innovative minimally invasive surgery," *The Lancet*, vol. 353, pp. S12–S15, Apr. 1999.

[90] H. Seeck, and M.R. Diehl, "A literature review on HRM and innovation – taking stock and future directions", *Int. J. Hum. Resour. Manage.,* vol. 28, no. 6, pp. 913-944, 2017.
[http://dx.doi.org/10.1080/09585192.2016.1143862]

SUBJECT INDEX

www.ingramcontent.com/pod-product-compliance
Lightning Source LLC
Chambersburg PA
CBHW050803220326
41598CB00006B/103